COPING AND SUBSTANCE USE

COLUMBIA COLLEGE
616.86C782S   C1   V 0
COPING AND SUBSTANCE USE$ ORLANDO
3 2711 00003 7382

COPING AND SUBSTANCE USE

Edited by

Saul Shiffman
Department of Psychology
University of Pittsburgh
Pittsburgh, Pennsylvania

Thomas Ashby Wills
Department of Public Health
Cornell University Medical College
New York, New York

With a foreword by Rudolf H. Moos

1985

ACADEMIC PRESS, INC.
(Harcourt Brace Jovanovich, Publishers)
Orlando San Diego New York London
Toronto Montreal Sydney Tokyo

616.86 C782s

Coping and substance use

COPYRIGHT © 1985 BY ACADEMIC PRESS, INC.
ALL RIGHTS RESERVED.
NO PART OF THIS PUBLICATION MAY BE REPRODUCED OR
TRANSMITTED IN ANY FORM OR BY ANY MEANS, ELECTRONIC
OR MECHANICAL, INCLUDING PHOTOCOPY, RECORDING, OR
ANY INFORMATION STORAGE AND RETRIEVAL SYSTEM, WITHOUT
PERMISSION IN WRITING FROM THE PUBLISHER.

ACADEMIC PRESS, INC.
Orlando, Florida 32887

United Kingdom Edition published by
ACADEMIC PRESS INC. (LONDON) LTD.
24-28 Oval Road, London NW1 7DX

LIBRARY OF CONGRESS CATALOGING IN PUBLICATION DATA

Main entry under title:

Coping and substance use.

Includes index.
1. Drug abuse.   2. Adjustment (Psychology)
3. Social adjustment.   I. Shiffman, Saul.
II. Wills, Thomas Ashby.   [DNLM: 1. Adaptation,
Psychological.   2. Social Adjustment.   3. Stress,
Psychological.   4. Substance Abuse—psychology.
WM 270 C783]
RC564.C677   1985   616.86   85-1323
ISBN 0-12-640040-7 (alk. paper)
ISBN 0-12-640041-5 (paperback)

PRINTED IN THE UNITED STATES OF AMERICA

85 86 87 88   9 8 7 6 5 4 3 2 1

CONTENTS

Contributors	xi
Foreword	xiii
Preface	xxi

Part I
CONCEPTUAL FRAMEWORK 1

1. Coping and Substance Use: A Conceptual Framework
   THOMAS ASHBY WILLS and SAUL SHIFFMAN

Introduction	3
Psychosocial Stress	4
Coping Processes	6
Substance Use as a Coping Mechanism	13
Coping and Stages of Involvement in Substance Use	15
Summary	21
References	21

2. Biological Commonalities of Stress and Substance Abuse
   NEIL E. GRUNBERG and ANDREW BAUM

Introduction and Overview	25
Stress and the Stress Response	26
Drugs of Abuse	33
Endogenous Opioid Peptides	45
Stress and Drug Abuse: The Search for Commonalities	48
Conclusion	53
Appendix: More Details about Endogenous Opioid Peptides	53
References	54

Part II
COPING AND SUBSTANCE USE INITIATION 63

3. Stress, Coping, and Tobacco and Alcohol Use
   in Early Adolescence
   THOMAS ASHBY WILLS

Introduction	67
Method	68
Results	74
Intervention Program	87
General Discussion	90
References	92

4. Coping with Social Influences to Smoke
   ANTHONY BIGLAN, WENDY WEISSMAN, and HERBERT SEVERSON

Introduction	95
Social Influences to Smoke among Adolescents	96
Teaching Teenagers to Cope with Pressures to Smoke	101
The Assessment of Refusal Skills	102
Effects of the Refusal Skills Training Program on Smoking	109
Future Directions	110
Conclusion	114
References	114

5. Social Competence and Self-Efficacy as Determinants of
   Substance Use in Adolescence
   MARY ANN PENTZ

Introduction	117
Social Competence as a Predictor of Drug Use	121
Social Competence Training for Prevention of Drug Use	127
Implications for Future Research	137
References	139

Part III
COPING AND ONGOING SUBSTANCE USE IN ADULT
SAMPLES 143

6. Coping and Drug Use among Heroin-Addicted
   Women and Men
   M. BELINDA TUCKER

Introduction	147

	Women's Use of Drugs: Prevalence and Research	148
	Psychological Perspectives on Female Addiction	149
	A Model of Stress and Coping Relevant to Female Addiction	151
	Methods	155
	Results	157
	Discussion	164
	References	168

7. **Life Stress, Helplessness, and the Use of Alcohol and Drugs to Cope: An Analysis of National Survey Data**
   SUSAN GOFF TIMMER, JOSEPH VEROFF, and MARY ELLEN COLTEN

Introduction	171
Theory of Moderating Effects	171
Methods	176
Results	183
Summary and Conclusions	195
References	197

8. **Daily Coping and Alcohol Use in a Sample of Community Adults**
   ARTHUR A. STONE, SHELLEY LENNOX, and JOHN M. NEALE

Introduction	199
Transactional Model of Stress and Coping	200
Method	203
Results	208
Discussion	216
References	219

Part IV
COPING AND CESSATION OF SUBSTANCE USE   221

9. **Coping with Temptations to Smoke**
   SAUL SHIFFMAN

Introduction	223
A Model of Smoking Cessation Maintenance	223
Method	225
Results	227
Discussion	235
Conclusions	239
References	240

10. Unaided Quitters' Strategies for Coping
    with Temptations to Smoke
    SUSAN GOLDSTEIN CURRY and G. ALAN MARLATT

Introduction	243
Methods	245
Results	248
Discussion	260
Conclusion	264
References	265

11. Coping in Opiate Addicts Maintained on Methadone
    EDMUND F. CHANEY and DOUGLAS K. ROSZELL

Introduction	267
Coping, Substance Abuse, and an Adaptive Orientation	267
Relapse and Coping Models	268
Coping and Relapse in Alcoholism	269
Coping in Opiate Addicts	270
Prospective Study of Coping in Opiate Addicts	274
General Discussion	288
References	291

12. Self-Change Strategies for the Control of Smoking,
    Obesity, and Problem Drinking
    MICHAEL G. PERRI

Overview	295
College Students' Coping with Smoking and Obesity	296
Adults' Coping with Problem Drinking	301
Implications for Theory and Practice	311
References	315

13. Processes and Stages of Self-Change: Coping and
    Competence in Smoking Behavior Change
    CARLO C. DICLEMENTE and JAMES O. PROCHASKA

Introduction	319
Method	326
Results	329
Conclusions	337
Appendix: Processes of Change Questionnaire	340
References	342

14. Common Processes of Self-Change in Smoking, Weight Control, and Psychological Distress
JAMES O. PROCHASKA and CARLO C. DICLEMENTE

Introduction	345
Method	348
Results	353
Discussion	358
References	362

Part V
SUMMARY AND INTEGRATION 365

15. Coping and Substance Abuse: Implications for Research, Prevention, and Treatment
G. ALAN MARLATT

Introduction	367
Theoretical Perspectives	367
Stages of Change in Substance Use	370
Stress, Temptation, and High-Risk Situations	372
Expectancies and Decision Making	374
Coping, Self-Efficacy, and Motivation for Change	376
Stages of Coping	379
Motivation and Coping	380
Issues for Future Research	381
References	385

Author Index	387
Subject Index	399

CONTRIBUTORS

Numbers in parentheses indicate the pages on which the authors' contributions begin.

ANDREW BAUM (25), Department of Medical Psychology, Uniformed Services University of the Health Sciences, Bethesda, Maryland 20814–4799

ANTHONY BIGLAN (95), Oregon Research Institute, Eugene, Oregon 97401

EDMUND F. CHANEY (267), Psychology Service, Seattle Veterans Administration Medical Center; and Department of Psychiatry and Behavioral Sciences, University of Washington, Seattle, Washington 98108

MARY ELLEN COLTEN (171), Center for Survey Research, Boston, Massachusetts 02116

CARLO C. DICLEMENTE (319, 345), Texas Research Institute of Mental Sciences, Houston, Texas 77030

SUSAN GOLDSTEIN CURRY (243), Addictive Behaviors Research Center, Department of Psychology, University of Washington, Seattle, Washington 98195

NEIL E. GRUNBERG (25), Department of Medical Psychology, Uniformed Services University of the Health Sciences, Bethesda, Maryland 20814–4799

SHELLEY LENNOX (199), Department of Psychiatry and Behavioral Science, State University of New York at Stony Brook, Stony Brook, New York 11794

G. ALAN MARLATT (243, 367), Addictive Behaviors Research Center, Department of Psychology, University of Washington, Seattle, Washington 98195

JOHN M. NEALE (199), Department of Psychiatry and Behavioral Science, State University of New York at Stony Brook, Stony Brook, New York 11794

MARY ANN PENTZ (117), Health Behavior Research Institute, University of Southern California, Los Angeles, California 90033

MICHAEL G. PERRI[1] (295), Psychology Service, Richard L. Roudebush Veterans Administration Medical Center; and Indiana University School of Medicine, Indianapolis, Indiana 46202

JAMES O. PROCHASKA (319, 345), Department of Psychology, University of Rhode Island, Kingston, Rhode Island 02881

DOUGLAS K. ROSZELL (267), Psychiatry Service, Seattle Veterans Administration Medical Center, Seattle, Washington 98108

HERBERT SEVERSON (95), Oregon Research Institute, Eugene, Oregon 97401

SAUL SHIFFMAN (3, 223), Department of Psychology, University of Pittsburgh, Pittsburgh, Pennsylvania 15260

ARTHUR A. STONE (199), Department of Psychiatry and Behavioral Science, State University of New York at Stony Brook, Stony Brook, New York 11794

SUSAN GOFF TIMMER (171), Survey Research Center, Institute for Social Research, University of Michigan, Ann Arbor, Michigan 48106

M. BELINDA TUCKER (147), Center for Afro-American Studies, University of California, Los Angeles, California 90024

JOSEPH VEROFF (171), Survey Research Center, Institute for Social Research, University of Michigan, Ann Arbor, Michigan 48106

WENDY WEISSMAN (95), Oregon Research Institute, Eugene, Oregon 97401

THOMAS ASHBY WILLS (3, 67), Department of Public Health, Cornell University Medical College, New York, New York 10021

---

[1]Present addresses: Department of Psychology, Fairleigh Dickinson University, Teaneck, New Jersey 07666; and Franklin Delano Roosevelt Veterans Administration Hospital, Montrose, New York 10548.

FOREWORD*

NEW PERSPECTIVES ON COPING AND SUBSTANCE USE

Remarkable progress is being made in our understanding of coping processes and of the underlying causes of substance use and abuse. Such progress stems from new information about the development and human costs of substance abuse, conceptual and empirical advances in the behavioral and social sciences, and the application of effective prevention and treatment programs. This book integrates some of the trends that underlie these advances and identifies common issues involved in understanding different types of substance use.

At the broadest level, behavioral medicine has sparked renewed interest in the role of personal and social factors in health and health-related behavior. By emphasizing the active role of the individual in the development, management, and prevention of illness, behavioral medicine has taken a valuable step beyond the biomedical model. As a field, however, it has tended to neglect psychosocial and personality factors and to limit itself to a somewhat restricted perspective on coping processes. The biopsychosocial model presented by the introductory chapters in this book captures the trend toward systems approaches in behavioral medicine and health psychology. These chapters point to the value of developing a biopsychosocial approach to clarifying the development and course of substance use. Two other major perspectives have shaped current approaches to the study of coping and substance use: stress and coping theory, and an emerging framework of process-oriented evaluation research.

---

*Preparation of the foreword was supported by NIAAA Grant AA02863 and by Veterans Administration Medical and Health Services Research and Development Service Research Funds.

STRESS AND COPING THEORY

Recent interest in human competence and coping has been sparked by in-depth studies of adaptation in life crises and transitions. The extensive research in this area has examined such events as divorce or bereavement, forced migration, internment in a prisoner of war or concentration camp, and victimization by rape or kidnapping. Some studies have described how individuals cope with serious illness or injury and with life-threatening surgery and other painful medical treatment, as well as how parents and other family members confront serious illness and the death of their loved ones. This body of research emphasizes the adaptive aspects of individual and group coping. It highlights the hopeful fact that many persons cope effectively with crises of such magnitude.

A related empirical trend grew from an emphasis on life changes as predictors of health and illness. The basic idea is that life events and transitions may foreshadow the development of illness and maladaptive behavior. But the direct link between life stress and illness is a relatively modest one. How is it that the majority of people function effectively in the face of omnipresent stressors? In addressing this issue, theorists have identified two related sets of "resistance resources" that enable individuals to prevent stress or to confront it effectively: social network resources and coping processes. Moos and Mitchell (1982) provide more information about the antecedents of research on social network resources. Current formulations of coping processes have been influenced by the three main historical trends described next.

Psychoanalytic Theory and Ego Psychology

Freud believed that ego processes served to resolve conflicts between an individual's impulses and the constraints of external reality. Their posited function was to reduce tension by enabling the individual to express sexual and aggressive impulses indirectly without recognizing their true intent. These ego processes are cognitive coping mechanisms (though their expression may include behavioral components) whose main functions are defensive (reality distorting) and emotion focused (oriented toward tension reduction). Subsequently, ego psychologists emphasized reality-oriented processes of the "conflict free" ego sphere, such as attention, perception, and memory. These ideas led to the formulation of broad theories of ego processes and of the mechanisms involved in coping and defense.

Evolutionary Theory and Behavior Modification

Charles Darwin's evolutionary perspective on adaptation provided the basis for a behaviorally oriented counterpoint to the psychoanalytic concern with intrapsychic and cognitive factors. This orientation led to an emphasis on behavioral problem-solving activities that contribute to individual and species survival. Initial applications of the behaviorist tradition emphasized the functional aspects of problem-solving behavior, but more recent theoretical approaches have highlighted the value of cognition in effective adaptation. Cognitive behaviorism is concerned with an individual's cognitive appraisal of the meaning of an event, as well as with behavioral problem-solving skills. Current developments in this area focus on the importance of a sense of self-efficacy as a coping resource. Effective coping is predicted to promote future expectations of efficacy, which, in turn, lead to more vigorous and persistent efforts to master new tasks and situations.

Life-Cycle Perspectives

Aside from emphasizing the processes of defense and coping, psychoanalysis and ego psychology spawned a developmental perspective that focused on the gradual accumulation of personal coping resources over an individual's life span. Erik Erikson (1963) described eight life-cycle stages, each of which represents a new challenge or crisis that must be negotiated successfully to enable an individual to cope adequately with the next stage. Personal coping resources (such as the development of trust and autonomy) accrued during the adolescent and young adult years are integrated into the self-concept and shape the process of coping in adulthood. Adequate resolution of the transitions and crises that occur at each point in the life cycle leads to coping resources that can help resolve subsequent crises. These ideas provide the rationale for "crisis theory" and the development of interventions to help individuals progress through life transitions more effectively.

CONTRIBUTIONS TO STRESS AND COPING THEORY

In addition to drawing from these historical trends in stress and coping, this book furthers future progress in this area. The editors develop a conceptual framework that views the link between stressful life circumstances and functioning as mediated by personal and environmental coping resources, as well as by cognitive appraisal and coping responses and their interconnections. This model is applied to different substance use problems (smoking, drinking, heroin use) and to the stages involved in the initiation and cessation of substance use and abuse. Some of the most important findings point to the link between drug use and high stress or inadequate social resources, to the interconnection of coping resources (self-efficacy) and coping skills (assertiveness) in forestalling relapse and lessening the chance that intermittent or mild substance use will develop into regular or heavy use, and to the specificity of the links between high-risk situations and the coping responses most likely to be used in them. In this regard, the findings provide little solace for those who wish to extol the positive or social reinforcement aspects of drug use. Instead, drug use compounds prior stress and foreshadows a decline in self-efficacy and personal functioning.

One unresolved problem involves the identification and measurement of coping domains. Several of the chapters make major contributions to this issue by formulating new categorizations of coping responses and change processes or by applying existing concepts in new ways. There is a refreshing emphasis on cognitive as well as behavioral coping and there is broad concern with diverse assessment methods such as structured interviews and questionnaires, as well as behavioral and role play procedures. Moreover, some of the contributors have tackled such difficult issues as the degree of structure that should be imposed on the assessment of coping, the need for fine-grained repeated measurements, and estimation of the reliability and validity of individuals' reports of their coping processes. Resolution of these issues is essential to future progress in this area.

CONTRIBUTIONS TO KNOWLEDGE ABOUT COPING IN PREVENTION AND RELAPSE

The findings highlight the value of cognitive and behavioral coping responses in reducing the likelihood of initiating substance use and moving to regular use, as well as in forestalling the chance of relapse after a period of reduced use or abstinence. Such findings emphasize the importance of coping and social skills training programs, as does evidence that these programs can help adolescents resist peer pressure to smoke. Social skills training may be most effective with assertive individuals and with those undergoing multiple life transitions. Thus, current intervention programs may need to be targeted to specific groups, while alternate skills training procedures should be developed for less assertive individuals.

The book includes valuable information on self-initiated change as well as on the personal characteristics of successful self-changers and on the coping strategies they use (e.g., overt and covert self-reinforcement procedures, stimulus control methods, and seeking social support). The specification of a small set of common coping or change processes involved in handling a diversity of substance use problems may help to identify the common sources of benefit in varied intervention procedures. Thus, prevention programs could concentrate on teaching generalizable coping skills that enable clients to learn an all-inclusive model of change and apply it to a diversity of problems. A major contribution here is the emphasis on different stages of substance use (initiation, maintenance, cessation) and the explicit consideration of tertiary prevention (i.e., the prevention of relapse) as well as primary and secondary prevention.

Process-Oriented Evaluation Research

Until recently, most evaluation researchers were guided by an idealized paradigm in which individuals were assessed, assigned to intervention (or control) conditions, and then reevaluated at follow-up to identify changes in their functioning and behavior. This summative paradigm is being expanded in several ways. Since intervention programs typically are neither implemented completely as planned nor delivered to recipients in a fixed standard manner, one area of development is the measurement of treatment implementation. Researchers are beginning to develop a more differentiated view of intervention processes and to examine the relationship between intervention processes and outcome. Evaluators are also realizing that powerful external experiences or life-context factors (e.g., major life events or social network resources) can affect the relative benefits of intervention programs.

A process-oriented framework for evaluation research embodies these trends in two ways. First, it reflects an emphasis on a better understanding of treatment and prevention, that is, on documenting the implementation and delivery of intervention programs and on assessing their quality. Second, it considers life-context factors as central determinants of program entry, duration, and outcome. This approach acknowledges the fact that an intervention program is only one among many sets of factors that influence subsequent adaptation. The framework can be used to examine the effects of a broad range of interventions, such as social skills training and milieu therapy, as well as to identify the factors involved in self-initiated recovery.

CONTRIBUTIONS TO EVALUATION RESEARCH

Several of the chapters reflect these concerns by considering the adequacy of implementation of intervention programs, the value of change processes and their implications for planning effective treatment, and the link between the overall context of an intervention program and its long-term efficacy and generalizability. For instance, an implementation check of a skills training program showed that students in the program actually learned and used refusal skills more often. A related point involves the finding that a decision skills program was more successful in one school context than in another. The speculation that a negative "school atmosphere" can deter program effectiveness illustrates the idea that the social context of an intervention can dramatically affect its outcome. Similarly, the emphasis on high risk for relapse situations is consistent with the idea that posttreatment or life-context factors influence the outcome of treatment and intervention programs.

Several of the contributors embody the applied orientation of evaluation research by using their findings to identify practical treatment alternatives. Information about effective self-change strategies points to the value of an initial phase of decision making and planning, of multifacted self-management programs tailored to the target problem, and of the special importance of cognitive self-reinforcement strategies, such as reminding oneself that one is doing well. Ironically, individuals who have been in treatment for smoking cessation are less likely to use cognitive coping strategies, even though such strategies may be more reliable and less vulnerable to environmental disruption. Since most skills training programs focus more heavily on behavioral than on cognitive coping, they may have detrimental consequences which must be identified and changed.

FUTURE DEVELOPMENTS

This book formulates a stress and coping framework and identifies some common domains of coping resources and processes implicated in substance use and abuse. Some future research directions include specification of basic types of coping processes, evaluation of the cross-situational consistency of coping, and clarification of the connections between coping processes and adaptational outcomes. Another high priority issue is to specify the long-term adaptive consequences of experiencing and coping successfully with life stressors and to clarify the personal and social resources that promote such consequences. Such personal resources as self-efficacy and internal control may enable individuals to confront stress effectively and to reappraise potentially traumatic events as opportunities for personal growth. The evolution of a general theory of stress and coping can promote a better understanding of the influence of coping processes on adaptation and can foster more effective intervention programs.

Research on substance use and abuse is being integrated into the mainstream of basic advances in the behavioral and social sciences. Analogous conceptual developments are taking place in related areas such as evaluation research. As the resulting new knowledge is organized within a biopsychosocial perspective, behavioral and social scientists will make more definitive contributions to clarifying the underlying nature of substance use and abuse. Such advances can spark new perspectives on the causes of these disorders and on the role of stress and coping processes in modifying them. This book exemplifies the search for new knowledge that will lead to the formulation of more effective intervention procedures and ultimately to fresh ideas that can be applied in primary as well as secondary and tertiary prevention.

REFERENCES

Erikson, E. (1963). *Childhood and society*. New York: Norton.
Moos, R. H., & Mitchell, R. E. (1982). Social network resources and adaptation: A conceptual framework. In T. A. Wills (Ed.), *Basic processes in helping relationships*. New York: Academic Press.

Rudolph H. Moos
Social Ecology Laboratory
Department of Psychiatry and Behavioral Sciences
Veterans Administration and Stanford University Medical Centers
Palo Alto, California

PREFACE

The purpose of this book is to present empirical studies that combine two important lines of investigation: research on coping and research on substance use. Research on drug use traditionally has tended to focus on biological factors, but in recent years there has been a shift toward viewing substance use as a maladaptive attempt to deal with life stresses. In this revised formulation of substance use, research on stress and coping has become increasingly relevant. From this perspective, persons are viewed as active agents who try to cope with the stressors and temptations they experience, rather than reacting passively to biological impulses or psychological temptations.

The contributors present current research relating coping processes to substance use and abuse. The central question addressed in each chapter is, What types of coping mechanisms enable individuals to avoid substance use? This issue, which has important implications for both basic research and drug-abuse prevention and treatment programs, is addressed here in detail for the first time.

This book began when the editors discovered interesting linkages between their respective areas of research at an American Psychological Association meeting. One area (Shiffman's) considers how people attempt to achieve self-control in the face of temptations to engage in undesirable behaviors; the other (Wills's) focuses on the means that persons use to deal with the demands of life stress. Recognizing that the two areas had some striking consistencies in methods and findings, with important implications for research and treatment, we began with equal editorship to prepare a volume that would integrate the two domains.

The volume presents current research on three phases of substance use: initiation, maintenance, and relapse. The chapters focus largely on tobacco and alcohol use because these are the most prevalent and widely studied substance use problems, but the chapters also touch on weight control, opiate addiction, and the use of prescription drugs. Evidence is presented from a variety of populations ranging from adolescents to adults, from small clinical samples to large community populations, and from normal populations to addicts in intensive treatment. The intent is to identify common processes in various types of substance use while recognizing distinctive characteristics in usage of particular substances.

The book is organized into five parts. Part I focuses on theoretical foundations. The first chapter approaches the topic from the perspective of social and clinical psychology, proposing a comprehensive model of the relationships among psychosocial stress, coping, and substance use. The second chapter is written from the perspective of physiological psychology and pharmacology, reviewing current knowledge about the physiological bases of stress and substance use and their relationship. While this single chapter cannot provide complete coverage of the area, it is intended as an introduction to biological considerations in a volume generally focused on psychosocial aspects of substance use. We feel that the study of substance use requires a biopsychosocial perspective and that full understanding of substance use is possible only by considering both psychosocial and biological factors.

Each chapter in the three parts that follow presents original empirical research relating coping and substance use. Although the contributors review relevant literature, that is not their major aim. We felt that presentation of original work would better meet the reader's needs than a book devoted to review. Several pertinent outcome studies are presented, the focus throughout being on the *process* of behavior change.

Parts II through IV each concentrate on a particular stage of substance use. Some common themes emerge in all stages of substance use—initiation, ongoing use, and cessation—and each part addresses the issues from a somewhat different perspective. The chapters in Part II are concerned with the initiation of substance use in adolescence. They consider the hypothesis that substance use is most likely when coping resources are limited for dealing with stressors encountered by adolescents.

Part III deals with the effects of stress and coping on variations in ongoing substance use. This section is shorter than the others, not because it is less important, but because of the paucity of empirical work on the topic. Part IV covers cessation of substance use and the maintenance of abstinence. Although several chapters address the impact of stress and attempts to cope with it, the primary focus is on how substance users cope with temptations or pressures to relapse. The final part summarizes and integrates the work presented in the chapters.

This book will be of value to professionals concerned with substance abuse problems, including psychologists, psychiatrists, sociologists, public health personnel, epidemiologists, social workers, and health educators.

Faculty members will find the book useful as a text for a graduate or postgraduate seminar on substance use or as a supplementary text for a course on stress and coping. Although this is not intended as a "how-to" guide for working clinicians, they will find a number of clinical implications in the chapters. Finally, and foremost, researchers involved in studies of stress, coping, or substance use will find the presentations stimulating and useful for developing new research in the area.

We express our appreciation to the contributors to this volume, who responded gracefully to the combined comments of two editors on initial drafts of their chapters. We also thank the staff of Academic Press for their help through the many phases of the production process. The editors' work on the volume was aided by grants from the University of South Florida College of Social and Behavioral Sciences and from the University of Pittsburgh Faculty of Arts and Sciences.

Part I

CONCEPTUAL FRAMEWORK

In this part, two chapters provide theoretical frameworks that address the relationship between stress, coping, and substance use from psychological and biological perspectives. We think that both perspectives are necessary for a complete understanding of how coping factors may be related to substance use and abuse. Knowledge about the biological mechanisms of drug action is a necessary component for a theory of substance use. From a complementary viewpoint we note that biological processes are ultimately expressed in psychological states (of stress, discomfort, or positive feeling), and knowledge about the psychosocial context of substance abuse seems necessary for understanding the typical behavioral patterns of substance use and their psychological correlates. Together, these chapters provide a broad perspective on coping and the addictions. Although there are probably some stress and coping factors that vary across different substances of abuse (e.g., tobacco vs. alcohol), the authors emphasize what they see as important commonalities.

In Chapter 1, Wills and Shiffman present a theoretical model of coping and substance use at the psychological level of analysis. They present a multiphasic model of affect management through substance use, positing that substances may be used both to reduce negative affect and to increase positive affect. Drawing on evidence from studies of coping and from studies of substance use, which have generally been conducted independently of each other, they outline cognitive and behavioral coping responses that are relevant for decreasing the probability of substance use in problematic situations. The authors distinguish between responses used for coping with general life stresses and responses employed to cope with temptation to use substances. The model is developed and discussed with reference to three different phases of substance use: initiation, maintenance, and cessation. Using evidence from studies of smoking and alcohol use, they show that a stress-coping framework is consistent with the available evidence on substance use and relapse, and suggest a number of questions for clinical and epidemiological research on coping and substance use.

In Chapter 2, Grunberg and Baum present an original conceptual framework of biological commonalities in stress–substance use relationships. They outline how stress affects functioning at the physiological level and then discuss mechanisms through which psychoactive substances may change stress-related physiological effects at either central or peripheral levels. Using the general model of addictive processes, they then provide a detailed discussion of current biochemical knowledge about the action of common drugs of abuse: opioids, alcohol, nicotine, amphetamines, and tranquilizers. While Grunberg and Baum are careful to point out possible differences in the mechanism of action of various substances, they emphasize biological concepts and principles that may represent important commonalities for addictive processes. Ultimately this approach may be useful for both pharmacological and psychological theories of substance abuse. The model presented here suggests a number of hypotheses than can be further tested in basic laboratory research. At the same time, the authors' integration of current biological knowledge can be useful for generating tests of constructs at the psychological level.

Chapter 1

Coping and Substance Use: A Conceptual Framework*

THOMAS ASHBY WILLS
SAUL SHIFFMAN

INTRODUCTION

Substances such as tobacco and alcohol are used by some persons at some times to deal with the stress of modern society. The purpose of this chapter is to delineate why stress is related to substance use, why substance use may be adopted as a coping mechanism, and what kinds of strategies enable persons to give up addictive or problematic substance use. Although we recognize that substance use is a multifactorial process, involving social, psychological, and biological factors, our goal is to relate propositions about stress and coping to the theory of substance use. This theoretical framework is set out to integrate the research reported in the chapters that follow and to generate hypotheses about the operation of various processes in stress, coping, and substance use. Our focus is on the most common drugs of abuse (tobacco, alcohol, and opiates), emphasizing the commonality of processes underlying the use, or cessation of use, of these substances. Occasional extensions are made to other types of substance abuse or problem behaviors, such as abuse of prescription drugs or overeating.[1]

*The authors thank David B. Abrams, Tom Kamarck, Edward Lichtenstein, Robert Millman, and John Neale for their comments on a draft of this chapter.

[1] The focus is mainly on cigarettes and alcohol because more empirical evidence is available in those areas. Evidence on opiate addiction also suggests that opiate use serves a coping or adaptive function by fulfilling psychological needs (Alexander & Hadaway, 1982), although support for this proposition is largely indirect. Evidence on stress and psychotropic drug use (Cafferata, Kasper, & Bernstein, 1983) and on the relation between emotional states and overeating (Baucom & Aiken, 1981; Doell & Hawkins, 1982; Leon & Chamberlain, 1973; Sjöberg & Persson, 1979) is consistent with the theoretical framework, but these behaviors are not discussed in detail because of the lack of a substantial body of literature in these areas.

This conceptual framework of coping and substance use is based on two central postulates. The first is that substances may be used as a coping mechanism for two independent reasons: They can reduce negative affect or can increase positive affect. Although these dual functions of substance use may appear paradoxical, there is reason to posit that substance use can accomplish both functions for a person. The second postulate is that it is useful to distinguish between *stress-coping skills,* which are cognitive or behavioral responses relevant for dealing with the stress evoked by negative life events or enduring strains, and *temptation-coping skills,* which are responses used to cope with temptations for substance use that occur in particular situations. In this sense, we distinguish between skills relevant for coping with stress and skills relevant for coping with temptation. The empirical basis for these two postulates and their applicability to the theory of stress, coping, and substance use is developed in detail in subsequent sections of this chapter.

The following sections outline the basic nature of psychosocial stress and the coping process and present a framework for understanding the psychological mechanisms of substance use. The framework is discussed with respect to initiation, regular use, and cessation of substance use, showing what we think are some essential commonalities in the operation of coping processes for these three aspects of substance use.

PSYCHOSOCIAL STRESS

In theory, stress could be construed in terms of three different levels of stressors. The first level represents coping with major life events, such as a heart attack or the death of a spouse (see, for example, Dohrenwend & Dohrenwend, 1981). These events usually occur suddenly, require major readjustments in life-style, and typically represent an initial period of shock followed by a period of gradual readjustment. The second category represents enduring life strains (see Pearlin & Schooler, 1978): difficulties in occupational, societal, or interpersonal relationships that persist over time and are not quickly or easily resolved. Examples of these kinds of stresses are dissatisfaction in a marital relationship or unhappiness with one's job or work conditions. This type of strain may be to some extent self-induced (e.g., a person may have chosen a bad position) or may be part of a socioeconomic environment in which the individual is a victim (e.g., the individual may be forced into a poor job because of discrimination). A third level of stress concerns everyday problems (DeLongis, Coyne, Dakof, Folkman, & Lazarus, 1982; Lewinsohn & Amenson, 1978), the small hassles of everyday life that come up, are resolved, and are soon replaced by others. It can be hypothesized that stress at any of these levels will increase the probability of substance use, although we would expect that enduring strains,

1. COPING AND SUBSTANCE USE: A CONCEPTUAL FRAMEWORK

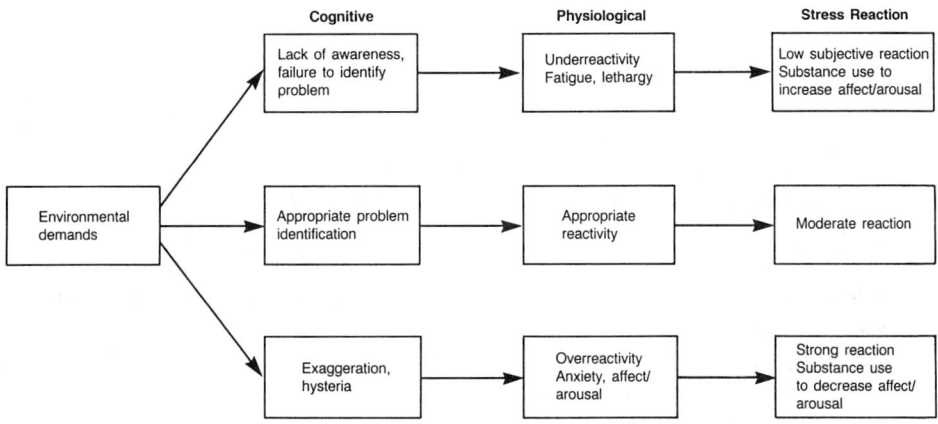

Figure 1.1 Components of the stress appraisal process.

because of their long-term nature, would be most likely to create risk for habitual substance abuse.[2]

Current research on stress suggests that a comprehensive model of stress perception is necessary to predict how stressful events will affect behavior. Such a model, diagrammed in Figure 1.1, posits that several processes may intervene between the occurrence of a potentially stressful event and the occurrence of an adverse reaction. At a cognitive level, individuals may differ in problem appraisal; some persons may fail to recognize potential problems until a bad situation exists, some may appropriately identify major and minor potential problems, and some may exaggerate minor situations and engage in inappropriate reactions. At the physiological level, individuals may differ in physiological reactivity to stimuli. Because of genetic or environmental effects on sympathetic nervous system activity, some individuals may be chronically underreactive to potentially arousing stimuli, some may be appropriately reactive, and some may be generally overreactive to stimulation. In this model, the eventual occurrence of a subjective (stress) reaction to a particular event is posited to depend on both the individual's appraisal of the event and on the individual's physiological reactivity to the stimulation resulting from the problem appraisal. Three possible pathways are included in Figure 1.1, representing some of the many permutations of processes that may mediate between environmental occurrences and subjective stress reactions.

This model of stress and substance use posits that substances may be used to reduce negative affect or increase positive affect. Given an elevated level

[2]Although these three levels of stressors are conceptually distinct, it is not clear whether they are statistically independent. For example, major negative events may be correlated with enduring strains and possibly with everyday events. At present, however, there is little empirical evidence on this issue (see Wills, 1985b).

of objective negative events, accompanied by problem appraisals and physiological reactions of stress, we predict that some individuals will engage in substance use in order to reduce negative affect. Alternatively, persons who were experiencing few enjoyable events, or were chronically underreactive to stimulation, might be expected to use substances in order to increase their level of positive affect. These propositions are consistent with evidence on the biphasic effects of nicotine and alcohol, indicating that these substances may act either to reduce negative or increase positive affect, depending on the rate of consumption and the physiological level of the substance (e.g., Gilbert, 1979; Russell & Mehrabian, 1975). Individuals may use a substance to reduce negative affect when they are anxious or overaroused, or they may also use the same substance to enhance positive affect when they are fatigued, depressed, or underaroused.[3]

COPING PROCESSES

Coping can be defined with respect to both stress-coping skills, which are relevant for coping with general life stressors, and to temptation-coping skills, which are relevant for coping with a situation where there is a specific temptation for substance use. With respect to stress-coping skills, coping is defined as activities or behaviors a person uses in the attempt to maintain a balance between demands from the environment and resources currently available to meet those demands (Coyne & Lazarus, 1980). In theory, the goal of such coping is to maintain an appropriate balance of positive and negative affect (Stone, Lennox, & Neale, Chapter 8; Wills, Chapter 3, this volume). From this perspective, substance use is one coping response (of several potential alternatives) that people could use to achieve affect management. Typical demands for persons in the general population are for career preparation, performance, and advancement, economic stability, harmonious relationships with significant others, and reasonably health-promoting behavior (implying nonabuse of substances). From this perspective the basic goal of the coping process is to achieve a sense of self-esteem and self-efficacy, and a feeling of predictability and stability in one's life situa-

---

[3] It should be noted that there is still some confounding of the concepts of affect and arousal in the literature. In principle these concepts are separable, generating four possible conditions based on combinations of affect and arousal: negative affect, high arousal—stress; negative affect, low arousal—depression; positive affect, high arousal—joy; positive affect, low arousal—relaxation. Although the literature on substance use has generally focused on affect management, it is possible that individuals are concurrently trying to manage both affect and arousal. Some drugs (e.g., amphetamines) may be used both to increase positive affect and to increase arousal among individuals who feel chronically underaroused.

1. COPING AND SUBSTANCE USE: A CONCEPTUAL FRAMEWORK

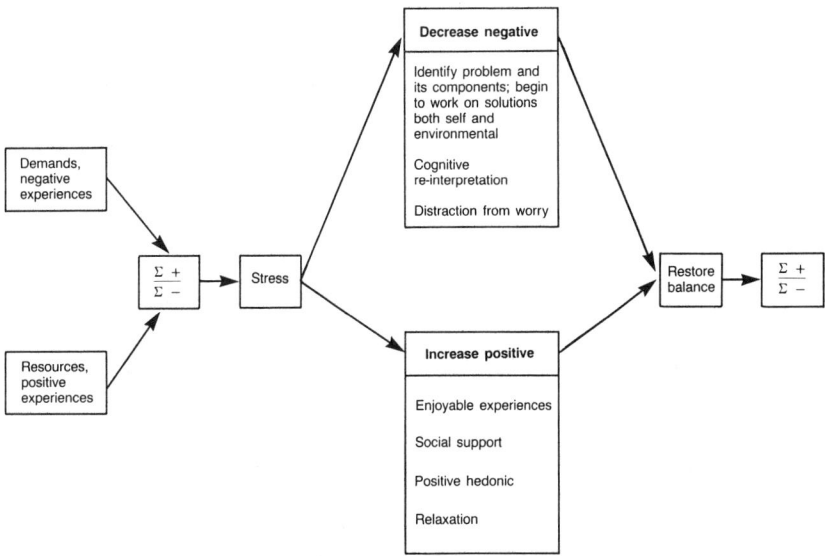

Figure 1.2 Outline of the stress–coping process.

tion.[4] To summarize the process of coping with generalized life stressors, an outline of the coping process is presented in Figure 1.2.

With respect to temptation-coping skills, we consider how individuals deal with demands created by various kinds of temptations: from cognitive expectations about the effects of substances, from explicit social pressure to use substances, from biologically rooted impulses, or (among regular users) from the pull of habit. Coping responses relevant to these demands include self-control processes (Shiffman, Chapter 9, this volume) and skills to cope with problematic social situations (Chaney & Roszell, Chapter 11, this volume). Background resources relevant to problems with substance use include motivation to change and perceived efficacy for dealing with temptations for substance use. The immediate goal of such coping is to avoid substance use; its long-term goals include the promotion of physical health together with feelings of self-efficacy arising from demonstrated success in controlling one's own undesirable behaviors.

---

[4]In this sense certain types of stable resources (e.g., financial assets, education, trait self-esteem) are relevant for psychological well-being (see Wills & Langner, 1980) but technically these are not defined as coping because they are not specific activities (cognitive or behavioral) undertaken by the individual. These types of resources may support or assist the coping process, but they are not in themselves coping behaviors.

Before discussing particular coping responses, we note two conceptual points about the coping process. First, coping may be performed in response to any of the three levels of stressors described previously. Stress-coping skills are probably most relevant for dealing with major life events and enduring strains, and temptation-coping skills are probably most relevant for situations in which substance use, or temptation to use substances, is present.

The second point concerns the effectiveness of coping. Although this is still an area with little theoretical or empirical development, in principle we would expect some coping responses to be more effective than others. For coping with major life events, some coping responses may lead to gradual adaptation and eventual resolution of life changes, whereas other responses may lead to unresolved grief patterns, depression, and social alienation. For coping with enduring strains, constructive coping patterns would lead to gradual change of the self and the environment, whereas less constructive coping would produce hostility, conflictual interpersonal behavior, and eventual characterological disturbances. At the level of everyday problems, some types of coping may lead to immediate and nonemotional resolution of problems, whereas others may lead to anger, arguments, and accumulations of resentment and unresolved details. In this context, we predict that substance use as a coping mechanism would have generally nonproductive consequences. Although substances may provide short-term changes in affect, a reliance on this approach for dealing with environmental stressors reduces the probability of learning and practicing alternative coping responses; in the long run this would tend to reduce social competence and increase overall stress levels (see Pentz, Chapter 5, this volume). Additionally, drug-abusing behavior may gradually alienate potential social supporters, leading to increasing social isolation and increased dependency on the use of substances to cope (see Tucker, Chapter 6, this volume).

Coping Responses

From basic psychological theory one can distinguish several different coping patterns that might apply to various types of problems and could be construed either in terms of stress-coping skills or in terms of skills for coping with specific temptations (see Lazarus, 1977; Moos & Billings, 1982; Pearlin & Schooler, 1978). In the following sections these coping responses are grouped into three categories: cognitive, behavioral, and acceptance. This classification is not meant to be restrictive, because the theory of coping responses is not well developed, and the overall process of coping may involve cognitive, behavioral, and other components. Rather, this categorization is intended as a general framework for discussion of different types of possible coping responses.

Responses in the category of cognitive coping involve an attempt to deal with problems through cognitive mechanisms. Persons may assure themselves that the problem or temptation is not worth getting upset about or that it will be over in a short time (*minimization*). They may focus on positive aspects of the situation or may turn their attention to other things (*distraction* or ignoring). They may use selective comparison processes to assure themselves that things could be worse or that in some ways they are better off than other people (*downward comparison*). They may try to reinterpret the situation so that it is perceived as nonproblematic (*restructuring*). Self-control processes for coping with temptation may involve reminding oneself of previous successes (*efficacy enhancement*), thinking about the positive or negative consequences of performing an undesired behavior (*thoughts of consequences*), or in some cases just telling oneself not to do something (*willpower*).

Responses in the category of behavioral coping involve an active attempt to make a decision and change the problematic situation. The coping pattern termed *decision-making* or *problem solving* involves gathering information relevant to the problem, evaluating alternative courses of action, and making a decision to pursue a particular course. *Direct action* involves making attempts to change a problematic situation, either through direct action or through negotiation or compromise with other persons. A strategy termed *withdrawal* involves physically leaving a problematic situation or avoiding such situations altogether. *Assertiveness* is a social coping skill with considerable relevance for many areas; the ability to apply appropriately assertive behavior in social situations is relevant both for overall well-being and for substance use, because substances are typically introduced and offered (often with some implicit pressure) in social situations. *Social support* is a process in which individuals actively seek help from other people, either through talking about their problems with someone they feel close to (emotional support or catharsis), or through seeking instrumental aid, advice, and guidance. Persons may intentionally engage in alternative behaviors that are incompatible with a problematic behavior (*alternative behaviors*). Another behavioral coping pattern, *relaxation,* involves various methods of achieving relaxation through muscle relaxation exercises, meditation, or stress control methods. Finally, a coping pattern termed *pleasure seeking* can be defined, involving an active attempt to provide positive experiences through entertainment or social and leisure activity.

The third category includes a coping pattern termed *acceptance,* based on the belief that nothing can or should be done about the problem in the short term and that the problem must simply be accepted and endured until the present situation is replaced eventually with better things (Veroff, Douvan, & Kulka, 1981). Although classification is somewhat arbitrary, religion is a coping approach found with considerable frequency in general-population samples (see Stone et al., Chapter 8, this volume; Timmer, Veroff, & Colten, Chapter 7, this volume). This involves coping with difficulties through praying for guidance and strength.

The coping responses defined above represent a potential repertoire of coping resources, any or all of which may be used by an individual to deal with a particular problem. The present model views coping as a multidimensional biopsychosocial process in which stressed individuals are attempting to solve practical problems, maintain a sense of positive self-esteem, and keep their biochemical and physiological state in optimal balance (i.e., affect management). From previous research on personality assessment, one would expect considerable variability in coping behavior across different situations and types of problems, and indeed, Folkman and Lazarus (1980) found that problem-solving coping was used more often for work-related problems compared with self- or family-related problems. It may be difficult to classify an individual's coping style in terms of a single distinct response, since individuals probably use several coping responses to deal with most problems (see Moos & Billings, 1982). It should be possible, however, to detect consistencies over time in the probability of using particular coping mechanisms, with some persons having a relatively broader repertoire of coping strategies and using them more frequently.

Stages of Coping

In the present theoretical framework, coping can be viewed either as an anticipatory response for stressful events that are expected to occur, as a means for management of events that are occurring, or as a restorative mechanism to help regain psychological equilibrium after an adverse event has occurred.[5] Although there are few data available on the application of these concepts to stress-coping skills, studies of individuals attempting to quit substance use have shown how these concepts are related to temptation-coping skills. Individuals may use various anticipatory strategies to

---

[5]This framework is similar to the model of coping self-statements developed by Meichenbaum for stress-inoculation training (e.g., Meichenbaum, 1977, Chapter 5), which involves separate strategies of preparing for the stressor, confronting and handling the stressful experience, and self-reinforcement to be used after successful performance in the stressful situation. Meichenbaum's model is primarily cognitive, however, and the present discussion points out behavioral and other coping responses that could be used in addition to cognitive techniques.

reduce the probability of temptation (Perri, Chapter 12, this volume), to avoid relapse in the middle of a temptation episode (Shiffman, Chapter 9; Curry & Marlatt, Chapter 10), or may use restorative coping responses to reward successful performance or minimize the negative impact of slips or relapses (DiClemente & Prochaska, Chapter 13).

Anticipatory coping involves problem-solving behavior that could help to prepare for a demanding event, cognitive efforts to alter the interpretation or perceived importance of an upcoming situation, and efforts to avoid the occurrence of temptations. It has also been suggested that individuals may use drugs before a stressful situation so that any substandard performance can then be attributed to the drug rather than to personal inadequacy, and some evidence for this process has been obtained in laboratory studies (e.g., Tucker, Vuchinich, & Sobell, 1981).

Immediate coping involves the use of cognitive or behavioral strategies to deal with difficulties as they are occurring. This could include use of direct problem solving or social skills to deal effectively with problematic situations, and use of cognitive strategies to minimize unproductive emotional reactions or to exercise self-control in the face of acute temptations.

Restorative coping could involve a variety of strategies that deal with the aftermath of problematic occurrences. Problem solving might be applied to limit the damage caused by the event, and cognitive reevaluations of the event may be applied to restore self-esteem or perceived efficacy. In addition, problem-solving actions might be used to help prevent the reoccurrence of the stressor, or individuals could engage in activities that would distract them from worrying about the problem. Pleasure-seeking activities could be used to redress the balance of positive experiences, which had been temporarily altered by the adverse effects of the stressor. Restorative coping may be especially important for dealing with lapses or slips in which a person succumbs temporarily to a specific temptation but still strives to avoid undesirable behavior and maintain self-control (Mermelstein & Lichtenstein, 1983). On theoretical grounds one would expect some variation in the types of coping responses used in different phases of coping, but at present there are no studies bearing on this issue.

Selection of Coping Response

In theory, selection of a particular coping mechanism has been hypothesized to depend on several factors (see Coyne & Lazarus, 1980; Stone et al., Chapter 8, this volume). Perceived stress is hypothesized to be based on an extensive appraisal process in which individuals compare the current environmental demands with the coping skills and background resources available to meet those demands. Given that significant stress is perceived, one determinant of coping behavior is the perceived severity of the stressor, with stressors that are more severe and more directly relevant to an individual's personal goals predicted to evoke a greater variety of coping responses. Another factor is the perceived changeability of the stressor; situations regarded as relatively changeable should evoke coping responses oriented toward problem solving and direct resolution of the situation, whereas problem situations that are perceived as relatively unchangeable should evoke coping strategies oriented toward cognitively reinterpreting the situation and minimizing the negative affect evoked by the stressor (e.g., substance use). It is worth noting also that a number of important stressors derive from difficulties in interpersonal relationships (see Wills, 1985a). To the extent that such difficulties were perceived as remediable, we would expect coping to occur through problem solving and compromise, social support seeking, or outside counseling (professional helpers). If such coping skills and resources were lacking, individuals might turn to substance use as a coping mechanism (Timmer et al., Chapter 7; Tucker, Chapter 6, this volume).

Persons coping with temptation must also choose whether to cope with the cause of the temptation or only with the temptation itself. When interpersonal conflict leads to a temptation to drink, for example, a person might address the underlying distress through interpersonal discussion and negotiation or through personal stress management techniques; alternatively, the person could deal with drinking temptation by cognitively coping in situations where alcohol is present. How individuals make these choices has yet to be explored, but they may be related to predominant modes of coping. It is also possible that coping varies with the nature of the problem situation, for example, social situations versus solitary situations (see Curry & Marlatt, Chapter 10, this volume).

Another possible factor in determining choice of a coping response is essentially an instrumental consideration, namely, the difficulty or cost of the coping response. Some responses require more effort, thought, or perseverance than others. Other things being equal, we would expect people to choose a response that involved less effort over one that involved more effort. Analogously, some responses (e.g., leaving a situation) are probably more visible than others, and people probably prefer courses of action that are less visible to those that may cause social disapproval; this has been suggested as a factor that deters help-seeking behavior in everyday contexts (Wills, 1983). These factors have direct extensions to the study of coping behavior, and there are grounds for expecting that response–cost considerations may be an important influence on people's choices of alternative coping patterns.

SUBSTANCE USE AS A COPING MECHANISM

For developing the theoretical basis of substance use as a mechanism for coping with life stress, it is necessary to consider a basic proposition about the structure of psychological well-being: Overall well-being is determined by independent dimensions of positive affect and negative affect. This proposition is supported by research in a variety of settings (for a review, see Diener, 1984). It is important to note the implication that positive mood is not simply the absence of negative mood, or vice versa; instead, each appears to derive from different types of variables and occurrences.

The evidence suggests that substance use may indeed accomplish both functions: minimizing negative mood and maximizing positive mood. A considerable body of evidence indicates that cigarette smoking or alcohol use, for example, serve a direct stress-reduction function (see Abrams, 1983; Leventhal & Cleary, 1980). In addition, this evidence also indicates that substance use may serve to increase positive affect through providing physically pleasurable sensations and achieving feelings of relaxation. Similar dynamics have been found generally for ongoing use of substances and in relapse episodes among persons who are trying to cease substance use (Shiffman, 1982, in press). To illustrate the role of a substance for both reducing negative affect and increasing positive affect, evidence on smoking is considered in detail.

Motivations for Smoking Behavior

One body of evidence derives from studies of smoking motivation, where investigators ask smokers about the reasons for their smoking. Remarkable consistency has been found across studies that have factor-analyzed such reports (Gottlieb, 1983; Ikard, Green, & Horn, 1969; Leventhal & Avis, 1976; McKennel, 1970); these have found two higher order dimensions of smoking motivation, each comprising several related motives concerning negative- or positive-affect management. One higher order dimension includes subscales indicating that smoking is used to reduce anxiety, tension, nervous irritation, and stress. This dimension has been given labels such as *negative emotional reaction, inner need,* or *pharmacological smoking.* The second general dimension is based on subscales indicating that smoking is used for stimulation, in social situations, or to provide pleasure or taste. This dimension has been termed *positive emotional reactions,* or, because of its frequent association with social situations, *social smoking.*[6]

---

[6]Sometimes a third factor termed *habit* is found, representing automatic smoking, repetitive behavior, and sensorimotor stimulation.

It is important to note that these factor-analytic studies identify different motives for smoking, not necessarily different types of smokers. The general failure to find easily discriminable subgroups of cigarette smokers (Leventhal & Cleary, 1980) suggests that people smoke for both reasons, probably at different times and in different situations. Individuals may experience negative affect situations and positive affect situations at different times but may smoke in both of them. Also, individuals may self-regulate the physiological level of a particular substance (e.g., nicotine) to produce affect management effects that are consistent with their momentary mood, producing arousing effects or tranquilizing effects as needed. This proposition is consistent with physiological evidence from human and animal studies, which show that nicotine can produce either arousal or relaxation states depending on the dose, the time since administration, the situation, and perhaps the temporary emotional state of the individual (see Gilbert, 1979). Correspondent to studies of people's stated motives for smoking, similar findings have obtained in studies that examine the situations in which people smoke (Best & Hakstian, 1978; Frith, 1971) or relapse (Shiffman, in press). These show two higher order dimensions, one group representing stressful, negative, or highly arousing situations, the other group representing relaxing, happy, or social situations.

Motivations for Alcohol Use

A similar two-dimensional process is indicated by studies of alcohol use. Epidemiological research (Neff & Husaini, 1982; Pearlin & Radabaugh, 1976) has indicated a relationship between stress and heavy alcohol use. Pearlin and Radabaugh (1976) found this effect primarily for individuals who were low in perceived self-efficacy, which suggests a limited repertoire of coping responses. Studies of expectancies of the effects of alcohol consumption (Christiansen, Goldman, & Inn, 1982; Southwick, Steele, Marlatt, & Lindell, 1981) indicate a group of expected effects similar to that observed for smoking situations. One major group of factors represents the expectation that alcohol will reduce tension, provide relaxation, and divert a person from worrying about problems, a dimension that has usually been termed *tension reduction*. A more diverse group of factors represents pleasurable effects of alcohol use, including positive physical effects and increased enjoyment of social situations, together with some cognitive effects such as enhanced sense of personal power and optimism about the future. Laboratory research on tension-reduction models of alcohol action, like studies of nicotine, have produced somewhat complex results, indicating that alcohol may either minimize negative affect or enhance positive mood depending on the point on the blood alcohol curve, the subject's temporary mood state, and possibly some personality variables (see Abrams, 1983). For example, Russell and Mehrabian (1975) have related positive affect to a rising blood alcohol level (BAL) and a pattern of slow sipping of alcohol in order to prolong the affect, while negative affect is related to a falling blood alcohol curve and to rapid gulping of drinking to get quickly to the depressing CNS effects produced by the BAL.

Analogous to research on smoking, studies of relapse among problem drinkers who are attempting to abstain from alcohol (e.g., Van Hasselt, Hersen, & Milliones, 1978) indicated both stressful and positive experiences as determinants of relapse episodes. Marlatt and Gordon (1980) interviewed relapsed drinkers and found that the majority of relapse situations were directly attributable to stress or frustration, but a number of relapses occurred in what were essentially positive social situations. DiClemente, Gordon, and Gibertini (1983) applied factor analysis to reports of situations that caused temptations to drink. They found that negative affect and positive affect emerged as independent dimensions of drinking temptation. In summary, the literature on alcohol use also indicates a dual function, in which alcohol may serve either to reduce negative affect or to increase positive affect.

COPING AND STAGES OF INVOLVEMENT IN SUBSTANCE USE

From epidemiological and clinical research it is possible to distinguish three separate stages of involvement in substance use. Initiation of substance use, which typically occurs during adolescence, begins with a period of initial awareness and development of favorable attitudes toward a particular substance, followed by a few experiments with actual use, which typically occur in situations with close friends or peer group members (see Botvin & McAlister, 1981; Leventhal & Cleary, 1980; Biglan, Weissman, & Severson, Chapter 4, this volume). After initial trials of cigarettes or other substances, some individuals go on to become regular (i.e., weekly or daily) users, a process that may take 1–2 years for cigarettes and perhaps longer for alcohol. When regular use becomes established, physiological dependence may become important, with substance use governed in part by cyclic mechanisms that act to maintain the level of a particular biochemical (see Grunberg & Baum, Chapter 2, this volume). At some point many individuals become motivated to cease regular use of a substance, either because of perceived negative health consequences, social pressure to quit, or other factors. At this stage, the person is in a state of ambivalence or conflict, desiring abstinence (with its long-term benefits) but frequently confronting

Table 1.1
COPING PROCESSES FOR THREE PHASES OF SUBSTANCE USE

Coping response	Phase and response[a]		
	Initiation	Maintenance	Relapse
Cognitive coping			
Minimization, ignoring, restructuring	Minimize negative aspects of problems (−)	Minimize negative aspects of life events (−)	Minimize discomfort of cessation (−)
Efficacy enhancement	Build confidence for resisting offers of SU (−)	Build confidence for reducing rate of regular SU (−)	Build confidence for resisting temptations for SU (−)
Thoughts of consequences	Increase awareness of negative aspects of SU (−)	Increase awareness of negative aspects of continued SU (−)	Increase awareness of positive aspects of abstinence (−)
Willpower	Resist offers of SU (−)	Resist temptations for heavy SU (−)	Resist urges and temptations for SU (−)
Behavioral coping			
Decision making or problem solving	Make decision about cost–benefit of SU (−)	Decide whether to continue SU (?−)	Formulate plans and strategies for quitting (−)
Direct action	Acquire effective strategies for stress reduction	Change problematic situations or interaction patterns	Remove temptations or create more favorable situations
Withdrawal	Minimize contact with peer users (−)	Not known (?−)	Leave situations that provide temptation for SU (−)
Assertiveness	Resist social pressure for SU (−)	Resist social pressure (?−)	Resist social offers of substance (−)
Social support	Depends on attitudes of social network (±)	Reduces negative impact of stress (−)	Reduces stress, reinforces cessation (−)
Pleasure-seeking	Seek out peer users (+)	Not known (?+)	Stronger probability of seeking out SU (+)
Acceptance coping			
Passive responding	Accept offers of SU (+)	Engage in high level of SU (+)	Succumb to temptation for SU (+)
Religion	Values unfavorable toward SU (−)	Values, possible stress reduction (−)	Stress reduction, social support (?−)

[a]Signs indicate predicted direction of effect: − indicates decreased use; + indicates increased use, ?− indicates direction unknown, probably negative; ?+ indicates direction unknown, probably positive. SU denotes substance use.

situations that evoke impulses to obtain immediate distress relief or positive reinforcement through substance use (see Prochaska & DiClemente, Chapter 14, this volume). Coping behaviors may deter or promote substance use at each of these stages of involvement. A summary of the postulated operation of various coping responses at different stages of involvement is presented in Table 1.1.

Coping and Substance Use Initiation

The role of coping in the initiation of substance use probably depends on both stress-coping and temptation-coping skills. Deficits in general coping ability, reflected in poor academic performance, family conflict, and low self-esteem, appear to predispose young persons to substance abuse (e.g., Bachman, Johnston, & O'Malley, 1981; Kandel, Kessler, & Margulies, 1978). The perceptions that substance use will help reduce tension, that it will enhance the user's social image and perhaps gain access to desirable peer groups by making him or her appear tougher and more mature (Chassin, Presson, Sherman, Corty, & Olshavsky, 1981), and that it will provide positive physical sensations, may increase the probability of substance use for particular subgroups of adolescents. Thus the model suggests that teens who are comparatively low in basic coping skills will be more likely to experiment with substances such as tobacco or alcohol, or that, once having experimented, they will be more affected by the stress-reducing aspect of substance use (Wills, Chapter 3, this volume).

With respect to skills for coping with substance-related situations, the analysis notes that individuals who have more favorable attitudes toward a substance are likely to gravitate toward groups of users of that substance, and most introduction to substances occurs in social situations (see Biglan et al., Chapter 4, this volume). Avoidance of substance use in such situations probably depends on abilities to cognitively weigh the costs and benefits of substance use, exercise relevant self-control skills, and effectively refuse offered cigarettes or alcohol without alienating members of the peer group. Although these coping responses are probably correlated with stress-coping skills, they are by no means identical, and it is possible to hypothesize individuals who represent all combinations of the two domains of coping. Persons may have good stress-coping skills but poor temptation-coping skills or may have good stress-coping skills plus good temptation-coping skills. As a working assumption it is reasonable to predict that each type of coping will make an independent contribution to the probability of substance use.

Coping patterns are probably relevant also for the transition from experimentation to regular substance use. Some individuals who try cigarettes or alcohol lose interest after one or two trials while others go on to regular use. At present there are few sound data on variables that affect the transition to regular use, but the present framework suggests a major hypothesis. It has been proposed that there is a shift in determining factors, with the property of substances for increasing positive affect being the dominant factor for initial attraction and early experimentation, whereas the property of substances for reducing negative affect may become the dominant factor for more regular users (McKennel & Thomas, 1967; Ashton & Stepney, 1982). It follows that individuals who are experiencing more negative affect will be more likely to make the transition to regular use. Initially, their probable need for increasing positive affect may lead to a greater probability of experimentation, and once semiregular use has become established, these individuals may be more susceptible to the stress-reducing effects of the substance.

Another derivation from coping theory concerns the transition from experimentation to multiple substance use. It has been found consistently in adolescent samples that there is a marked intercorrelation between cigarette smoking, heavy drinking, and other substance use (e.g., Jessor, Chase, & Donovan, 1980; Wills, 1985b). Moreover, longitudinal investigations have shown that for a subgroup of teens there is a consistent sequence of substance use adoptions, beginning with smoking, progressing to alcohol use and smoking, followed by addition of marijuana use, and (for a small subgroup) proceeding to use of opiates and other "hard" drugs (see Kandel, 1975). These findings suggest that similar mechanisms underlie the use of these different substances. The present framework suggests that such mechanisms may lie largely in the domain of general coping skills, which might account for the variables of poor academic performance and alienation from family and social institutions that seem to be characteristic of heavy substance users (Kandel, Kessler, & Margulies, 1978; Kaplan, Martin, & Robbins, 1982). The substantial commonality in the determinants of heavy substance use in adolescence may derive from the fact that various substances are used to decrease stress (caused by poor role performance) and to increase positive affect enhancement and perhaps to enhance self-esteem through social image management.

Coping Behavior and Maintenance of Substance Use

Once regular use of a substance has become established, the rate and frequency of use may be related to stress and coping factors. Persons who are experiencing a greater level of generalized stress are hypothesized to be more likely to continue using substances and particularly to pursue heavy substance use such as addictive smoking, problem drinking, or dependence on opiates or tranquilizers (see Timmer et al., Chapter 7, this volume). This stress may derive from problems in work conditions or performance (Conway, Vickers, Ward, & Rahe, 1981), difficulties in relationships with family members (Cafferata, Kasper, & Bernstein, 1983), or general economic difficulties (Pearlin & Radabaugh, 1976). One would expect this phase of substance use to show some cyclicity (see DiClemente & Prochaska, Chapter 13, this volume). As individuals enter problematic periods of their lives and encounter increased stress, substance use is predicted to increase. For persons who successfully resolve problems that arise, the prediction is that substance use will diminish; in contrast, if they are unable to resolve and manage problems, it is likely that substance use will continue and perhaps develop into problematic use.

Social support may be particularly relevant for this phase of substance use because the capacity of social networks for providing supportive functions that help to reduce or buffer the potentially adverse impact of negative life events such as unemployment, divorce, or illness (see Cohen & Wills, in press; Tucker, Chapter 6, this volume). A coping formulation also predicts that at this stage of involvement the breadth or variety of a person's coping repertoire is most important for determining the ongoing rate of substance use. People with more support or better coping skills are predicted to be less likely to engage in heavy substance use. Unlike initiation or cessation stages, where specific situational skills may be particularly important, temptation-coping skills probably are not as relevant for the maintenance period. A possible exception is self-control skills, which would be relevant for situations in which an individual is under high stress and is subject to strong temptations for problematic substance use (e.g., drinking that leads to inebriation or difficulties in social relationships). These skills would enable individuals to maintain moderate substance use even in periods of high stress.

Coping Behavior and Cessation of Substance Use

Persons attempting to end an established pattern of substance use (e.g., individuals attempting to quit smoking or stop drinking) must apply coping responses from several different domains. They must deal with background stressors that raise the overall level of negative affect; they must deal with the temporary discomfort presented by withdrawal symptoms; and they must find alternative sources of positive affect to replace gratifications previously supplied by the substance habit. In addition they must cope with specific temptations to relapse that are evoked by stress, by associations with pleasurable activities, or by social stimuli such as observing substance use by other persons.

With regard to general life stress, there is considerable evidence that negative life events increase the probability of relapse among exsmokers, exdrinkers, and opiate addicts (Abrams, 1983; Gunn, 1983; Krueger, 1981; Litman, Eiser, Rawson, & Oppenheim, 1979; Mermelstein, Cohen, & Lichtenstein, 1983; Pomerleau, Adkins, & Pershuck, 1978; Rhoads, 1983; Rosenberg, 1983; Shiffman, 1982). Not much is known, however, about how generalized coping skills are related to relapse probability. One relevant study (Cronkite & Moos, 1980) found that alcoholic patients with more effective general coping skills were more likely to remain abstinent at a 2-year follow-up after treatment, and a clinical study by Chaney, O'Leary, and Marlatt (1978) showed that training in coping skills reduced the probability of relapse among alcoholic clients. The same kinds of constructive coping patterns that are relevant for reducing generalized stress levels (e.g., problem solving, cognitive coping, social support) would be expected to decrease the probability that episodes of serious temptation to relapse would occur.

Many coping strategies used in cessation are designed to prevent or minimize temptation. Anticipatory stimulus control strategies, such as removing ashtrays or liquor from the home, are meant to avoid the arousal of temptation by specific cues. Avoidance strategies (e.g., leaving a room when someone begins to smoke or avoiding situations where it is known that alcohol will be consumed) involve a similar approach because they anticipate the operation of social influences. Efficacy enhancement strategies, such as congratulating oneself for successfully handling difficult situations, may be applied to build confidence and self-efficacy for resisting subsequent temptations. Only a few of these anticipatory or preventive strategies have been studied in any detail.

More is known about immediate coping in specific situations where there is a strong temptation for relapse. Work by several investigators (Shiffman, 1984, Chapter 9, this volume; Curry & Marlatt, Chapter 10, this volume) has identified several coping patterns that may be used to cope with temptation. These can be classified into broad categories of behavioral coping, where the individual performs some action to cope with the temptation (e.g., assertiveness, relaxation, physical exercise, leaving the situation), and cognitive coping, where the individual engages in cognitive activity to forestall a relapse (e.g., thinking about positive consequences of abstaining, distracting attention from the temptation). The use of either cognitive or behavioral coping strategies has been shown to reduce the probability of relapse, and coping that combines both cognitive and behavioral responses is more effective than either used alone (Shiffman, Chapter 9; Curry & Marlatt, Chapter 10). Other studies (see Perri, Chapter 12, this volume; Sjöberg & Johnson, 1978; Sjöberg & Olsson, 1981) have indicated that the more coping responses a person uses over the course of an entire cessation effort, the greater the probability of success. This suggests that a broad repertoire of coping responses may be an effective deterrent to relapse.

To note some specific hypotheses, cognitive coping may be particularly important for dealing with slips: instances where a person has succumbed to temptation and taken a single drink or cigarette. Here, effective coping seems to involve minimizing the importance of the momentary lapse, generating confidence about ability to resist temptation in the future, and emphasizing one's previously successful performance (Curry & Marlatt, Chapter 10). Support from spouses or family members may also help individuals to cope effectively with temporary relapses and build confidence for long-term cessation (Mermelstein, Lichtenstein, & McIntyre, 1983). Problem-solving skills are probably important for planning the cessation effort. Social coping skills are probably relevant throughout the process of cessation. An individual can generate and maintain support for cessation efforts through discussion with social network members, can receive approval from others for successful cessation, and must deal assertively with social situations where persons offer cigarettes, liquor, or other temptations. Again, a broad range of coping responses is relevant for the eventual success or failure of persons who are attempting to cease substance use.

SUMMARY

A coping model appears to have considerable value for the area of substance use and its prevention. We hope that the present theoretical framework and the following chapters suggest new hypotheses about the processes involved in substance use and new treatment intervention techniques that may help individuals to successfully manage substance dependence or other problematic behavior. The book is intended to serve as a stimulus for further research in the area, which would build upon the current work in this field.

REFERENCES

Abrams, D. B. (1983). Psychosocial assessment of alcohol and stress interactions: Bridging the gap between laboratory and treatment outcome research. In L. A. Pohorecky & J. Brick (Eds.), *Stress and alcohol use*. New York: Elsevier.

Alexander, B. K., & Hadaway, P. F. (1982). Opiate addiction: The case for an adaptive orientation. *Psychological Bulletin, 92*, 367–381.

Ashton, H., & Stepney, R. (1982). *Smoking: Psychology and pharmacology*. New York: Tavistock Publications.

Bachman, J. G., Johnston, L. D., & O'Malley, P. M. (1981). Smoking, drinking, and drug use among American high school students: Correlates and trends, 1975–1979. *American Journal of Public Health, 71,* 59–69.

Baucom, D. H. & Aiken, P. A. (1981). Effect of depressed mood on eating among obese and nonobese dieting and nondieting persons. *Journal of Personality and Social Psychology, 41,* 577–585.

Best, J. A., & Hakstian, A. R. (1978). A situation-specific model for smoking behavior. *Addictive Behaviors, 3,* 79–92.

Botvin, G., & McAlister, A. (1981). Cigarette smoking among children and adolescents: Causes and prevention. In C. B. Arnold, L. H. Kuller, & M. R. Greenlick (Eds.), *Advances in disease prevention* (Vol. 1). New York: Springer.

Cafferata, G. L., Kasper, J., & Bernstein, A. (1983). Family roles, structure, and stressors in relation to sex differences in obtaining psychotropic drugs. *Journal of Health and Social Behavior, 24,* 132–143.

Chaney, E. F., O'Leary, M. R., & Marlatt, G. A. (1978). Skill training with alcoholics. *Journal of Consulting and Clinical Psychology, 46,* 1092–1104.

Chassin, L., Presson, C. C., Sherman, S. J., Corty, E., & Olshavsky, R. W. (1981). Self-images and cigarette smoking in adolescence. *Personality and Social Psychology Bulletin, 7,* 670–676.

Christiansen, B. A., Goldman, M. S., & Inn, A. (1982). Development of alcohol-related expectancies in adolescents: Separating pharmacological from social-learning influences. *Journal of Consulting and Clinical Psychology, 50,* 336–344.

Cohen, S., & Wills, T. A. (in press). Social support, stress, and the buffering hypothesis. *Psychological Bulletin.*

Conway, T. L., Vickers, R. R., Jr., Ward, H., & Rahe, R. H. (1981). Occupational stress and variation in cigarette, coffee, and alcohol consumption. *Journal of Health and Social Behavior, 22,* 155–165.

Coyne, J. C., & Lazarus, R. S. (1980). Cognitive style, stress perception, and coping. In I. L. Kutash & L. B. Schlesinger (Eds.), *Handbook on stress and anxiety: Contemporary knowledge, theory, and treatment.* San Francisco: Jossey-Bass.

Cronkite, R. C., & Moos, R. H. (1980). Determinants of the posttreatment functioning of alcoholic patients: A conceptual framework. *Journal of Consulting and Clinical Psychology, 48,* 305–316.

DeLongis, A., Coyne, J. C., Dakof, G., Folkman, S., & Lazarus, R. S. (1982). Relationship of daily hassles, uplifts, and major life events to health status. *Health Psychology, 1,* 119–136.

DiClemente, C. C., Gordon, J. R., & Gibertini, M. (1983, August). *Self-efficacy and determinants of relapse in alcoholism treatment.* Paper presented at the meeting of the American Psychological Association, Anaheim, CA.

Diener, E. (1984). Subjective well-being. *Psychological Bulletin, 95,* 542–575.

Doell, S. R., & Hawkins, R. C., II. (1982). Pleasures and pounds: An exploratory study. *Addictive Behaviors, 7,* 65–69.

Dohrenwend, B. S., & Dohrenwend, B. P. (Eds.). (1981). *Stressful life events and their contexts.* New York: Prodist.

Folkman, S., & Lazarus, R. S. (1980). Analysis of coping in a middle-aged community sample. *Journal of Health and Social Behavior, 21,* 219–239.

Frith, C. D. (1971). Smoking behavior and its relation to the smoker's immediate experience. *British Journal of Social and Clinical Psychology, 10,* 73–78.

Gilbert, D. G. (1979). Paradoxical tranquilizing and emotion-reducing effects of nicotine. *Psychological Bulletin, 86,* 643–661.

Gottlieb, N. H. (1983). The determination of smoking types: Evidence for a sociological-pharmacological continuum. *Addictive Behaviors, 8,* 47–51.
Gunn, R. C. (1983). Smoking clinic failures and recent life stress. *Addictive Behaviors, 8,* 83–87.
Ikard, F. F., Green, D. E., & Horn, D. A. (1969). A scale to differentiate between types of smoking as related to management of affect. *International Journal of the Addictions, 4,* 649–659.
Jessor, R., Chase, J. A., & Donovan, J. E. (1980). Psychosocial correlates of marijuana use and problem drinking in a national sample of adolescents. *American Journal of Public Health, 70,* 604–613.
Kandel, D. B. (1975). Stages of adolescent involvement in drug use. *Science, 190,* 912–914.
Kandel, D. B., Kessler, R. C., & Margulies, R. Z. (1978). Antecedents of adolescent initiation into stages of drug use: A developmental analysis. In D. B. Kandel (Ed.), *Longitudinal research on drug use: Empirical findings and methodologic issues.* New York: Wiley.
Kaplan, H. B., Martin, S. S., & Robbins, C. (1982). Application of a general theory of deviant behavior: Self-derogation and drug use. *Journal of Health and Social Behavior, 23,* 274–294.
Krueger, D. W. (1981). Stressful life events and the return to heroin use. *Journal of Human Stress, 7,* 3–8.
Lazarus, R. S. (1977). Cognitive and coping processes in emotion. In A. Monat & R. S. Lazarus (Eds.), *Stress and coping: An anthology.* New York: Columbia University Press.
Leon, G. R., & Chamberlain, K. (1973). Emotional arousal, eating patterns, and body image as differential factors associated with varying success in maintaining weight loss. *Journal of Consulting and Clinical Psychology, 40,* 474–480.
Leventhal, H., & Avis, N. (1976). Pleasure, addiction, and habit: Factors in verbal report on factors in smoking behavior. *Journal of Abnormal Psychology, 85,* 478–488.
Leventhal, H., & Cleary, P. D. (1980). The smoking problem: A review of the research and theory in behavioral risk modification. *Psychological Bulletin, 88,* 370–405.
Lewinsohn, P. M., & Amenson, C. S. (1978). Some relations between pleasant and unpleasant mood-related events and depression. *Journal of Abnormal Psychology, 87,* 644–654.
Litman, G. K., Eiser, J. R., Rawson, N. S. B., & Oppenheim, A. N. (1979). Differences in relapse precipitants and coping behavior between alcohol relapsers and survivors. *Behavioral Research and Therapy, 17,* 89–94.
Marlatt, G. A., & Gordon, J. R. (1980). Determinants of relapse: Implications for the maintenance of behavior change. In P. O. Davison & S. M. Davison (Eds.), *Behavioral medicine: Changing health lifestyles.* New York: Brunner/Mazel.
McKennell, A. C. (1970). Smoking motivation factors. *British Journal of Social and Clinical Psychology, 9,* 8–22.
McKennel, A. C., & Thomas, R. K. (1967). *Adults' and adolescents' smoking habits and attitudes.* London: British Ministry of Health.
Meichenbaum, D. (1977). *Cognitive-behavior modification: An integrative approach.* New York: Plenum Press.
Mermelstein, R., Cohen, S., & Lichtenstein, E. (1983, August). Perceived and objective stress, social support, and smoking cessation. In S. Shiffman (Chair), *Stress and smoking: Effects on initiation, maintenance, and relapse.* Symposium presented at the meeting of the American Psychological Association, Anaheim, California.
Mermelstein, R., & Lichtenstein, E. (1983, March). *Slips vs. relapses in smoking cessation: A situational analysis.* Paper presented at the meeting of the Western Psychological Association, Los Angeles.

Mermelstein, R., Lichtenstein, E., & McIntyre, K. (1983). Partner support and relapse in smoking-cessation programs. *Journal of Consulting and Clinical Psychology, 51,* 465–466.
Moos, R. H., & Billings, A. G. (1982). Conceptualizing and measuring coping resources and processes. In L. Goldberger & S. Breznitz (Eds.), *Handbook of stress: Theoretical and clinical aspects.* New York: Macmillan.
Neff, J. A., & Husaini, B. A. (1982). Life events, drinking patterns and depressive symptomatology: The stress-buffering effect of alcohol consumption. *Journal of Studies on Alcohol, 43,* 301–318.
Pearlin, L. I., & Radabaugh, C. W. (1976). Economic strains and the coping functions of alcohol. *American Journal of Sociology, 82,* 652–663.
Pearlin, L. I., & Schooler, C. (1978). The structure of coping. *Journal of Health and Social Behavior, 19,* 2–21.
Pomerleau, O., Adkins, D., & Perschuck, M. (1978). Predictors of outcome and recidivism in smoking cessation treatment. *Addictive Behaviors, 3,* 65–70.
Rhoads, D. L. (1983). A longitudinal study of life stress and social support among drug abusers. *International Journal of the Addictions, 18,* 195–222.
Rosenberg, H. S. (1983). Relapsed vs. nonrelapsed alcohol abusers: Coping skills, life events, and social support. *Addictive Behaviors, 8,* 183–186.
Russell, J. A., & Mehrabian, A. (1975). The mediating role of emotions in alcohol use. *Journal of Studies on Alcohol, 36,* 1508–1536.
Shiffman, S. (1982). Relapse following smoking cessation: A situational analysis. *Journal of Consulting and Clinical Psychology, 50,* 71–86.
Shiffman, S. (1984). Coping with temptations to smoke. *Journal of Consulting and Clinical Psychology, 52,* 261–267.
Shiffman, S. (in press). A cluster-analytic classification of smoking relapse episodes. *Addictive Behaviors.*
Sjöberg, L., & Johnson, T. (1978). Trying to give up smoking: A study of volitional breakdowns. *Addictive Behaviors, 3,* 149–164.
Sjöberg, L., & Olsson, G. (1981). Volitional problems in carrying through a difficult decision: The case of drug addiction. *Drug and Alcohol Dependence, 7,* 177–191.
Sjöberg, L., & Persson, L. O. (1979). A study of attempts by obese patients to regulate eating. *Addictive Behaviors, 4,* 349–359.
Solomon, R. L. (1980). The opponent-process theory of acquired motivation: The costs of pleasure and the benefits of pain. *American Psychologist, 35,* 691–712.
Southwick, L., Steele, C., Marlatt, A., & Lindell, M. (1981). Alcohol-related expectancies: Defined by phase of intoxication and drinking experience. *Journal of Consulting and Clinical Psychology, 49,* 713–721.
Tucker, J. A., Vuchinich, R. E., & Sobell, M. B. (1981). Alcohol consumption as a self-handicapping strategy. *Journal of Abnormal Psychology, 90,* 220–230.
Van Hasselt, V. B., Hersen, M., & Milliones, J. (1978). Social skills training for alcoholics and drug addicts: A review. *Addictive Behaviors, 3,* 221–233.
Wills, T. A. (1983). Social comparison in coping and help-seeking. In B. M. DePaulo, A. Nadler, & J. D. Fisher (Eds.), *New directions in helping*: Vol. 2. *Help-seeking.* New York: Academic Press.
Wills, T. A. (1985a). Supportive functions of interpersonal relationships. In S. Cohen & L. Syme (Eds.), *Social support and health.* New York: Academic Press.
Wills, T. A. (1985b). *Objective stress, subjective stress, and substance use in adolescence.* Unpublished manuscript, Cornell University Medical College, 1985.
Wills, T. A., & Langner, T. S. (1980). Socioeconomic status and stress. In I. L. Kutash & L. B. Schlesinger (Eds.), *Handbook on stress and anxiety.* San Francisco: Jossey-Bass.

Chapter 2

Biological Commonalities of Stress and Substance Abuse*

NEIL E. GRUNBERG
ANDREW BAUM

INTRODUCTION AND OVERVIEW

Stress and substance abuse seem to go together—but why? Individuals commonly report that drugs are sometimes taken to relieve stress. This implies that drugs of abuse decrease stress or in some way relieve associated upset and tension. Alternatively, stress may lead to increased drug taking because stress induces particular psychological or biological effects that alter the pharmacological effects of drugs of abuse. Possibly, the drug effects of a given dose are diminished under stress, so an increased dosage or increased frequency of administration may be required to have the same effects as taking the drug when stress is not present. Another possibility is that administration of drugs of abuse may come to be associated with stressors. The effects of these drugs may become identified with the similar effects of stressful stimuli or situations, and drug taking therefore may increase under stress. In contrast, it could be that cessation of administration of drugs acts as a stressor because of physiological disequilibrium or psychological discomfort, and leads to continued drug taking. Regardless, psychological, behavioral, social, pharmacological, and physiological factors must be considered in order to understand the relationship between stress and drug abuse.

This chapter presents and discusses biological factors involved in stress and drug abuse and emphasizes possible commonalities. The idea that there may be biological commonalities in substance abuse and habitual behavior

---

*The opinions or assertions contained herein are the private ones of the authors and are not to be construed as official or reflecting the views of the Department of Defense or the Uniformed Services University of the Health Sciences.

is not new. For example, panels of reputable investigators and scholars have addressed this issue (see National Research Council, 1977). The results of such conferences tend to be lists of interesting questions that need to be answered, accompanied by some intriguing speculation. However, individual authors who discuss this question usually emphasize only one biological system (e.g., endogenous opioids) and do not address the role of other physiological factors, such as the autonomic nervous system, respiratory function, gastric function, and so on (see Bloom, 1983; McClearn, 1983; Weisz & Thompson, 1983). We have been struck by the relative silence in the literature regarding possible commonalities of biological effects, other than endogenous opioids, across drugs of abuse. In contrast to those who examine biological effects of drugs, some behavioral pharmacologists (e.g., Falk, 1983; Barrett & Witkin, 1985) emphasize nonpharmacological explanations of the effects of drugs of abuse. However, it may be that the sometimes overriding importance of behavioral variables on drug self-administration (including history, response rates, and schedules of reinforcement) attests to underlying behavioral commonalities in responses to drugs that overshadow the differences in biological effects across drugs. These are some of the questions we address in this chapter.

In addition to discussing biological commonalities in drug abuse, this chapter considers biological factors in stress. Fairly successful attempts have been made to determine some biological commonalities in response to different stressors (see Selye, 1976), but we know of no synthesis of biological commonalities in stress and drug abuse. The chapter presents brief overviews of biological effects of stress and then biological effects of drugs of abuse. There is a separate section describing endogenous opioid peptides, because many investigators and theorists are searching for commonalities within this rapidly expanding field. Finally, we discuss possible biological commonalities between stress and drug abuse.

STRESS AND THE STRESS RESPONSE

Overview

Recent studies and discussions of stress emphasize integration of psychological and biological perspectives for its measurement, mechanisms of action, and consequences (Baum, Grunberg, & Singer, 1982; Jenkins, 1979). These analyses typically consider psychological activation of physiological processes that occur during and after stress, following Mason's (1975) position that psychological awareness of danger, threat, and/or harm is necessary for these responses to occur.

The stress response appears to be similar in many ways to the emergency response first described by Cannon (1915, 1929). This biological change suggested a general arousal response that accompanied threat or danger. More commonly known as the fight-or-flight response, this arousal involved the sympathetic nervous system and was viewed as adaptive in preparing the organism to resist (by making it stronger and less vulnerable) or to flee (by making it faster). The presence or threat of danger was accompanied by an increase in adrenal secretion of epinephrine; increases in heart rate, blood pressure, and respiration; decreases in blood flow to the viscera and skin; and increases in blood flow to skeletal muscles and in general muscle tone.

Cannon's work suggested the importance of adrenal hormones in emotional response and stress. Subsequent work by Selye (1976) called attention to a different neuroendocrine pathway and to different adrenal hormones. Because the adrenal glands appear to be central to the stress response, we briefly discuss features of these glands relevant to the stress response.

The Adrenal Glands

The adrenal glands are located at the superior poles of the two kidneys. Each of the adrenal glands is composed of medullary and cortical tissue. These two parts of the adrenal gland secrete different hormones, and their activity may be stimulated by different events. The adrenal medulla, containing cells that synthesize, store, and release epinephrine (adrenaline) and norepinephrine, are also rich with secretors for endogenous opioids. (This feature is important for reasons that are discussed later.) Generally, epinephrine and norepinephrine have effects throughout the body similar to stimulation of the sympathetic nervous system (SNS). Stimulation of the SNS causes arousal throughout the body opposed by the effects of parasympathetic stimulation, which generally reduces arousal and brings the body back toward resting levels of functioning. The adrenal cortex also secretes two major types of hormones: glucocorticoids and mineralocorticoids. The glucocorticoids (mostly cortisol in humans) affect carbohydrate, protein, and fat metabolism, altering the availability of glucose and other nutrients. Mineralocorticoids affect the essential electrolytes (especially sodium and potassium).

Selye and the Adrenal Cortical Response

Selye's studies of stress described a response syndrome that he believed could account for the observation of common pathology caused by divergent noxious agents: the general adaptation syndrome (GAS) (Selye, 1956,

1976). The GAS emphasizes the role of corticosteroids in generating the stress-induced responses and has a few other characteristic features. First, the syndrome is nonspecific. That is, it is caused by any stressor. Extreme cold, stressful anticipation, and injection of organ extract all cause the same responses by the organism. Selye rejected the view that different events might cause similar but distinct responses and argued that the GAS was associated with all insults or injuries. It is important to note, however, that the GAS is specific in the sense that it is a particular, general response to all stressful stimuli.

Another characteristic of the GAS is that it is divided into three phases. During the first phase, the alarm, the body mobilizes and prepares to counter whatever threat is posed. During the resistance phase that follows, the body deals with the stressor and usually overcomes it. If this does not occur, a third phase follows. During this phase of exhaustion, the organism depletes its ability to cope and is at risk for organ damage and disease. The actual mechanisms by which these phases occur are presumed to be based in the pituitary–adrenal cortical system. According to Selye, the alarm phase of the GAS is centered on secretion of adrenocorticotropic hormone (ACTH) by the pituitary which, among other effects, evokes secretion of cortisol from the adrenals. This increase is maintained as long as resistance is required, within the limits of the glands' ability to do so. If a stressor persists long enough, the adrenals may become exhausted, and secretion of corticoids then decreases rapidly.

A number of studies have shown that a wide variety of stressors give rise to response by the pituitary–adrenocortical axis and that this response follows the general pattern outlined by the GAS (Selye, 1976). Exposure to stress is characterized by increases in plasma levels of ACTH as well as depletion of pituitary ACTH, increased secretion of glucocorticoids (such as cortisol), and increased secretion of mineralocorticoids, most notably aldosterone (Elmadjian, 1962; Ingle, 1950; Rochefort, Rosenberger, & Saffran, 1959).[1] It should be considered, however, that some investigators argue that cortisol levels have limited value as indicators of arousal because this endocrinological response and behavioral arousal may be dissociated (Natelson, Krasnegor, & Holaday, 1976).

The Adrenal Medullary Response

A number of developments during the past 25 years, including refinements in assay procedures and the discovery of norepinephrine, influenced some investigators to reconsider the role of the medulla in the stress re-

---

[1] The adrenal glands' role in response to stress or shock also is suggested by their extensive vasculature. Blood flow in and out of the adrenals has been estimated at 5 ml per minute. Each gland is supplied by up to 50 arteries (Bethune, 1974).

sponse. Mason (1968) found that adrenal medullary hormones—the catecholamines, epinephrine and norepinephrine—increased during stress in much the same ways as did the corticosteroids, and Frankenhaeuser (1972, 1975) found evidence of adrenal medullary activity in response to a range of psychological stressors. Research evidence from studies of humans and animals has continued to accumulate indicating that epinephrine and norepinephrine play a central role in stress (Baum et al., 1982; Campbell & Singer, 1983).

Present evidence suggests that levels of epinephrine in the periphery are derived entirely from medullary activity. In contrast, peripheral levels of norepinephrine are affected by other sources in addition to the adrenal. Sympathetic nerve endings secrete norepinephrine throughout the body, and concentrations of norepinephrine-bearing cells also have been located in vascular beds. Therefore, during periods of heightened SNS activity, there should be a rise in levels of norepinephrine, independent of adrenomedullary response.

Unlike adrenal cortical stimulation, the medullae are not activated by the pituitary but rather are innervated by the SNS. Arousal of the SNS results in the kinds of responses described by Cannon, and it appears that the secretion of catecholamines supports and extends these responses over longer periods of time. Epinephrine, among other things, increases heart rate. Norepinephrine constricts blood vessels and extends the length of SNS arousal. Adrenomedullary response during stress is best viewed as an integrated part of SNS arousal.

Other Endocrine Responses

In addition to corticosteroids, norepinephrine, and epinephrine, other endocrine responses are involved in stress. Mason (1968) reported that increases in corticosteroids and catecholamines during stress are accompanied by increases in thyroid hormones and growth hormone and by decreases in insulin, testosterone, and estrone. These findings led Mason (1975) to propose that endocrine activity during stress reflected one of two general processes: Some activity is catabolic, increasing energy availability, while some activity is anabolic, inhibiting tissue synthesis. Corticosteroid and catecholamine levels (which increase during exposure to stress) facilitate arousal and energy release, while insulin (which is more important for storing energy) decreases during exposure to stress but increases after exposure ends. Unfortunately, research is not consistent on some aspects of this response pattern.[2]

[2]Stress also affects secretion of growth hormone; most studies report increases during stress. However, a recent animal study reported that stress suppresses growth hormone secretion (Kant, Meyerhoff, Bunnell, & Lenox, 1982). Luteinizing hormone (LH) and follicle-stimulat-

Cholesterol, a precursor of corticosteroids, also appears to vary with stress. Most studies suggest that stress depletes levels of adrenal cholesterol while increasing plasma levels (e.g., Kasl, Cobb, & Brooks, 1968). There also is evidence of changes in vasopressin during stress. Studies have suggested that vasopressin has effects that are similar to those of ACTH (e.g., DeWied, Bohus, & Wimersma Greidanus, 1974), that administration of vasopressin acts to maintain stress-mediated responses beyond the period of exposure (Bohus, Gispen, & DeWied, 1973), and that vasopressin is released during stress (Fendler, Rakoczi, & Zibotics, 1966).

In describing the stress response, we have focused on autonomic responses and the endocrine system as a central component of autonomic arousal. SNS activity appears to be an important aspect of bodily response to stress, and pituitary–adrenocortical activity also appears to play a significant role. The role of other hormones is less clear, though Mason (1968) has suggested that they fit as part of an integrated, central nervous system (CNS)-mediated stress response. More recently, interest in other modes of stress response has increased, particularly the role of endogenous opioids.

Endogenous Opioid Peptides and Stress

Recent discoveries of endogenous opioid peptides (EOPs) have altered scientific perspectives on a number of issues. Receptors for EOPs have been found throughout the CNS and in a number of peripheral organs and ganglia including the adrenal medulla. Initial studies of the morphine-like effects of EOPs concentrated on pain threshold, but findings also suggested effects on behavior as well as on the functioning of other organs (Millan & Emrich, 1981).

A number of factors point to a role for EOPs in stress. Findings of animal studies suggested that stress produced an analgesic-like effect (i.e., increased pain tolerance) that could be explained by stress-linked secretion of EOPs (Kelly, 1982). The presence of opiate receptors in the adrenal and the finding that EOPs altered pituitary activity also suggested that EOPs might be involved in stress (Chavkin, Cox, & Goldstein, 1979; Gibson, Ginsburg, Hall, & Hart, 1979).

Studies have indicated that stress is associated with changes in levels of EOPs in both the CNS and in the periphery (Amir, Brown, & Amit, 1979; Millan & Emrich, 1981; Kant, Mougey, Pennington, & Meyeroff, 1983).

---

ing hormone (FSH) show inconsistent changes during stress. Cartensen, Amér, Wide, and Amér (1973) found decreases in LH and no changes in FSH during the first 24 hours after surgical stress, while Euker, Meites, and Riegle (1975) reported increases in these hormones during stress. Neill (1970) found increases in prolactin during stress but reported no changes in LH levels.

Stress-induced analgesia can be blocked by administration of opiate antagonists such as naloxone (Bodnar, Glusman, Brutus, Spiaggia, & Kelley, 1980), further suggesting that this effect is mediated by EOPs secreted during stress. Research also indicates that morphine affects activity by the adrenal medulla and suggests that EOPs may affect epinephrine secretion during stress. Gibson et al. (1979) reported that naloxone can prevent or reduce plasma increases in corticosteroids during exposure to a stressor. Therefore, EOP activity is associated with corticosteroid increases. In addition, clinical research has indicated that naloxone blocks some stress effects while exacerbating others (Millan & Emrich, 1981).

EOPs deserve particular attention in this chapter because they also may be involved in the effects and mechanisms of action of drugs of abuse. A fuller discussion of EOPs is presented in the section, "Endogenous Opioid Peptides," after the effects of drugs of abuse are described.

Systemic and Organ System Effects of Stress

Stress has a number of other physiological consequences, some of which are mediated by the effects we already have considered. Basal metabolic rate decreases during severe stress (Cannon, 1929). However, studies have suggested that initial response to stress (i.e., during the alarm phase) includes increased metabolic rate (Kirschner, Prosser, & Quastler, 1949; Selye, 1976). Changes in gastrointestinal function have been noted. Stress hormones, including ACTH and corticosteroids, have been linked to basal nocturnal gastric hydrochloric acid and pepsin secretion, but this ulcerative condition can be blocked by vagotomy. Although the reasons for stress-induced ulcers are not clear, acid secretion and hormonal factors appear to be the most probable cause (Gray, Ramsey, Reifenstein, & Benson, 1953; Selye, 1937).

Hepatic function appears to be affected by stress—a fact that is important in the present context because drugs are metabolized in the liver. Chronic stress has been associated with decreases in liver size, congestion of peripheral hepatic lobules, and degeneration and necrosis of liver tissue (MacMahon, 1929; Moon, 1948). The distribution of necrosis in the liver is irregular. Destroyed tissue may be scattered widely or limited to small sections. The consequences of these effects, therefore, are unclear.

Cardiovascular and respiratory function are affected by stress. Sympathetic arousal includes, among other things, increases in heart rate and respiration rate. Epinephrine causes dilation of the bronchi, increasing the amount of oxygen that can be taken in and the carbon dioxide that can be released. Pulmonary circulation also may be affected (Szidon & Fishman, 1971). Stress appears to cause myocardial necroses, changes in blood pressure, arteriosclerotic lesions, and increased cardiac output (Hauss, 1973; Raab, Chaplin, & Bajusz, 1964). Stress is typically associated with increased blood pressure and heart rate, but severe stress may cause blood pressure and heart rate to fall (Border, Gallo, & Schenk, 1966; Morris, 1941; Mordkoff, 1964).

Enzymes

Stress appears to affect many enzymes but research on this topic is limited.[3] Stress facilitates drug metabolism via corticosteroid secretion (Rupe, Bousquet, & Miya, 1963). For example, the length of time needed to metabolize hexobarbital, pentobarbital, and meprobamate is reduced by stress, and this effect can be regulated by adrenalectomy and administration of corticosteroids (Bousquet, Rupe, & Miya, 1965; Driever, Bousquet, & Miya, 1966). This effect has not been noted with phenobarbital, and Stitzel and Furner (1967) have suggested that stress-induced stimulation of microsomal metabolism is additive to the effects of phenobarbital. Additional research attention concerning the effects of particular stressors on enzymes in the liver that metabolize exogenous agents (such as drugs of abuse) may provide valuable information to help understand the relationship between stress and drug abuse.

Summary

This brief review of biological aspects of stress depicts bodily responses occurring in a vacuum. However, environmental and psychological contexts in which these responses occur are crucial. For instance, whether stimuli or situations are perceived as stressful and whether the individual successfully copes with a stressor alter the physiological response to the stressor

---

[3]Stress increases the concentration and secretion of salivary amylase (Groza, Zamfir, & Lungu, 1971), adrenal adenosine nucleotide-metabolizing enzymes (ATPase), and decarboxylases (Hilf, Breuer, & Borman, 1961; Schayer, 1960). Stress also augments enzymes that participate in the synthesis of adrenal hormones, facilitating the production of catecholamines, for example, by increasing levels of tyrosine hydroxylase (Kvetnansky & Kopin, 1972).

Stress-related increases in glucocorticoids stimulate production of hepatic enzymes (Knox, 1962; Nemeth & Jurani, 1974). There is evidence that clearing factor lipase production is inhibited during stress (Ham & Slack, 1969; Seifter & Baeder, 1954). Reduction in lipase activity impairs elimination of blood lipids and is probably caused by increased catecholamine levels (Oehler, Wolf, Schmahl, & Roka, 1974). Studies suggest that there is stress-related release of plasminogen activator from hepatic lysosomes (Beard, Carroll, & Danos, 1969) and that changes in levels of tyrosine aminotransferase (TAT) in the liver also may be related to stress (Nemeth, Strakova, & Vigas, 1973; Nemeth & Jurani, 1974). Further, stress may reduce levels of tryptophan pyrrolase activity in the liver (Nomura, 1965; Green & Curzon, 1975).

(Lazarus, 1966). It is not possible to determine clearly whether stress patterns are situation-specific or nonspecific, but most stressors appear to evoke activity by the SNS and the pituitary–adrenocortical axis. Challenge to the organism is met by readying responses that prepare the organism to cope and with resistance by integrated psychoneuroendocrine-mediated responses.

DRUGS OF ABUSE

Overview

Most drugs of abuse can be categorized into eight pharmacological groups: opioids; general central nervous system (CNS) depressants; CNS sympathomimetics (including cocaine); nicotine and tobacco; cannabinoids; psychedelics (hallucinogens, psychotomimetics, psychotogens); arylcyclohexylamines (e.g., phencyclidine); and inhalants (e.g., nitrous oxide, ethyl ether, volatile solvents) (Jaffe, 1980). "*Drug abuse* refers to the use, usually by self-administration, of any drug in a manner that deviates from the approved medical or social patterns within a given culture" (Jaffe, 1980, p. 535). Substances may be abused for psychological, sociological, or biological reasons (Lettieri, Sayers, & Pearson, 1980; Levison, 1981). The biological reasons for abuse have been broadly characterized as (1) a "liking" factor, and (2) the effects of tolerance and physical dependence. The liking factor has been separated into two processes: mood elevation and relief of anxiety or tension (Way, 1978). The influence of these processes on drug abuse might be considered in psychological terms as positive and negative reinforcement.

Self-administration and the reinforcing function of abused drugs have been highlighted as important commonalities in substance abuse (Brady, 1981). Although self-administration is a behavior, the reinforcement that maintains it is a commonality that may be biologically based. Some investigators have argued that brain-stimulation reward (intracranial self-administration) is a model for the euphoric effects of abused drugs and may suggest biological commonalities for the behavior of self-administration (Kornetsky & Bain, 1982). Other investigators argue that reinforcement involves particular chemicals in the brain, particularly catecholamines and endogenous opioid peptides (see the sections, "Endogenous Opioid Peptides" and "Stress and Drug Abuse: The Search for Commonalities"), and the reinforcement effects of these chemicals help to explain the behavior of drug self-administration.

In addition to these biobehavioral effects, addictive drugs of abuse typically have three biological effects: physical dependence, tolerance, and withdrawal.[4] Physical dependence exists when continued drug administration is required to prevent the withdrawal or abstinence syndrome. Tolerance exists when a given drug dosage results in a decreased effect or when increasingly larger dosages are required to have the effects of the original dose (Jaffe, 1980).

With regard to the association between physical dependence and withdrawal, Jaffe (1980, p. 539) writes:

> Physical dependence has been studied after chronic administration of opioids, general depressants of the CNS (alcohol, barbiturates, and related hypnotics), amphetamines, cannabinoids, nicotine, and opioid antagonists. The withdrawal symptoms associated with many of these classes of agents are characterized by rebound effects in those same physiological systems that were modified initially by the drug (*rebound hyperexcitability*). For example, general depressants elevate the seizure threshold, but spontaneous seizures are seen during withdrawal; morphine depresses the flexor and crossed extensor reflexes, but these same polysynaptic reflexes are hyperexcitable during morphine withdrawal. Amphetamines alleviate fatigue, suppress appetite, and elevate mood; amphetamine withdrawal is characterized by lack of energy, hyperphagia, and depression. Nicotine tends to suppress anger and produce an alerting pattern in the EEG; irritability and drowsiness are common complaints following abrupt cessation in heavy smokers.

Considering the diversity of drug effects and withdrawal effects following cessation of different drugs, it may seem that a search for biological commonalities is a quixotic quest. However, the fact that there are differences between drugs in their direct and withdrawal effects does not obviate the possibility that there are underlying similarities in mechanisms and processes. The search is more difficult than simply finding similar gross effects. The fact that one drug can replace another drug in terms of physically dependent effects (cross-dependence) and that experience with one drug can alter the effects of another drug (cross-tolerance) suggests that there are some biological commonalities. But only certain drugs show these effects with each other and they usually are within the same or similar pharmacological classes. However, there are examples of cross-tolerance between drugs of different classes, such as alcohol and opiates (see Levine, Hess, & Morley, 1983). Also, it has been reported that naloxone (an antagonist that blocks or reduces the effects of opiates) blocks the threshold-decreasing effects of *d*-amphetamine and cocaine on intracranial self-stimulation (Esposito, Perry, & Kornetsky, 1980; Kornetsky, Bain, & Riedl, 1981). In addition, Griffiths, Bigelow, and Henningfield (1980) maintain

---

[4]Physical dependence and tolerance are not inseparable characteristics. Tolerance develops with many drugs that are not self-administered. However, most theories of physical dependence and the effects of most self-administered drugs of abuse involve physical dependence and tolerance, and these conditions usually develop and decay at similar rates.

that there are experimental manipulations that show similarities across drugs of abuse. Generally, drug self-administration is increased with increasing dose up to a point (examples include pentobarbital, diazepam, and ethanol). In addition, increases in the response requirement (or response cost) result in decreases in the total amount of drug consumed (e.g., ethanol, pentobarbital, diazepam, methadone, tobacco). These similarities may involve biological commonalities, behavioral commonalities, or both.

The withdrawal or abstinence syndrome is important for clinical and scientific reasons. One reason many people maintain their drug habit is to avoid the unpleasantness of withdrawal. This explanation has been used for self-administration of drugs ranging from opiates (Wikler, 1948, 1973) to tobacco (Schachter, 1977). Similar to cross-dependence and cross-tolerance, some drugs suppress the withdrawal effects resulting from cessation of other drugs. For example, pentobarbital can suppress withdrawal from alcohol (Jaffe, 1980). However, not all drugs of abuse can be substituted for all others, so there is no single, obvious commonality. Although withdrawal effects differ for different drugs, there is one notable similarity across drugs. That is, "the withdrawal syndrome is in many respects the mirror image of the 'primary effects of the drug'" (Lasagna, 1981, p. 24). This mirror image, which is similar to the point made by Jaffe (1980) regarding rebound, suggests that there may be an underlying biological commonality in that repeated exposure to a drug results in an opposite or opponent effect that becomes obvious only after cessation of drug administration (see Solomon & Corbit, 1973, for one version of this theory).

Biological scientists often reject such general notions as commonalities when the specific mechanisms are not stipulated or when clear biological differences can be identified (as is the case for effects of drugs and withdrawal effects). In contrast, physical scientists assume that "laws" operate as underlying commonalities despite differences in observed details. Gravity is a physical science mechanism (law) although its cause is unknown. By analogy, one biological law might be the relationship between the effects of drugs of abuse and the rebound effects of withdrawal.

Nonpharmacological Explanations of Effects of Drugs of Abuse

PSYCHOLOGICAL FACTORS IN BIOLOGICAL EFFECTS OF DRUGS OF ABUSE

The biological effects of dependence and withdrawal are accompanied by psychological and behavioral factors. For example, the emergence of the withdrawal syndrome from mild to extreme physical symptoms is accompanied by increasingly intense self-reports of craving for the drug of abuse (Henningfield, Griffiths, & Jasinski, 1981). Moreover, psychological effects may come to cause biological effects. It is now clear that conditioned responses play a role in the effects of administration of drugs of abuse and cessation of these drugs. There are clinical examples and experimental evidence for biological effects that are a result of conditioned drug effects. For example, habitual opiate users display opiate-like effects with saline injections (that they think are opiate injections). Also, opiate addicts experience withdrawal symptoms when shown films of themselves using drugs or drug-related pictures (O'Brien, Ternes, Grabowski, & Ehrman, 1981).

There are at least three nonbiological explanations of tolerance and physical dependence. According to the classical (Pavlovian) conditioning approach, repeated drug administration and the environmental cues associated with drugs and drug self-administration become conditioned stimuli that eventually cause (as a conditioned response) the physiological responses that result from repeated administration of the drug. Another view is that tolerance is the result of a behavioral cost associated with use of a drug, such as a decrease in reinforcement frequency or an increase in the frequency of punishment. This situation provides a stimulus to correct the drug-affected behavior to regain the reward or avoid the punishment. A third position holds that tolerance is a homeostatic physiological response to the functional disturbance produced by the drug (and not to the drug itself), and that conditioning and reinforcement also are involved (Kalant, 1978).

There are ample demonstrations of conditioned effects and drugs of abuse to be convinced that this is a real phenomenon. For example, Siegel (1976) reported that analgesic tolerance to morphine occurs in rats in environments in which they previously received morphine but not in an environment where morphine had not been given. There also have been reports that conditioning is involved in tolerance to the hyperthermic effect of morphine (Siegel, 1976), the lethal effects of opiates (Siegel, Hinson, & Krank, 1979; Siegel, Hinson, Krank, & McCully, 1982), and hypothermic tolerance to pentobarbital and ethanol (Cappell, Roach, & Poulos, 1981; Crowel, Hinson, & Siegel, 1981; Mansfield & Cunningham, 1980). In addition to these animal studies, there have been demonstrations that conditioned stimuli paired with opiate abstinence precipitated by opiate antagonists (e.g., naloxone) elicit classic abstinence symptoms including increased respiration, increased heart rate, yawning, lacrimation, rhinorrhea, complaints of cramps, and nausea (Griffiths et al., 1980). These conditioning mechanisms in drug tolerance and withdrawal may themselves be important commonalities among drugs of abuse (Brady, 1981).

IMPORTANCE OF BEHAVIOR COMPARED TO BIOLOGICAL EFFECTS

The effects of drugs on behavior are altered by the rate and pattern of responding, the type of event controlling behavior, and the animal's behavioral and pharmacological history (Barrett, 1981; Barrett & Witkin, 1985). The effects of a given stimulus (e.g., electric shock, nicotine) can be positive reinforcement, negative reinforcement, or punishment (Barrett, 1983; Goldberg & Spealman, 1982; Mello & Mendelson, 1978). Therefore, there is not a simple identity between pharmacological agents and their behavioral effects. (For detailed discussions of these issues, see McKearney & Barrett, 1978.)

Falk (1983) has argued strongly against the relative importance of biological effects in drug dependence: "Popular thinking about drug dependence all but equates it with physical dependence, a physiological need state producing a reputed zombie-like uncontrolled drive for the needed drug. The role of physical dependence in drug taking is in most respects a minor one" (p. 389). In addition, there is evidence that drug abuse may be so situation-specific that it disappears in another situation regardless of the biological effects of the drug. An example is provided by the observation that many U.S. soldiers who apparently became addicted to narcotics in Viet Nam did not exhibit addiction when they returned home (Robins, Helzer, & Davis, 1975).

Demonstrations that environmental factors, schedules of reinforcement, drug history, and so on, can dramatically alter behavioral responses to drugs (including self-administration of drugs of abuse) suggest that biological effects of these drugs can be swept away or overshadowed by behavioral and psychological factors. Physical dependence may not be necessary to generate drug-seeking behavior, and a particular biological effect may not be the key to understanding drug abuse (Falk, Dews, & Schuster, 1983). The fact that animals will self-administer noxious electric shocks argues against simple pleasure-driven motivation for self-administration of particular substances (Falk et al., 1983). According to Thompson (1981, p. 9): "It seems unlikely that a useful single common reductionistic mechanism can be identified accounting for the reinforcing property of such diverse drugs as toluene, heroin, phencyclidine, tobacco, and cocaine."

It is most likely that both behavioral and biological effects are involved in drug abuse. For instance, there are certain properties of pharmacologic agents that are important if the drug is to be abused: rapid onset of action and brief duration of effect (e.g., belts of liquor, snorts of cocaine, hits of heroin, and drags on smoked substances) (Falk, 1983). Possibly, biological effects of pharmacologic agents are necessary but not sufficient conditions for abuse. Psychological and situational factors alter the interpretation and experience of drug effects and thereby affect abuse. The nonbiological factors and biological effects together may be necessary to result in drug abuse. Although there are different biological effects of particular pharmacologic agents, some general change in physiologic arousal or state coupled with situational and psychological cues may be crucial for drug abuse. This interpretation could fit the demonstrations of the importance of behavioral and environmental variables without ruling out a crucial role for biological factors. Most psychologists will recognize this analysis as an application or extension of Schachter and Singer's (1962) theory of emotions.

The different effects of drugs under different schedules of reinforcement, environmental stimuli, and so on, might involve alterations in biological mechanisms that mediate drugs' effects. That is, the psychological variable may cause biological changes that alter the effects of drugs on behavior and on other biological changes. These types of possibilities are now being examined (e.g., comparisons of central levels of neurotransmitters and their metabolites in animals responding under different schedules of reinforcement). The importance of psychological and behavioral factors in drug abuse does not rule out biological factors. Instead, it highlights the need for interdisciplinary studies and analyses. With these concerns in mind, we proceed to the biological effects of specific drugs of abuse.

Specific Drugs of Abuse

OPIOIDS

The opioid drugs, or narcotics, are commonly considered to be prototypical drugs of abuse. The term *opioid* includes naturally occurring substances from the opium poppy and synthetic drugs that are pharmacologically similar (Woolf, 1983a). The term *narcotics* is derived from *narcosis*, indicating the sedative or tranquilizing effect of these substances (Brecher, 1972). Opioids include opium, morphine, heroin, meperidine, methadone, and codeine. These substances are abused by humans and are self-administered by animals (Griffiths et al., 1980). There also are opioids that are naturally present in the body—endogenous opioids (see the section, "Endogenous Opioid Peptides").

Opioids produce their major effects on the CNS and the bowel (Jaffe & Martin, 1980). Opioids have analgesic, euphoric, sedative, and addictive effects. They cause respiratory depression, emesis, a warm flushing of the skin, and sensations in the lower abdomen (described by addicts as similar to sexual orgasm). These latter effects are particularly pronounced about 45 seconds after rapid intravenous injection of an opioid and are known as the "rush," "kick," or "thrill" (Jaffe, 1980). Opioids decrease intestinal contractions, delay gastric emptying, and decrease gastric contractile activity (Konturek, 1978). They also decrease heart rate and blood pressure (by increasing parasympathetic tone and decreasing sympathetic tone) and may cause orthostatic hypotension (Holaday, 1983). Other effects include constriction of pupils, changes in temperature (increases after low doses, decreases after higher doses), and inhibition of norepinephrine release from sympathetic neurons (Cox & Baizman, 1982). Acute narcotic administration to animals has been shown to result in increased secretion of glucocorticoids from the adrenals. Chronic administration results in an eventual decrease in glucocorticoid secretion (Fishman, 1978). Corroborating these effects are reports that morphine increases levels of ACTH and decreases hypothalamic levels of norepinephrine (Holaday & Loh, 1979).

Tolerance develops to the analgesic, sedative, emetic, and euphoric effects of opioids (Haertzen & Hooks, 1969; Jaffe, 1980). There is some decrease in the pupillary constriction and respiratory depression with repeated opioid administration, but these effects continue (Martin & Jasinski, 1969). Little tolerance seems to develop to the gastrointestinal effects that cause constipation (Woolf, 1983a).

Abstinence from opioids by chronic users results in withdrawal symptoms, including nausea, cramps, lacrimation, rhinorrhea, yawning, sweating, tremors, and increased respiration (Donegan, Rodin, O'Brien, & Solomon, 1983; Jaffe, 1980). Other signs and symptoms of opioid withdrawal are dilated pupils, anorexia, gooseflesh, restlessness, irritability, insomnia, tremor, weakness, increased heart rate, increased blood pressure, and diarrhea. CNS hyperexcitability may include ejaculation in men and orgasm in women. Also, there may be increased urinary concentrations of 17-ketosteroids and leukocytosis (resulting in high white blood cell counts) (Jaffe, 1980). Some of these withdrawal symptoms (compared to the direct effects of opioids) indicate physiological rebound (see the section, "Drugs of Abuse—Overview"). In addition, some of these symptoms are reminiscent of the effects of stress (see the section, "Stress and Stress Response").

The pilomotor activity occurring in withdrawal from opioids—waves of gooseflesh—explains the derivation of the term *cold turkey*. Muscle spasms and kicking movements that sometimes occur during withdrawal may partially account for the phrase "kicking the habit" (Jaffe, 1980). The central role of opioids as a model of drug addiction and abuse is reflected in the application of these phrases to other drugs (e.g., tobacco). Withdrawal from morphine, methadone, meperidine, codeine, semisynthetic and synthetic opioids are similar, except the effects follow different time courses (Jaffe, 1980).

ALCOHOL

Alcohol (ethanol) causes a general depression of the CNS (Ritchie, 1980; Woolf, 1983b). Although the immediate effects on circulation are rather minor, alcohol enhances cutaneous and gastric blood flow and thereby results in a feeling of warmth. Alcohol can stimulate the release of adrenocortical hormones, and it produces an increase in urinary excretion of epinephrine and norepinephrine (Ritchie, 1980).

Chronic use of alcohol increases hepatic microsomal enzyme activity (Jaffe, 1980) and affects sleep patterns, EEG, and evoked responses (Donegan et al., 1983). Prolonged alcohol use may result in fatty liver, cirrhosis of the liver, damage to cardiac and skeletal muscle, and cerebral atrophy (Jaffe, 1980; Ritchie, 1980). Chronic use also results in pharmacodynamic tolerance and an increased capacity to metabolize alcohol. Tolerance to alcohol commonly shows cross-tolerance to general anesthetics and benzodiazepines (Jaffe, 1980).

Repeated administration of alcohol can result in dependence, and cessation of drinking by an alcoholic results in particular withdrawal signs and symptoms (Mello & Mendelson, 1978). The typical progression of withdrawal symptoms are tremulousness, nausea, weakness, anxiety, sweating, cramps, vomiting, hyperreflexia, hallucinations, and possibly grand mal seizures (Victor & Adams, 1953). Withdrawal after minimal dependence includes sleep disturbances, nausea, weakness, anxiety, and mild tremors. After more severe physical dependence, withdrawal includes the tremulous syndrome, alcohol-related seizure disorders, and delirium tremors (Jaffe, 1980). Other signs include dysrhythmia in EEG, a rebound increase in rapid eye movement (REM) sleep (that is depressed by alcohol), and hyperthermia (Donegan et al., 1983; Jaffe, 1980; Victor & Adams, 1953).

NICOTINE AND TOBACCO

Nicotine (or one of its metabolites) probably is the pharmacologic agent of addiction in tobacco. Nicotine has ganglionic-stimulating actions and excites the sympathetic nervous system. It increases heart rate by excitation of the sympathetic or paralysis of the parasympathetic cardiac ganglia. It also alters heart rate by affecting chemoreceptors of the carotid and aortic bodies and by acting on medullary centers. In small to moderate dosages it causes release of catecholamines from a number of isolated organs. Large doses prevent catecholamine release from the adrenal medulla in response to splanchnic nerve stimulation. It increases respiration via its CNS effects (Taylor, 1980).

Nicotine induces vomiting by stimulating the emetic chemoreceptor trigger zone in the area postrema of the medulla oblongata (central effects) and by stimulating vagal and afferent nerves in the sensory input of the reflex pathway involved in the vomiting response (peripheral effects). In addition, nicotine stimulates the hypothalamic–neurophyseal system to release antidiuretic hormone (ADH) and affects the gastrointestinal system via parasympathetic stimulation (Taylor, 1980). Nicotine also has been shown to cause an alerting EEG pattern (low voltage, fast activity), decrease skeletal muscle tone, decrease amplitude in EMG, decrease deep-tendon reflexes, and increase plasma levels of growth hormone, cortisol, and glycerol (Jaffe, 1980).

Nicotine acts on specific receptors for nicotine and on dopaminergic pathways. Mecamylamine blocks nicotine, but muscarinic cholinergic or adrenergic-blocking agents do not block nicotine (Jaffe, 1980). There is some evidence that nicotine increases plasma glucose levels (Glauser, Glauser, Reidenberg, Rusy, & Tallarida, 1970), circulating levels of endogenous opioids (Pomerleau, 1981), and acts to decrease body weight or keep normal gains in body weight down (Grunberg, 1982; Wack & Rodin, 1982). Tolerance develops to nicotine (Donegan et al., 1983; Jarvik, 1979). The harmful physical and physiological effects of tobacco—including cardiovascular damage, pulmonary damage, and a wide variety of cancers—are well documented (U.S. Department of Health, Education and Welfare, 1979; U.S. Department of Health and Human Services, 1982, 1983).

Cessation of habitual tobacco use has a withdrawal syndrome. The effects may include nausea, headache, constipation, irritability, insomnia, inability to concentrate, decreased heart rate and blood pressure, a decrease in high-frequency EEG activity and an increase in low-frequency activity, and weight gain (Shiffman, 1979).

AMPHETAMINES AND COCAINE

These sympathomimetic drugs stimulate the CNS and increase synaptic levels of norepinephrine and dopamine. These drugs act on adrenergic receptors and increase norepinephrine levels at the synapse by inhibiting the actions of monoamine oxidase and by inhibiting norepinephrine reuptake into the nerve endings. Therapeutic dosages of these drugs usually increase blood pressure, cause a reflexive decrease in heart rate, relax bronchial smooth muscle, and decrease gastrointestinal motility (Holbrook, 1983a). They also produce sleeplessness and decrease appetite (Weiner, 1980). Acute intoxication with high dosages of amphetamines may result in dizziness, tremor, irritability, confusion, tachycardia, headache, hallucinations, chest pain, heart palpitations, hypertension, sweating, and cardiac arrhythmias (Jaffe, 1980; Holbrook, 1983a). Toxic symptoms to high dosages may include bruxism, touching and picking the face and extremities, suspiciousness, and a feeling of being watched (Jaffe, 1980).

Amphetamines usually elevate mood; alleviate fatigue; increase alertness;

result in a sense of physical strength, energy, and mental capacity; decrease appetite; and cause insomnia. However, some individuals report that amphetamines result in anxiety, irritability, loquaciousness, and drowsiness. The environment and other nonbiological factors seem to alter the effects of these drugs (Jaffe, 1980). In fact, subjects taking high doses in experimental settings often exhibit depression and irritability (Griffith, Cavanaugh, Held, & Oates, 1972).

The effects of cocaine are similar to the amphetamines, except that cocaine has a shorter half-life and therefore shorter duration of action (Holbrook, 1983a). Cocaine stimulates the CNS, blocks the initiation or conduction of the nerve impulse, potentiates responses of sympathetically innervated organs to norepinephrine, and seems to block uptake of catecholamines at adrenergic nerve endings (Ritchie & Green, 1980).

Tolerance usually develops to some of the central effects of amphetamines, including the euphoric, anorectic, and lethal effects. Cessation of amphetamines or cocaine results in craving for the drug, prolonged sleep, general fatigue, lassitude, hyperphagia, and possibly depression (Jaffe, 1980).

HYPNOTICS AND SEDATIVES (EXCLUDING ETHANOL)

The important hypnotics and sedatives that may be abused (excluding ethanol) are the barbiturates (including amobarbital, barbital, pentobarbital, secobarbital) and the benzodiazepines (e.g., diazepam). The barbiturates are CNS depressants that are associated with abuse by humans and maintain self-administration in animals (Griffiths et al., 1980). These drugs depress transmission in the sympathetic ganglia and result in decreased respiratory drive and a slight decrease in blood pressure and heart rate. They competitively interfere with the biotransformation of other drugs by the microsomal drug-metabolizing enzyme system of the liver. In addition, the barbiturates induce synthesis of these microsomal enzymes and therefore can result in increased metabolism of other drugs (Harvey, 1980).

In contrast to the barbiturates, the benzodiazepines are not general neuronal depressants. The benzodiazepines act on the CNS to cause sedation, muscle relaxation, anticonvulsant activity, and decreased action. Their mechanism of action seems to be related to metabolism or action of gamma aminobutyric acid (GABA). The benzodiazepines have minor effects on the respiratory and cardiovascular systems (Harvey, 1980).

The effects of barbiturates include thick, slurred speech, diplopia (seeing two images), vertigo, ataxic gait, and decreased superficial reflexes. Intoxication with barbiturates may result in general sluggishness, difficulty in thinking, poor comprehension and memory, emotional lability, irritability, quarrelsomeness, and moroseness. In general, the subjective and intoxication effects of barbiturates and related substances are similar to the effects of ethanol (Jaffe, 1980).

Tolerance develops to the barbiturates and benzodiazepines. Most sedative-hypnotics show some cross-dependence with each other (including barbiturates and alcohol) (Jaffe, 1980). There is some evidence that the depressant effects of barbiturates are partially reduced by naloxone (an opiate antagonist) (Cox & Baizman, 1982).

There is a "general depressant withdrawal syndrome" after cessation of habitual use of barbiturates, benzodiazepines, and other sedative-hypnotics. The effects include restlessness, anxiety, tremulousness, paroxysmal EEG abnormalities, insomnia, and anorexia. There may also be abdominal cramps, nausea, vomiting, orthostatic hypotension, and convulsions (Jaffe, 1980).

CANNABINOIDS

This class of psychoactive agents refers to cannabis (obtained from the flowering tops of hemp plants) and its products. This group includes marijuana (general term that also refers to the plant *Cannabis sativa*), hashish (dried resinous exudate of the plant tops), bhang (dried leaves and flowering shoots), and ganja (resinous mass from the small leaves and brackets of inflorescence) (Jaffe, 1980). These substances are either smoked or eaten. There is good evidence that the primary psychoactive component of marijuana is l-Δ^9-tetrahydrocannabinol (Δ^9-THC, or THC) (Holbrook, 1983b; Jaffe, 1980).

THC usually results in an increased sense of well-being, impairs short-term memory, decreases balance and stability of stance, decreases muscle strength and head steadiness, and alters time perception (time seems to pass slowly). THC has its major effects on the CNS and cardiovascular system. There may be an increase in heart rate and systolic blood pressure, but the cardiovascular and CNS effects vary depending on dosage, route of administration, setting, and prior experience of the subjects. Cannabinoids also decrease intraocular pressure, have some antiemetic effects, may cause bronchodilation, and have some anticonvulsant actions. Chronic high dosages in females decrease concentrations of luteinizing hormone (LH) and follicle-stimulating hormone (FSH) and may result in anovulatory cycles. THC has some actions similar to barbiturates: It raises threshold for EEG and behavioral arousal, depresses polysynaptic reflexes, has anticonvulsant activity, and prolongs hexobarbital sleeping time. Δ^9-THC and Δ^8-THC produce sedation and decrease aggressive behavior in monkeys. Humans often report increases in hunger, more vivid visual imagery, and a sharpened sense of hearing (Jaffe, 1980).

Tolerance to the effects of cannabinoids can develop to the mood changes, decreased intraocular pressure, changes in EEG, tachycardia, changes in skin and body temperature, and impairment of psychomotor performance. There is some cross-tolerance with alcohol but not with the hallucinogens. Abrupt cessation of chronic use of high dosages of these drugs commonly results in irritability, restlessness, nervousness, decreased appetite, weight loss, insomnia, a rebound increase in REM sleep, tremor, increased body temperature, and chills (Jaffe, 1980).

PSYCHEDELICS

This group of drugs has been called psychedelics, hallucinogens, psychotomimetics, psychotogens, and a variety of other names. They include the indolealkylamines (e.g., lysergic acid diethylamide or LSD, psilocybin, psilocin, dimethyltryptamine or DMT, diethyltryptamine or DET), the phenylethylamines (e.g., mescaline), and the phenylisopropylamines (e.g., 2,5-dimethoxy-4-methylamphetamine or DOM or STP). They include synthetic chemicals (e.g., LSD) and chemicals from naturally occurring plants (e.g., mescaline from peyote cactus and psilocin from mushrooms). These substances affect the peripheral and central CNS. There is some evidence that LSD and related psychedelics have agonistic actions to serotonin.

These drugs commonly increase blood pressure, increase body temperature, produce mydriasis, distort perceptions of time and distance, and may produce euphoria, depression, and visual hallucinations. Reported effects of LSD include pupillary dilation, increased blood pressure and heart rate, hyperreflexia, tremor, nausea, piloerection, muscular weakness, increased body temperature and respiratory rate, dizziness, euphoria and mood lability, perception that time passes slowly, and synesthesias (e.g., hearing visual stimuli, seeing auditory stimuli) (Holbrook, 1983b; Jaffe, 1980).

Tolerance develops to some of the effects of LSD. Also, cross-tolerance has been demonstrated among LSD, mescaline, and psilocybin. There does not seem to be any cross-tolerance between LSD-like drugs and the amphetamines or Δ^9-THC. There does not seem to be any clear withdrawal syndrome after cessation of these drugs. However, these drugs are not usually self-administered repetitively over prolonged periods of time (Jaffe, 1980).

ARYLCYCLOHEXYLAMINES

The primary drug of abuse of this group is phencyclidine (PCP). PCP is also known as angel dust, crystal, horse tranquilizer, and peace pill. It is self-administered orally, by inhalation, and sometimes by intravenous injection (Holbrook, 1983b; Jaffe, 1980).

PCP and related arylcyclohexylamines have CNS stimulant, CNS depressant, hallucinogenic, and analgesic effects. PCP could be classified as a nonspecific CNS depressant (like ethanol or the barbiturates), as an anesthetic, as a tranquilizer, or as a psychedelic. It was first used as an anesthetic for animals and, for a brief time, as an anesthetic for humans. However, human patients experienced delirium after the anesthetic effects (Holbrook, 1983b; Jaffe, 1980). PCP is structurally similar to norepinephrine and to serotonin. It can increase acetylcholine levels and it has anticholinergic actions. Its actions could be related to any or all of these neurotransmitters (Holbrook, 1983b).

Specific effects of PCP include staggering gait, slurred speech, nystagmus, numbness of the extremities, increased heart rate, increased blood pressure, hypersalivation, increased sensitivity to external stimuli, a sense of intoxication, restlessness, and changes in mood. There may also be sweating, fever, repetitive movements, disorganized thought, disorientation, drowsiness, apathy, and catatonic muscular rigidity. Animals, as well as humans, self-administer PCP. Tolerance seems to develop to this drug, but it is presently unclear whether or not a withdrawal syndrome follows cessation of PCP administration (Jaffe, 1980).

INHALANTS

This broad group of drugs includes nitrous oxide, ethyl ether, the nitrites (especially amyl and butyl nitrite), and glue. Inhalation of nitrous oxide or ethyl ether produces intoxicating and euphorigenic effects. These effects were recognized before the anesthetic effects of these substances were realized. Animals will self-administer nitrous oxide, chloroform, toluene, and other solvents (Vourakis, 1983).

Among the inhalants there is some cross-tolerance and cross-dependence between chloroform and the barbiturates (Jaffe, 1980). Also, tolerance develops to the effects of the nitrites (Vourakis, 1983). Little is known about withdrawal effects of these pharmacologic agents. Whether these drugs have any actions and mechanisms in common with the most frequently abused drugs (i.e., tobacco, alcohol) is yet to be determined.

ENDOGENOUS OPIOID PEPTIDES

Background and General Information

The fact that particular exogenous substances (e.g., opiates) bind to receptor sites in the brain and result in biological actions led investigators to wonder why the body responds to plant alkaloids and other naturally occurring and synthetic pharmacologic agents. It was hypothesized that there may be endogenous substances in the body that are involved in important processes (e.g., pain) and that the exogenous drugs interfere or interact with the normal functioning and sites of action of these endogenous substances. The research attention to and discoveries regarding these endogenous substances have been extraordinary during the last 10 years. Tens of endogenous peptides have been identified, and their effects on physiological systems (e.g., cardiovascular, respiratory), pain, hunger, and drug abuse are being examined and considered.

In 1975 the term *endorphin* (from *endo*genous m*orphin*e) was accepted as a common label for the endogenous substances that were being isolated and examined (Simon, 1982). However, that term now refers to only some specific endogenous peptides (those derived from pro-opioimelanocortin). Currently, the best general term for these substances is "endogenous opioid peptides" (Cox, 1982).

There are three major groups of endogenous opioid peptides (EOPs): peptides related to β-endorphin, enkephalins, and peptides related to dynorphin. There are five different opioid receptors: μ (mu), δ (delta; formerly called peptide receptor), κ (kappa), σ (sigma), and ϵ (epsilon). Generally, the names of these receptors are derived from the drugs that bind to them. (More details about endogenous opioid peptides are given in the appendix.) Opiate binding sites are in the CNS and in the innervation of certain smooth muscles (e.g., the gut) (Simon, 1983). However, the distribution of the EOPs differs from the distribution of opiate receptors (Bloom, 1983). These differences indicate that not all the functions of the EOPs are necessarily related to opiate drugs.

Effects of Endogenous Opioid Peptides

EOPs have a number of effects similar to those of opiates. For example, EOPs produce analgesia and have an antinocisponsive effect (i.e., reduces responsiveness to noxious stimuli) (Bloom, 1983; Holaday, Wei, Loh, & Li, 1978). In addition, intravenous β-endorphin administration to human opiate addicts after cessation of exogenous opiates markedly attenuates the withdrawal syndrome (Su et al., 1978) and attenuates withdrawal responses in animals (Bhargava, 1978; Tseng, Loh, & Li, 1976). Intracerebroventricular injection of EOPs (particularly β-endorphin) to rodents results in akinesia, hypothermia, and hyperglycemia (Bloom, 1983). However, the effects of different EOPs are clearly different. For instance, there is evidence that intraventricular administration of met-enkephalin or α-endorphin in rats results in hyperthermia (Malick & Goldstein, 1982). It has been suggested that EOPs play a role in thermoregulation (Holaday, Loh, & Li, 1978).

EOPs also affect the cardiovascular and respiratory systems. For example, β-endorphin and met-enkephalin produce bradycardia (Bolme, Fuxe, Agnati, Bradley, & Smythies, 1978); enkephalins increase arterial pressure (Holaday, 1983); β-endorphin, leu-enkephalin, and met-enkephalin have vasopressor effects (Bolme et al., 1978); and baroreceptor systems seem to be opiate-sensitive (Holaday, 1983). EOPs cause respiratory depression (Bloom, 1983; Malick & Goldstein, 1982), sedation and catalepsy (Cox & Baizman, 1982). β-endorphin causes insomnia in cats, an EEG arousal pattern, and salivation (Malick & Goldstein, 1982).

There is good evidence that EOPs (especially certain fragments of dynorphin) affect food intake and may play an important role in the regulation of eating and hunger (Levine & Morley, 1983; Morley & Levine, 1983a). EOPs also affect hormonal release, including vasopressin, prolactin, and growth hormone (Bloom, 1983). EOPs seem to regulate luteinizing hormone and ACTH. Also, there are indications that enkephalins function as neurotransmitters in the brain (Cox & Baizman, 1982). In addition, it appears that EOPs modulate carbohydrate homeostasis, modulate immune function (including immune responses to stress), and play a role in the pathogenesis of stress ulceration (Morley, 1983; Morley, Levine, & Silvis, 1982). These last two effects are particularly noteworthy when considering possible biological commonalities in stress and drug abuse.

Like morphine and heroin, EOPs may produce dependence and tolerance. Naloxone (an opioid antagonist) infused intraventricularly to animals along with β-endorphin or met-enkephalin produces morphine-like withdrawal symptoms. Also, cross-tolerance develops between EOPs (especially β-endorphin and met-enkephalin) and morphine (Weisz & Thompson, 1983). Based on these and similar findings, it has been suggested that EOPs are involved in the effects of and addiction to opiate drugs (Kosterlitz & Hughes, 1978) and may help to explain alcohol addiction (Weisz & Thompson, 1983). However, according to Weisz and Thompson (1983): "It is premature to conclude that endogenous opioids are involved in the etiology of morphine and heroin addiction" (p. 306). In addition, "No evidence, very fragmentary evidence, and negative evidence have been found regarding interactions of the endogenous opioid system with a host of other substances including benzodiazepines (such as Valium), barbiturates, marijuana, and PCP" (p. 314).[5]

---

[5]Despite the current lack of empirical support, it is common to hear investigators speculate and even assume that EOPs are involved in opiate addiction in particular and drug abuse in general. One possible mechanism for an EOP–drug abuse link that is receiving increased research attention involves cyclic nucleotides (adenosine 3′, 5′-monophosphate or cyclic AMP and guanosine 3′,5′-monophosphate or cyclic GMP). These "second messengers" play a role in the control of cell metabolism and function, mediate the effects of neurotransmitters and hormones, and may be involved in the release and synthesis of pituitary hormones (Kant et al., 1982; Klee, 1978). Adenylate cyclase (the enzyme that converts ATP to cyclic AMP) seems to be involved in adaptive changes in tolerance (Cox & Baizman, 1982), and there is some evidence that suggests that cyclic AMP may be involved in dependence (Butt, Collier, Cuthbert, Francis, & Saeed, 1979).

Endogenous Opioids and Stress

In addition to the possibility that EOPs are somehow involved in drug abuse, it has been suggested that EOPs may be involved in the stress response. EOPs may act to reduce the effects of stress, decrease the aversiveness of stressful stimuli, or modulate responses to stress (such as conditioned fear) (Weisz & Thompson, 1983). The facts that EOPs are present in sites in the body (e.g., pituitary) that are involved in stress and that β-endorphin and ACTH are both secreted in response to stressors have been cited to support the hypothesis that there is a link between stress and the EOPs (Bloom, 1983; Holaday & Loh, 1979).

Animal research indicates that inescapable electric shock and limb fracture affect EOP levels. In addition to effects of painful stressors on EOPs, immobilization, transportation, and handling can affect EOP levels (Cox & Baizman, 1982). Other studies indicate that repeated exposure to a mild tail-pinch (a type of chronic stress) results in a naloxone-precipitable syndrome that resembles withdrawal from morphine (Morley & Levine, 1980).

Regarding stress and anxiety, it has been reported that naloxone can increase tension-anxiety scores in humans, and that naloxone can block the anxiolytic effects of chlordiazepoxide in animals (Malick & Goldstein, 1982). Therefore, EOPS may be involved in modulating this psychological response to stress.

STRESS AND DRUG ABUSE: THE SEARCH FOR COMMONALITIES

Introduction

Most instances of hypothesized links between stress and drug abuse are unidirectional, positing that stress leads to taking drugs and helps to maintain drug self-administration. It is implied that drugs of abuse can decrease the experience of stress. This idea is consistent with Lazarus's (1966) description of palliative coping (including drug use) that was designed to manage or reduce emotional responses to stressors. There are other possible points of interaction between stress and drug use. For example, our review of research on stress suggests that stress may increase the rate at which drugs are detoxified in the liver. Therefore, stress may increase need or result in larger required amounts of drug by changing the body's response to it. Our brief review of stress and drugs tried to highlight points of interface. Several systems are clearly involved in both, including EOPs, ACTH and adrenal hormones, and hepatic function. It is possible that these relationships also play a role in cessation of drug use and that part of withdrawal may be attributed to stress.

Former heroin addicts in methadone maintenance programs seem to be particularly vulnerable to relapse when they are under stress. In fact, they may exhibit withdrawal symptoms (pseudowithdrawal) despite the fact that they are receiving standard dosages of methadone (Whitehead, 1974). Alcohol intake by humans and animals may increase under stress (Donegan et al., 1983; Clark & Polish, 1960). Also, cigarette smoking increases under stress (Schachter, 1978). We have tried to point out some possible biological commonalities as we have summarized the biological effects of stress and of drugs of abuse. However, the major purpose of the sections "Stress and the Stress Response," "Drugs of Abuse," and "Endogenous Opioid Peptides" was to provide background information regarding biological effects of stress and drugs of abuse. Now we present some hypotheses about commonalities.

Catecholamines, Drugs, and Stress

ETHANOL, OPIATES, AND CATECHOLAMINES

Catecholamine depletion aggravates the alcohol withdrawal syndrome (Donegan et al., 1983). Alcohol increases the number of opiate receptors available for naloxone binding in vitro (Levine et al., 1983). These seemingly unrelated findings may speak to a common theme. Davis and Walsh (1970) proposed and later elaborated that ethanol and opiate abuse may be related and that some of the effects of ethanol may involve EOPs (Weisz & Thompson, 1983). More specifically, certain metabolites of ethanol combine with endogenous catecholamines to form tetrahydroisoquinolines (TIQs) (Davis & Walsh, 1970; Weisz & Thompson, 1983). These substances bind to opiate receptors (Greenwald, Fertel, Wong, Schwarz, & Bianchine, 1979; Weisz & Thompson, 1983). In addition, it has been reported that opiate antagonists decrease ethanol self-administration in ethanol-dependent monkeys (Altshuler, Phillips, & Feinhandler, 1980), attenuate ethanol-induced narcosis (Blum, Wallace, Eubanks, & Schwertner, 1975), and prevent ethanol-induced impairment of human reaction time (Jeffcoate, Herbert, Cullen, Hastings, & Walder, 1979).

The potential link between alcohol and opioids needs further research attention and careful analysis. However, we find it intriguing that the ethanol–opioid link involves catecholamines, a class of chemicals that are important in the stress response. We hope that future studies consider exactly which catecholamines combine with which drugs under what situations.

INTRACRANIAL SELF-STIMULATION, OPIOIDS, AND CATECHOLAMINES

Intracranial self-stimulation (ICSS) in particular areas of the brain appears to be rewarding—animals will repeatedly self-administer electric shocks to these sites. Some investigators have likened ICSS to drug self-administration and drug abuse. Interestingly, it has been suggested that catecholamines (especially dopamine) and EOPs are involved in ICSS. Also, naloxone attenuates the threshold-lowering effect that amphetamine, cocaine, and phencycline have on the threshold for rewarding brain stimulation (Kornetsky & Bain, 1982; Weisz & Thompson, 1983). These related effects of ICSS, catecholamines, and EOPs may play some role in a stress–drug abuse link.

OPIOIDS, CATECHOLAMINES, AND OTHER NEUROTRANSMITTERS

In addition to the observations and studies already cited, there are a variety of reasons to believe that catecholamines and EOPs are somehow related to one another. Opioids suppress activity in the locus coeruleus (a noradrenergic center in the brain); naloxone reverses this effect. Clonidine (an adrenergic agonist) inhibits activity at this site and suppresses the opioid withdrawal syndrome (Bloom, 1983). Opioids bind on dopaminergic neurons of the nigrostriatal pathway (Morley & Levine, 1982b) and catecholamines and enkephalins both are synthesized and stored within chromaffin granules of the adrenal medulla (Levine & Morley, 1983).

The adrenal gland appears to be involved in the antinociceptive actions of opioids and opiate-induced hyperthermia (Levine & Morley, 1983). Also, drugs that disturb catecholaminergic activity decrease opiate self-administration (Smith, Co, Freeman, & Lane, 1982). In addition, EOPs increase resistance to extinction of learned responses and this effect may involve catecholamines (Weisz & Thompson, 1983). Moreover, morphine, barbiturates, and ethanol alter brain levels of acetylcholine (Wahlstrom, 1978), and there are other data that suggest that EOPs play a role in the regulation of norepinephrine and acetylcholine release from the brain (Cox & Baizman, 1982; Jhamandas & Sutak, 1976; Taube, Borowski, Endó, & Starke, 1976). Whatever the exact mechanism, there appears to be some relationship between EOPs and neurotransmitters that may be relevant to the effects of stress and drugs.

Stress, Endogenous Opioid Peptides, and Eating

Although many of the interpretations of the early stress research have been modified, the classic studies of Cannon and Selye provided the impetus for decades of work. The discovery and investigation of EOPs may contribute substantially to understanding the stress response. It has been suggested that endogenous opioids are a logical extension of Cannon's concept of "fight-or-flight" and Selye's general adaptation syndrome (Morley & Levine, 1982a, 1982b).

STRESS AND EATING

Stress in humans affects eating behavior and mild tail-pinch to rats results in increased eating (Morley, Levine, & Rowland, 1983). According to Morley et al. (1983) EOPs are involved in the central regulation of stress-induced eating. Naloxone suppresses stress-induced eating by rats and adrenalectomy abolishes the anorectic effect of naloxone (Levine & Morley, 1983). Regarding the increases and decreases in eating observed in humans under stress, Morley and Levine (1983a) suggested that stress might produce overeating by activation of the EOP system or could produce decreased eating by increasing corticotropin-releasing factor (CRF) activity. CRF is involved in Selye's model as well. The possibility that CRF is involved with EOP effects is supported by evidence in animals that there is a physiological interplay between corticosteroids and EOPs (Holaday, Law, Loh, & Li, 1979). Opioids affect hypothalamic–pituitary hormonal function, and these hormones affect opioid-induced effects. For example, stress results in pituitary secretion of EOPs and ACTH (Holaday & Loh, 1979). Morley and Levine (1982b) take the strong position that the major effect of EOPs is to induce the feeding drive and that the analgesic effects are an epiphenomenon. Whether or not this is the case, it is clear that EOPs affect stress-induced eating behavior and that naloxone suppresses stress-induced eating.

FROM EATING TO DRUG ABUSE

The argument that EOPs may be involved in drug abuse is usually based on the similarities between the EOPs and opiates. Another link between EOPs and drug abuse is suggested by the reports of a relationship between EOPs and eating. Drug abuse may be related to eating, and the effects of drugs of abuse may somehow interact with or short-circuit neuronal pathways and biochemical systems involved in the regulation of eating. Drugs may be self-administered because they relieve the hunger drive or affect particular aspects of eating. For example, there is an inverse relationship between cigarette smoking and body weight (Grunberg, 1982; Wack & Rodin, 1982). Nicotine administration decreases normal gains in body weight and cessation of nicotine results in increased rates of body weight growth. These changes in body weight are partially explained by changes in consumption of sweet-tasting foods. Nicotine decreases consumption of sweet-tasting foods, and cessation of nicotine results in marked increases in consumption of these foods (Grunberg, 1982). In light of these findings, it is noteworthy that high glucose values induce sensitivity to naloxone-induced suppression of food intake. Therefore, glucose may alter the affinity and number of opiate receptors (Morley & Levine, 1982b). Also, "one component of some alcoholism treatment programs is to provide a high carbohydrate diet with ready access to sweets which is thought to reduce 'alcohol craving' in early stages of treatment" (Griffiths et al., 1980, p. 57). Moreover, food deprivation increases self-administration by animals of a variety of drugs (e.g., nicotine, ethanol, pentobarbital, and phencyclidine) (Griffiths et al., 1980). Additional investigations of the relationship between EOPs and stress, stress and eating, eating and drugs of abuse, should prove valuable.

Stress, Urinary pH, and Drug Taking

In a series of human studies, Schachter and colleagues established that stressful situations resulted in decreased urinary pH (i.e., greater acidity) and increased smoking (Schachter et al., 1977). They argued that habitual smokers smoke more under stress to maintain their internal level of nicotine and to avoid the unpleasantness of withdrawal. Stress had no effect on smoking if urinary pH was not allowed to vary. Schachter's interpretation has received support from animal research (Grunberg, Morse, & Barrett, 1983).

This line of investigation provides a biological explanation for the effects of stress on cigarette smoking. This mechanism also may help to explain the effects of stress on other drug taking. For example, in terms of the effects of urinary pH on excretion of drugs, opiates are similar to nicotine. Possibly, the pseudowithdrawal reported for ex-heroin addicts in methadone maintenance programs results from a depletion of methadone in the body in response to stress (R. E. Clymer, personal communication, 1981). Interestingly, decreased urinary pH also accelerates the excretion of amphetamines and phencyclidine (Jaffe, 1980). The effects of urinary pH on bioavailability of drugs and changes in drug taking deserve further research attention.

Withdrawal as a Stressor or Stress Response

There is another possible commonality that is worth considering. Some of the symptoms associated with withdrawal are similar to the stress response. Admittedly, abstinence from different drugs results in some similar and some different symptoms. However, there are a number of biological effects that commonly occur in both situations (e.g., changes in heart rate and respiration, stomach cramps, headache). It may be that the habitual drug user who experiences stress interprets the stress response as the effects of withdrawal and therefore increases drug taking to relieve the unpleasantness. Alternatively, the major effects of withdrawal and stress may be biologically similar enough that drug taking combats the biologically induced unpleasantness of both situations. In this context, it may be valuable to reconsider and extend Schachter and Singer's (1962) theory of emotions. According to this theory, the experience of emotions depends on changes in physiological arousal and situational or cognitive labels. Possibly, the relationship between stress and drugs of abuse similarly involve general changes in physiological state and contextual or psychological processes.

CONCLUSION

We have considered several biological commonalities of stress and drugs of abuse. Currently, it is not possible to reach any single, simple conclusion about these relationships. We have tried to provide summaries of substantive topics relevant to this theme, and we have briefly discussed some possibilities that we favor and that deserve more research attention. If nothing else, we hope our Reference section proves useful for those readers who would like to begin or continue their own search for biological commonalities of stress and drug abuse.

APPENDIX: MORE DETAILS ABOUT ENDOGENOUS OPIOID PEPTIDES

A number of different β-endorphins have been identified, including β-endorphin, β-endorphin (1–16) (α-endorphin), β-endorphin (1–17) (γ-endorphin), β-endorphin (1–27) (C'-fragment), and β-endorphin (1–26). β-endorphin binds to μ, κ, and σ receptors (Cox, 1982). There are high concentrations of β-endorphin in the pituitary gland and in certain hypothalamic neurons. At the amino terminal residue of β-endorphin is the pentapeptide sequence of methionine-enkephalin (Cox & Baizman, 1982).

Methionine-enkephalin (met-enkephalin or ME) and leucine-enkephalin (leu-enkephalin or LE) were isolated and characterized in 1975. These substances are distributed differently from β-endorphin in the brain and in the periphery. For instance, the adrenal gland contains high concentrations of the enkephalins and their precursors. Also, there is a wider distribution in the brain of enkephalins compared to β-endorphin (Cox, 1982). In fact, the term *enkephalin* literally means "in the head."

Dynorphin was isolated and partially characterized in 1979. Its name derives from its high potency (*dyn*amic end*orphin*) when measured in the isolated guinea pig ileum bioassay. It contains the leu-enkephalin sequence at the N- (amino) terminus. Dynorphin A is a heptapeptide containing the leu-enkephalin sequence. Dynorphin B is a tridecapeptide containing the leu-enkephalin sequence. Dynorphin-32 contains dynorphins A and B and is structurally similar to a component of pre-proenkephalin. α-neo-dynorphin is a decapeptide that is similar to dynorphin but different from both dynorphin A and B. It is likely that there is a gene (not pre-POMC or pre-proenkephalin) that directs the synthesis of dynorphin and its related peptides (Cox, 1982).

Morphine binds to the μ receptors; the enkephalins and closely related peptides especially bind to the δ receptors; ketocyclazocine (and the related drugs pentazocine and cyclazocine) bind to the κ receptors; SKF-10047 (N-allyl-normetazocine) binds to the σ receptors; the ε receptor is less well known (Cox, 1982; Simon, 1983).

REFERENCES

Altshuler, H. L., Phillips, P. E., & Feinhandler, D. A. (1980). Alteration of ethanol self-administration by naltrexone. *Life Sciences, 26,* 679–688.

Amir, S., Brown, Z. A., & Amit, Z. (1979). The role of endorphins in stress: Evidence and speculations. *Neuroscience Behavior Review, 4,* 77–86.

Barrett, J. E. (1981). Differential drug effects as a function of the controlling consequences. In T. Thompson & C. E. Johanson (Eds.), *Behavioral pharmacology of human drug dependence* (NIDA Research Monograph 37). Rockville, MD: Department of Health and Human Services.

Barrett, J. E. (1983). Interrelationships between behavior and pharmacology as factors determining the effects of nicotine. *Pharmacology Biochemistry & Behavior, 19,* 1027–1029.

Barrett, J. E., & Witkin, J. M. (1985). The role of behavioral and pharmacological history in determining the effects of abused drugs. In S. R. Goldberg & I. Stolerman (Eds.), *Behavioral analysis of drug dependence.* New York: Academic Press.

Baum, A., Grunberg, N. E., & Singer, J. E. (1982). The use of psychological and neuroendocrinological measurements in the study of stress. *Health Psychology, 1,* 217–236.

Beard, E. L., Carroll, G. F., & Danos, G. T. (1969). Release of plasminogen activator from rat liver lysomes induced by stress related enzymes. *Proceedings of the Society for Experimental Biology and Medicine, 131,* 438–442.

Bethune, J. E. (1974). *The adrenal cortex.* Kalamazoo, MI: Upjohn Co.

Bhargava, H. N. (1978). New *in vivo* evidence for narcotic agonist property of leucine-enkephalin. *Journal of Pharmaceutical Sciences, 67,* 136–137.

Bloom, F. E. (1983). Endorphins: Cellular and molecular aspects for addictive phenomena. In P. K. Levison, D. R. Gerstein, & D. R. Maloff (Eds.), *Commonalities in substance abuse and habitual behavior.* Lexington, MA: D. C. Heath.

Blum, K., Wallace, J. E., Eubanks, J. D., & Schwertner, H. H. (1975). Effects of naloxone on ethanol withdrawal, preference and narcosis. *Pharmacologist, 17,* 197.

Bodnar, R. J., Glusman, M., Brutus, M., Spiaggia, A., & Kelley, D. D. (1980). Analgesia induced by cold-water stress: Attenuation following hypophysectomy. *Physiology and Behavior, 23,* 53–62.

Bohus, B., Gispen, W. H., & DeWied, D. (1973). Effect of lysine vasopressin and ACTH 4-10 on conditioned avoidance behavior of hypophysectomized rats. *Neuroendocrinology, 11,* 137–143.

Bolme, P., Fuxe, K., Agnati, L. F., Bradley, R., & Smythies, J. (1978). Cardiovascular effects of morphine and opioid peptides following intracisternal administration in chloralose-anesthetized rats. *European Journal of Pharmacology, 48,* 319–324.

Border, J. R., Gallo, E., & Schenk, W. G. (1966). Alterations in cardiovascular and pulmonary physiology in the severely stressed patient. *Journal of Trauma, 6,* 176–193.

Bousquet, W. F., Rupe, B. D., & Miya, T. S. (1965). Endocrine modification of drug responses in the rat. *Journal of Pharmacology and Experimental Therapeutics, 147,* 376–379.

Brady, J. V. (1981). Common mechanisms in substance abuse. In T. Thompson & C. E. Johanson (Eds.), *Behavioral pharmacology of human drug dependence* (NIDA Research Monograph 37). Rockville, MD: Department of Health and Human Services.

Brecher, E. M. (1972). *Licit and illicit drugs.* Boston: Little, Brown.

Butt, N. M., Collier, H. O. J., Cuthbert, N. J., Francis, D. L., & Saeed, S. A. (1979). Mechanism of quasi-morphine withdrawal behaviour induced by methylxanthines. *European Journal of Pharmacology, 53,* 375–378.

Campbell, F., & Singer, G. (1983). *Stress, drugs and health: Recent brain-behaviour research.* Sydney, Australia: Pergamon.

Cannon, W. B. (1915). *Bodily changes in pain, hunger, and rage.* New York: Appleton.

Cannon, W. B. (1929). *Bodily changes in pain, hunger, fear, and rage.* Boston: Branford.

Cappell, H., Roach, C., & Poulos, C. X. (1981). Pavlovian control of cross-tolerance between pentobarbital and ethanol. *Psychopharmacology, 74,* 54–57.

Cartensen, H., Amér, I., Wide, L., & Amér, B. (1973). Plasma testosterone, LH, and FSH during the first 24 hours after surgical operations. *Journal of Steroid Biochemistry, 4,* 605–611.

Chavkin, C., Cox, B. M., & Goldstein, A. (1979). Stereospecific opiate binding in bovine adrenal medulla. *Molecular Pharmacology, 15,* 751–753.

Clark, R., & Polish, E. (1960). Avoidance conditioning and alcohol consumption in rhesus monkeys. *Science, 132,* 223–224.

Cox, B. M. (1982). Endogenous opioid peptides: A guide to structures and terminology. *Life Sciences, 31,* 1645–1658.

Cox, B. M., & Baizman, E. R. (1982). Physiological functions of endorphins. In J. B. Malick & R. S. Bell (Eds.), *Endorphins: Chemistry, physiology, pharmacology, and clinical relevance.* New York: Marcel Dekker.

Crowell, C. R., Hinson, R. E., & Siegel, S. (1981). The role of conditional drug responses in tolerance to the hypothermic effects of ethanol. *Psychopharmacology, 73,* 51–54.

Davis, V. E., & Walsh, M. J. (1970). Alcohol, amines, and alkaloids: A possible biochemical basis for alcohol addiction. *Science, 167,* 1005–1007.

DeWied, D., Bohus, B., & Wimersma Greidanus, T. (1974). The hypothalamoneurohypophyseal system and the preservation of conditioned avoidance behavior in rats. *Progress in Brain Research, 41,* 417–428.

Donegan, N. H., Rodin, J., O'Brien, C. P., & Solomon, R. L. (1983). A learning theory approach to commonalities. In P. K. Levison, D. R. Gerstein, & D. R. Maloff (Eds.), *Commonalities in substance abuse and habitual behavior.* Lexington, MA: D. C. Heath.

Driever, C. W., Bousquet, W. F., & Miya, T. S. (1966). Stress stimulation of drug metabolism in the rat. *International Journal of Neuropharmacology, 5,* 199–205.

Elmadjian, F. (1962). Epinephrine, norepinephrine, and aldosterone: Release and excretion. In K. E. Schaefer (Ed.), *Man's dependence on the earthly atmosphere.* New York: Macmillan.

Esposito, R. U., Perry, W., & Kornetsky, C. (1980). Effects of *d*-amphetamine and naloxone on brain stimulation reward. *Psychopharmacology, 69,* 187–191.

Euker, J. S., Meites, J., & Riegle, G. D. (1975). Effects of acute stress on serum LH and prolactin in intact, castrate, and dexamethasone-treated male rats. *Endocrinology, 96,* 85–92.

Falk, J. L. (1983). Drug dependence: Myth or motive? *Pharmacology Biochemistry & Behavior, 19,* 385–391.

Falk, J. L., Dews, P. B., & Schuster, C. R. (1983). Commonalities in the environmental control of behavior. In P. K. Levison, D. R. Gerstein, & D. R. Maloff (Eds.), *Commonalities in substance abuse and habitual behavior.* Lexington, MA: D. C. Heath.

Fendler, K., Rakoczi, I., & Zibotics, H. (1966). Effects of daily electroshock treatment on neurohypophyseal hormone content in the rat. *Acta Physiologica Academiae Scientiarum Hungaricae, 29,* 41–45.

Fishman, J. (1978). The opiates and the endocrine system. In J. Fishman (Ed.), *The bases of addiction.* Berlin: Dahlem Konferenzen.

Frankenhaeuser, M. (1972). *Biochemical events, stress, and adjustment.* Reports from the Psychological Laboratories, University of Stockholm, Sweden.

Frankenhaeuser, M. (1975). Sympathetic-adrenomedullary activity, behavior and the psychosocial environment. In P. H. Venables & M. J. Christie (Eds.), *Research in psychophysiology.* New York: Wiley.

Gibson, A., Ginsburg, M., Hall, M., & Hart, S. L. (1979). The effects of opioid drugs and of lithium on steroidogenesis in rat adrenal cell suspensions. *British Journal of Pharmacology, 65,* 671–676.

Glauser, S. C., Glauser, E. M., Reidenberg, M. M., Rusy, B. R., & Tallarida, R. J. (1970). Metabolic changes associated with the cessation of cigarette smoking. *Archives of Environmental Health, 20,* 377–381.

Goldberg, S. R., & Spealman, R. D. (1982). Maintenance and suppression of behavior by intravenous nicotine injections in squirrel monkeys. *Federation Proceedings, 41,* 216–220.

Gray, S. J., Ramsey, C., Reifenstein, R. W., & Benson, J. A., Jr. (1953). The significance of hormonal factors in the pathogenesis of peptic ulcer. *Gastroenterology, 25,* 156–172.

Green, A. R., & Curzon, G. (1975). Effects of hydrocortisone and immobilization on tryptophan metabolism in brain and liver of rats of different ages. *Biochemical Pharmacology, 24,* 713–716.

Greenwald, J. E., Fertel, R. H., Wong, L. K., Schwarz, R. D., & Bianchine, J. R. (1979). Salsolinol and tetrahydropapaveroline bind opiate receptors in the rat brain. *Federation Proceedings, 38,* 379.

Griffith, J. D., Cavanaugh, J., Held, J., & Oates, J. A. (1972). Dextroamphetamine. *Archives of General Psychiatry, 26,* 97–100.

Griffiths, R. R., Bigelow, G. E., & Henningfield, J. E. (1980). Similarities in animal and human drug-taking behavior. In N. K. Mello (Ed.), *Advances in substance abuse.* Greenwich, CT: JAI Press.

Groza, P., Zamfir, V., & Lungu, D. (1971). Post-operative salivary amylase changes in children. *Review of Roumanian Physiology, 8,* 307–312.

Grunberg, N. E. (1982). The effects of nicotine and cigarette smoking on food consumption and taste preferences. *Addictive Behaviors, 7,* 317–331.

Grunberg, N. E., Morse, D. E., & Barrett, J. E. (1983). Effects of urinary pH on the behavioral responses of squirrel monkeys to nicotine. *Pharmacology Biochemistry & Behavior, 19,* 553–557.

Haertzen, C. A., & Hooks, N. T. (1969). Changes in personality and subjective experience associated with the chronic administration and withdrawal of opiates. *Journal of Nervous and Mental Disease, 148,* 606–614.

Ham, J. M., & Slack, W. W. (1969). Lipoprotein lipase activity in patients before and after minor surgical operations. *Clinica Chimica Acta, 25,* 417–422.
Harvey, S. C. (1980). Hypnotics and sedatives. In A. G. Gilman, L. S. Goodman, & A. Gilman (Eds.), *The pharmacological basis of therapeutics* (6th ed.). New York: Macmillan.
Hauss, W. H. (1973). Tissue alterations due to experimental arteriosclerosis. In H. G. Vogel (Ed.), *Connective tissue and aging* (Int. Congr. Ser. No. 264). Amsterdam: Excerpta Medica.
Henningfield, J. E., Griffiths, R. R., & Jasinski, D. R. (1981). Human dependence on tobacco and opioids: Common factors. In T. Thompson & C. E. Johanson (Eds.), *Behavioral pharmacology of human drug dependence* (NIDA Research Monograph 37). Rockville, MD: Department of Health and Human Services.
Hilf, R., Breuer, C., & Borman, A. (1961). The effect of sarcoma 180 and other stressing agents upon adrenal adenine nucleotide-metabolizing enzymes. *Cancer Research, 21,* 1439–1444.
Holaday, J. W. (1983). Cardiovascular effects of endogenous opiate systems. *Annual Review of Pharmacology and Toxicology, 23,* 541–594.
Holaday, J. W., Law, P.-Y., Loh, H. H., & Li, C. H. (1979). Adrenal steroids indirectly modulate morphine and β-endorphin effects. *Journal of Pharmacology and Experimental Therapeutics, 208,* 176–183.
Holaday, J. W., & Loh, H. H. (1979). Endorphin-opiate interactions with neuroendocrine systems. In H. H. Loh & D. H. Ross (Eds.), *Neurochemical mechanisms of opiates and endorphins.* New York: Raven Press.
Holaday, J. W., Loh, H. H., & Li, C. H. (1978). Unique behavioral effects of β-endorphin and their relationship to thermoregulation and hypothalamic function. *Life Sciences, 22,* 1525–1536.
Holaday, J. W., Wei, E., Loh, H. H., & Li, C. H. (1978). Endorphins may function in heat adaptation. *Proceedings of the National Academy of Sciences, 75,* 2923–2927.
Holbrook, J. M. (1983a). CNS stimulants. In G. Bennett, C. Vourakis, & D. S. Woolf (Eds.), *Substance abuse: Pharmacologic, developmental and clinical perspectives.* New York: Wiley.
Holbrook, J. M. (1983b). Hallucinogens. In G. Bennett, C. Vourakis, & D. S. Woolf (Eds.), *Substance abuse: Pharmacologic, developmental, and clinical perspectives.* New York: Wiley.
Ingle, D. J. (1950). The biologic properties of cortisone: A review. *Journal of Clinical Endocrinology, 10,* 1312–1354.
Jaffe, J. H. (1980). Drug addiction and drug abuse. In A. G. Gilman, L. S. Goodman, & A. Gilman (Eds.), *The pharmacological basis of therapeutics* (6th ed.). New York: Macmillan.
Jaffe, J. H., & Martin, W. R. (1980). Opioid analgesics and antagonists. In A. G. Gilman, L. S. Goodman, & A. Gilman (Eds.), *The pharmacological basis of therapeutics* (6th ed.). New York: Macmillan.
Jarvik, M. E. (1979). Tolerance to the effects of tobacco. In N. A. Krasnegor (Ed.), *Cigarette smoking as a dependence process* (NIDA Research Monograph 23). Rockville, MD: Department of Health, Education and Welfare.
Jeffcoate, W. J., Herbert, M., Cullen, M. H., Hastings, A. G., & Walder, C. P. (1979). Prevention of effects of alcohol intoxication by naloxone. *Lancet, 2,* 1157–1159.
Jenkins, C. D. (1979). Psychosocial modifiers of response to stress. *Journal of Human Stress, 5,* 3–15.
Jhamandas, K., & Sutak, M. (1976). Morphine-naloxone interaction in the central cholinergic system: The influence of subcortical lesioning and electrical stimulation. *British Journal of Pharmacology, 58,* 101–107.

Kalant, H. (1978). Behavioral criteria for tolerance and physical dependence. In J. Fishman (Ed.), *The bases of addiction*. Berlin: Dahlem Konferenzen.

Kant, G. J., Meyeroff, J. L., Bunnell, B. N., & Lenox, R. H. (1982). Cyclic AMP and cyclic GMP response to stress in brain and pituitary stress elevates pituitary cyclic AMP. *Pharmacology Biochemistry & Behavior, 17*, 1067–1072.

Kant, G. J., Mougey, E. H., Pennington, L. L., & Meyeroff, J. L. (1983). Graded footshock stress elevates pituitary cyclic AMP and plasma β-endorphin, β-LPH, corticosterone and prolactin. *Life Sciences, 33*, 2657–2663.

Kasl, S. V., Cobb, S., & Brooks, G. W. (1968). Changes in serum uric acid and cholesterol levels in men undergoing job loss. *Journal of the American Medical Association, 206*, 1500–1507.

Kelley, D. D. (1982). The role of endorphins in stress-induced analgesia. *Annals of New York Academy of Sciences, 398*, 260–271.

Kirschner, L. B., Prosser, C. L., & Quastler, H. (1949). Increased metabolic rate in rats after irradiation. *Proceedings of the Society for Experimental Biology and Medicine, 71*, 463–467.

Klee, W. A. (1978). Dual regulation of adenylate cyclase: A biochemical model for opiate tolerance and dependence. In J. Fishman (Ed.), *The bases of addiction*. Berlin: Dahlem Konferenzen.

Knox, W. E. (1962). Adaptive enzymes in animals. In J. Monjar & A. deReude (Eds.), *Ciba Foundation Symposium on Enzymes and Drug Action*. London: Churchill.

Konturek, S. J. (1978). Endogenous opiates and the digestive system. *Scandinavian Journal of Gastroenterology, 13*, 257–261.

Kornetsky, C., & Bain, G. (1982). Biobehavioral bases of the reinforcing properties of opiate drugs. *Annals of the New York Academy of Sciences, 398*, 241–259.

Kornetsky, C., Bain, G., & Riedl, M. (1981). Effects of cocaine and naloxone on brain-stimulation reward. *Pharmacologist, 23*, 192.

Kosterlitz, H. W., & Hughes, J. (1978). Endogenous opioid peptides. In J. Fishman (Ed.), *The bases of addiction*. Berlin: Dahlem Konferenzen.

Kvetnansky, R., & Kopin, I. J. (1972). Activity of adrenal catecholamine producing enzymes and their regulation after stress. *Advances in Experimental Medicine and Biology, 33*, 517–533.

Lasagna, L. (1981). Towards a rapprochement between clinical pharmacology and behavioral pharmacology. In T. Thompson & C. E. Johanson (Eds.), *Behavioral pharmacology of human drug dependence* (NIDA Research Monograph 37). Rockville, MD: Department of Health and Human Services.

Lazarus, R. (1966). *Psychological stress*. New York: McGraw Hill.

Lettieri, D. J., Sayers, M., & Pearson, H. W. (Eds.). (1980). *Theories on drug abuse: Selected contemporary perspectives* (NIDA Research Monograph 30). Rockville, MD: Department of Health and Human Services.

Levine, A. S., Hess, S., & Morley, J. E. (1983). Alcohol and the opiate receptor. *Alcoholism: Clinical and Experimental Research, 7*, 83–84.

Levine, A. S., & Morley, J. E. (1983). Adrenal modulation of opiate induced feeding. *Pharmacology Biochemistry & Behavior, 19*, 403–406.

Levison, P. K. (1981). An analysis of commonalities in substance abuse and habitual behavior. In T. Thompson & C. E. Johanson (Eds.), *Behavioral phamacology of habitual drug dependence* (NIDA Research Monograph 37). Rockville, MD: Department of Health and Human Services.

MacMahon, H. E. (1929). Electric shock. *American Journal of Pathology, 5*, 333–347.

Malick, J. B., & Goldstein, J. M. (1982). Animal pharmacology of endorphins. In J. B. Malick

& R. M. S. Bell (Eds.). *Endorphins: Chemistry, physiology, pharmacology, and clinical relevance.* New York: Marcel Dekker.

Mansfield, J. G., & Cunningham, C. L. (1980). Conditioning and extinction of tolerance to the hypothermic effect of ethanol in rats. *Journal of Comparative and Physiological Psychology, 94,* 962–969.

Martin, W. R., & Jasinski, D. R. (1969). Physiological parameters of morphine dependence in man—tolerance, early abstinence, protracted abstinence. *Journal of Psychiatric Research, 7,* 9–17.

Mason, J. W. (1968). Organization of the multiple endocrine responses to avoidance in monkey. *Psychosomatic Medicine, 70,* 774–790.

Mason, J. W. (1975). Emotion as reflected in patterns of endocrine integration. In L. Levi (Ed.), *Emotions: Their parameters and measurement.* New York: Raven.

McClearn, G. E. (1983). Commonalities in substances use: A genetic perspective. In P. K. Levison, D. R. Gerstein, & D. R. Maloff (Eds.), *Commonalities in substance abuse and habitual behavior.* Lexington, MA: D. C. Heath.

McKearney, J. W., & Barrett, J. E. (1978). Schedule-controlled behavior and the effects of drugs. In D. E. Blackman & D. J. Sanger (Eds.), *Contemporary research in behavioral pharmacology.* New York: Plenum Press.

Mello, N. K., & Mendelson, J. H. (1978). Behavioral pharmacology of human alcohol, heroin and marihuana use. In J. Fishman (Ed.), *The bases of addiction.* Berlin: Dahlem Konferenzen.

Millan, M. J., & Emrich, H. M. (1981). Endorphinergic systems and the response to stress. *Psychotherapy and Psychosomatics, 36,* 43–56.

Moon, V. H. (1948). The pathology of secondary shock. *American Journal of Pathology, 24,* 235–273.

Mordkoff, A. M. (1964). The relationship between psychological and physiological responses to stress. *Psychosomatic Medicine, 26,* 135–150.

Morley, J. E. (1983). Neuroendocrine effects of endogenous opiod peptides in human subjects: A review. *Psychoneuroendocrinology, 8,* 361–379.

Morley, J. E., & Levine, A. S. (1980). Stress-induced eating is mediated through endogenous opiates. *Science, 209,* 1259–1261.

Morley, J. E., & Levine, A. S. (1982a). Corticotrophin releasing factor, grooming and ingestive behavior. *Life Sciences, 31,* 1459–1464.

Morley, J. E., & Levine, A. S. (1982b). The role of the endogenous opiates as regulators of appetite. *American Journal of Clinical Nutrition, 35,* 757–761.

Morley, J. E., & Levine, A. S. (1983a). The central control of appetite. *Lancet, 1,* 398–401.

Morley, J. E., Levine, A. S., & Rowland, N. E. (1983). Stress induced eating. *Life Sciences, 32,* 2169–2182.

Morley, J. E., Levine, A. S., & Silvis, S. E. (1982). Endogenous opiates and stress ulceration. *Life Sciences, 31,* 693–699.

Morris, D. P. (1941). Blood pressure and pulse changes in normal individuals under emotional stress; their relationship to emotional instability. *Psychosomatic Medicine, 3,* 389–398.

Natelson, B. H., Krasnegor, N., & Holaday, J. W. (1976). Relations between behavioral arousal and plasma cortisol levels in monkeys performing repeated free-operant avoidance sessions. *Journal of Comparative and Physiological Psychology, 90,* 958–969.

National Research Council (1977). *Common processes in habitual substance use: A research agenda* (Committee on Substance Abuse and Habitual Behavior, Assembly of Behavioral and Social Scientists). Washington, DC: National Academy of Sciences.

Neill, J. D. (1970). Effect of "stress" on serum prolactin and luteinizing hormone levels during the estrous cycle of the rat. *Endocrinology, 87,* 1192–1197.

Nemeth, S., & Jurani, M. (1974). Hepatic tyrosine aminotransferase (TAT) in stressed trouts and rats. *General and Comparative Endocrinology, 22,* 388.

Nemeth, S., Strakova, A., & Vigas, M. (1973). The role played by adrenal hormones in the increase of liver tyrosine aminotransferase activity of rats subjected to trauma. *Hormone and Metabolic Research, 5,* 204–207.

Nomura, J. (1965). Effects of stress and psychotropic drugs on rat liver tryptophan pyrrolase. *Endocrinology, 76,* 1190–1194.

O'Brien, C. P., Ternes, J. W., Grabowski, J., & Ehrman, R. (1981). Classically conditioned phenomena in human opiate addiction. In T. Thompson & C. E. Johanson (Eds.), *Behavioral pharmacology of human drug dependence* (NIDA Research Monograph 37). Rockville, MD: Department of Health and Human Services.

Oehler, G., Wolf, H., Schmahl, F. W., & Roka, L. (1974). Modification of the lipoprotein lipase after experimental fracture of the femur. *Research in Experimental Medicine, 163,* 31–38.

Pomerleau, O. F. (1981). Underlying mechanisms in substance abuse: Examples from research on smoking. *Addictive Behaviors, 6,* 187–196.

Raab, W., Chaplin, J. P., & Bajusz, E. (1964). Myocardial necroses produced in domesticated rats and in wild rats by sensory and emotional stresses. *Proceedings of the Society for Experimental Biology and Medicine, 116,* 665–669.

Ritchie, J. M. (1980). The aliphatic alcohols. In A. G. Gilman, L. S. Goodman, & A. Gilman (Eds.), *The pharmacological basis of therapeutics* (6th ed.). New York: Macmillan.

Ritchie, J. M., & Greene, N. M. (1980). Local anesthetics. In A. G. Gilman, L. S. Goodman, & A. Gilman (Eds.), *The pharmacological basis of therapeutics* (6th ed.). New York: Macmillan.

Robins, L. N., Helzer, J. E., & Davis, D. H. (1975). Narcotic use in Southeast Asia and afterward. *Archives of General Psychiatry, 32,* 955–961.

Rochefort, G. J., Rosenberger, J., & Saffran, M. (1959). Depletion of pituitary corticotrophin by various stresses and by neurohypophyseal preparations. *Journal of Physiology, 146,* 105–116.

Rupe, B. D., Bousquet, W. F., & Miya, T. S. (1963). Stress modification of drug response. *Science, 141,* 1186–1187.

Schachter, S. (1977). Nicotine regulation in heavy and light smokers. *Journal of Experimental Psychology: General, 106,* 5–12.

Schachter, S. (1978). Pharmacological and psychological determinants of smoking. *Annals of Internal Medicine, 88,* 104–114.

Schachter, S., Silverstein, B., Kozlowski, L. T., Perlick, D., Herman, C. P., & Liebling, B. (1977). Studies of the interaction of psychological and pharmacological determinants of smoking. *Journal of Experimental Psychology: General, 106,* 3–40.

Schachter, S., & Singer, J. E. (1962). Cognitive, social, and physiological determinants of emotional state. *Psychological Review, 69,* 379–399.

Schayer, R. W. (1960). Relationship of stress-induced histidine decarboxylase to circulatory homeostasis and shock. *Science, 131,* 226–227.

Seifter, J., & Baeder, D. H. (1954). Lipemia clearing by hyalurondase, hyaluronate, and desoxycorticosterone, and its inhibition by cortisone, stress, and nephrosis. *Proceedings of the Society for Experimental Biology and Medicine, 86,* 709–713.

Selye, H. (1937). Studies on adaptation. *Endocrinology, 21,* 169–188.

Selye, H. (1956). *The stress of life* (1st ed.). New York: McGraw-Hill.

Selye, H. (1976). *The stress of life* (2nd ed.). New York: McGraw-Hill.

Shiffman, S. M. (1979). The tobacco withdrawal syndrome. In N. A. Krasnegor (Ed.), *Ciga-*

rette smoking as a dependence process (NIDA Research Monograph 23). Rockville, MD: Department of Health, Education and Welfare.

Siegel, S. (1976). Morphine analgesic tolerance: Its situation specificity supports a Pavlovian conditioning model. *Science, 193,* 323–325.

Siegel, S., Hinson, R. E., & Krank, M. D. (1979). Modulation of tolerance to the lethal effect of morphine by extinction. *Behavioral and Neural Biology, 25,* 257–262.

Siegel, S., Hinson, R. E., Krank, M. D., & McCully, J. (1982). Heroin "overdose" death: Contribution of drug-associated environmental cues. *Science, 216,* 436–437.

Simon, E. J. (1982). History. In J. B. Malick & R. M. S. Bell (Eds.), *Endorphins: Chemistry, physiology, pharmacology, and clinical relevance.* New York: Marcel Dekker.

Simon, E. J. (1983). Opiate receptors: Properties and possible functions. In P. K. Levison, D. R. Gerstein, & D. R. Maloff (Eds.), *Commonalities in substance abuse and habitual behavior.* Lexington, MA: D. C. Heath.

Smith, J. E., Co, C., Freeman, M. E., & Lane, J. D. (1982). Brain neurotransmitter turnover correlated with morphine-seeking behavior of rats. *Pharmacology Biochemistry & Behavior, 16,* 509–519.

Solomon, R. L., & Corbit, J. D. (1973). An opponent-process theory of motivation: II. Cigarette addiction. *Journal of Abnormal Psychology, 81,* 158–171.

Stitzel, R. E., & Furner, R. L. (1967). Stress-induced alterations in microsomal drug metabolism in the rat. *Biochemical Pharmacology, 16,* 1489–1494.

Su, C.-Y., Lin, S.-H., Wang, Y.-T., Li, C.-H., Hung, L. H., Lin, C. S., & Lin, B. C. (1978). Effects of β-endorphin on narcotic abstinence syndrome in man. *Journal of the Formosan Medical Association, 77,* 133–141.

Szidon, J. P., & Fishman, A. P. (1971). Participation of pulmonary circulation in the defense reaction. *American Journal of Physiology, 220,* 364–370.

Taube, H. D., Borowski, E., Endó, J., & Starke, K. (1976). Enkephalin: A potential modulator of noradrenaline release in rat brain. *European Journal of Pharmacology, 38,* 377–380.

Taylor, P. (1980). Ganglionic stimulating and blocking agents. In A. G. Gilman, L. S. Goodman, & A. Gilman (Eds.), *The pharmacological basis of therapeutics* (6th ed.). New York: Macmillan.

Thompson, T. (1981). Behavioral mechanisms and loci of drug dependence: An overview. In T. Thompson & C. E. Johanson (Eds.), *Behavioral pharmacology of human drug dependence* (NIDA Research Monograph 37). Rockville, MD: Department of Health and Human Services.

Tseng, L.-F., Loh, H. H., & Li, C. H. (1976). β-endorphin: Cross tolerance to and cross physical dependence on morphine. *Proceedings of the National Academy of Sciences, 73,* 4187–4189.

United States Department of Health, Education, and Welfare (1979). *Smoking and health: A report of the Surgeon General* (DHEW Publication No. PHS 79-50066). Washington, DC: U.S. Government Printing Office.

United States Department of Health and Human Services (1982). *The health consequences of smoking: Cancer.* Rockville, MD: U.S. Public Health Service.

United States Department of Health and Human Services (1983). *The health consequences of smoking: Cardiovascular disease.* Rockville, MD: U.S. Public Health Service.

Victor, M., & Adams, R. D. (1953). The effect of alcohol on the nervous system. *Research Publications—Association for Research in Nervous and Mental Disease, 32,* 526–573.

Vourakis, C. (1983). Homosexuals in substance abuse treatment. In G. Bennett, C. Vourakis, & D. S. Woolf (Eds.), *Substance abuse: Pharmacocologic, developmental, and clinical perspectives.* New York: Wiley.

Wack, J. T., & Rodin, J. (1982). Smoking and its effects on body weight and the systems of caloric regulation. *American Journal of Clinical Nutrition, 35,* 366–380.

Wahlstrom, G. (1978). Addictive drugs and some neurotransmitters (acetylcholine and gamma-aminobutyric acid). In J. Fishman (Ed.), *The bases of addiction.* Berlin: Dahlem Konferenzen.

Way, E. L. (1978). Common and selective mechanisms in drug dependence. In J. Fishman (Ed.), *The bases of addiction.* Berlin: Dahlem Konferenzen.

Weiner, N. (1980). Norepinephrine, epinephrine, and the sympathomimetic amines. In A. G. Gilman, L. S. Goodman, & A. Gilman (Eds.), *The pharmacological basis of therapeutics* (6th ed.). New York: Macmillan.

Weisz, D. J., & Thompson, R. F. (1983). Endogenous opioids: Brain-behavior relations. In P. K. Levison, D. R. Gerstein, & D. R. Maloff (Eds.), *Commonalities in substance abuse and habitual behavior.* Lexington, MA: D. C. Heath.

Whitehead, C. C. (1974). Methadone pseudowithdrawal syndrome: Paradigm for a psychopharmacological model of opiate addiction. *Psychosomatic Medicine, 36,* 189–198.

Wikler, A. (1948). Recent progress in research on the neurophysiologic basis of morphine addiction. *American Journal of Psychiatry, 105,* 329–338.

Wikler, A. (1973). Conditioning of successive adaptive responses to the initial effects of drugs. *Conditional Reflex, 8,* 193–210.

Woolf, D. S. (1983a). Opioids. In G. Bennett, C. Vourakis, & D. S. Woolf (Eds.), *Substance abuse: Pharmacologic, developmental, and clinical perspectives.* New York: Wiley.

Woolf, D. S. (1983b). CNS depressants: Alcohol. In G. Bennett, C. Vourakis, & D. S. Woolf (Eds.), *Substance abuse: Pharmacologic, developmental, and clinical perspectives.* New York: Wiley.

Part II

COPING AND SUBSTANCE USE INITIATION

Initiation of substance use is an important area of research for the substance abuse field. The great majority of smoking and alcohol use initiation, for example, occurs during adolescence, and it appears likely that both expectations about the effects of substances and patterns of regular use are established during this period. The available evidence on initiation of cigarette smoking (Leventhal & Cleary, 1980) suggests that smoking initiation during adolescence is a complex process that typically takes about 2 years to complete. During this time, a person starts out with vague expectations about smoking, experiments in a few trial smoking situations, and in some cases continues, pursuing a pattern of semi-regular smoking. Although many adolescents discontinue cigarettes after one or two trials, a proportion of initial experimenters go on to become regular users by the age of 14–15 years (Botvin & McAlister, 1981). A similar process of initiation has been suggested for alcohol and other drug use (Gordon & McAlister, 1982; Kandel, 1978) although there have been few specific studies of initiation in these areas.

In the initiation of substance use during adolescence, coping processes may be involved in several ways. In terms of the present conceptual framework, a person's pattern of stress-coping skills (for dealing with general life stressors) may affect the long-term stress level so that he or she is more or less susceptible to the perceived stress-reducing function of cigarettes or alcohol. General social competence, defined as the types of social skills useful for coping with problematic interpersonal situations, may be related to overall stress level and to a person's capability for dealing with social situations where substance use occurs. Finally, temptation-coping skills are relevant for coping with specific situations where cigarettes or alcohol are offered.

The chapters in Part II deal with each of these aspects of coping. The studies were all conducted with school-age populations, typically surveying a large sample of students at about age 12, where levels of regular substance use are relatively low, and investigating the stress and coping variables that are related to an increased probability of smoking or alcohol use at this and subsequent time points. The methods used vary according to the research questions addressed. In Chapter 3, Wills examines the relationship between stress, coping, and substance use at relatively early time points (seventh and eighth grade), using data obtained with questionnaire scales indexing generalized life stress and generalized stress-coping patterns. Pentz, in Chapter 5, employs measures of social competence that address an intermediate level of coping; these include questionnaire scales of perceived efficacy for coping with typical interpersonal problem situations and role-play measures for assessing the level of social competence that an adolescent displays in some standard situations. Biglan, Weissman, and Severson in Chapter 4, concentrating on a role-play analogue assessment technique based on specific smoking initiation situations, study how adolescents deal with social influences for substance use. In this part the investigators address a number of questions, asking what types of coping are related to increased versus decreased rates of substance use, how use of substances for stress reduction may affect subsequent levels of coping, and what types of specific refusal skills are most effective for coping successfully with social influences for substance use. These investigators report a variety of new findings about the relationship between coping and substance use and describe in detail methodological approaches that will be useful for further research in this area.

In each case, these investigators also conducted field trials of skill-training programs that were implemented in real-world settings to test their effectiveness as primary prevention approaches to reduce the incidence of substance use initiation in adolescent populations. The intervention programs include components involving didactic instruction about the health consequences of smoking, guided modeling and rehearsal for teaching stress-coping and social competence skills, and role-play exercises to teach refusal skills for use in smoking situations. The researchers implemented the prevention programs with large populations of students in public school districts to determine the impact of the programs on actual rates of smoking and alcohol use in the population. These studies, conducted as a stringent test of coping concepts, have shown promising results suggesting that improved coping skills can be taught on a large-scale basis and that this can reduce the initiation of smoking and other substances in adolescent populations. This finding has significant implications because even small changes in rates of initiation at early ages may translate into a large effect on eventual rates of substance use during adulthood. Additionally, the investigators included measures of hypothesized mediating variables (e.g., coping patterns, social skills) in the evaluation design so that the effects of the intervention programs could be directly related to the mediators suggested by a stress-coping theoretical framework.

REFERENCES

Botvin, G. J., & McAlister, A. (1981). Cigarette smoking among children and adolescents. In C. B. Arnold, L. H. Kuller, & M. R. Greenlick (Eds.), *Advances in disease prevention* (Vol. 1). New York: Springer.

Gordon, N. P., & McAlister, A. (1982). Adolescent drinking: Issues and research. In T. J. Coates, A. C. Petersen, & C. Perry (Eds.), *Promoting adolescent health*. New York: Academic Press.

Kandel, D. B. (1978). Convergences in prospective longitudinal surveys of drug use in normal populations. In D. B. Kandel (Ed.), *Longitudinal research on drug use*. New York: Wiley.

Leventhal, H., & Cleary, P. D. (1980). The smoking problem: A review of research and theory in behavioral risk modification. *Psychological Bulletin, 88,* 370–405.

Chapter 3

Stress, Coping, and Tobacco and Alcohol Use in Early Adolescence*

THOMAS ASHBY WILLS

INTRODUCTION

This study is based on a formulation positing that stress predisposes adolescents to begin using substances such as tobacco and alcohol. It was recognized that initiation of substance use is a multifactorial process that involves substance-related knowledge and attitudes (Bentler & Speckart, 1979), social influences from parents and peers (Coates, Perry, Killen, & Slinkard, 1981), as well as various psychological characteristics that may increase susceptibility to smoking influences (Botvin & McAlister, 1981). The focus in this study, however, is on stress and coping factors that predispose students toward early experimentation with substances. This focus was suggested in part of a body of research with adults (e.g., Abrams, 1983; Leventhal & Cleary, 1980) suggesting that smoking or alcohol use serves a direct stress-reduction function. Although there was little evidence linking perceived stress with smoking in adolescence, the implication was that adolescents under stress are more likely to be regular smokers, presumably because they derive more psychological or physiological benefit from nicotine use (see Wills & Shiffman, Chapter 1, this volume). This formulation led to the development of measures to index stress and to investigation of the relationship between stress and substance use.

Another focus of this study is on the measurement of coping patterns relevant for substance use in early adolescence. This was suggested by epidemiological research indicating that adolescents who engage in prob-

---

*This research was supported by Grant #HRRP 80A-23 from the Centers for Disease Control. The author thanks Stephen Ramirez, Donna Spitzhoff, Roger Vaughan, and Aaron Warshawsky for their assistance in this project, Arthur Stone for several research suggestions, and Saul Shiffman for his comments on a draft of this chapter.

lematic substance use are characterized by a syndrome of variables including poor academic performance, social marginality or conflictual interpersonal relationships, low self-esteem, and a tendency to use substances to deal with negative mood states such as depression (see, e.g., Jessor, Chase, & Donovan, 1980; Kandel, Kessler, & Margulies, 1978). This evidence suggested that coping skills might be a common factor underlying various empirical predictors of substance use. This concept led to the use of several approaches to measure coping patterns that might be particularly relevant for substance use in adolescence. At the same time, it seemed prudent to be alert to possible differences between the dynamics of smoking and those of problematic alcohol use. Measures for both cigarette smoking and alcohol use were obtained, and results for these two substances were always analyzed separately.

In analyzing the data, attention was given not only to the direct main effect of stress and coping on substance use but also to the interaction between stress and coping. At the outset it seemed plausible that coping patterns were most relevant for persons under relatively high stress and less relevant (or perhaps even irrelevant to drug use) for persons who were experiencing little stress. Thus, analyses were performed to examine interactions between stress and various coping patterns, to determine whether a process similar to the buffering model of social support (Cohen & Wills, in press) might operate in relation to stress, coping, and substance use.

METHOD

Subjects

The subjects in this study were a cohort of public school students from a community school district in New York City that covers mid-Manhattan between Greenwich Village and the upper East and West Sides. This was basically a population sample, because the subjects were the entire seventh grades of three junior schools in the district. The original cohort, which was first surveyed at the beginning of their seventh-grade year in Fall 1981, consisted of 675 completed questionnaires out of a population of approximately 800 students. In a replication study, a second cohort, first surveyed in Fall 1982 at the beginning of their seventh-grade year, was a larger class and consisted of 901 completed questionnaires out of a population of approximately 1100 students. Ethnic backgrounds for both cohorts were comparable, with approximately 50% white, 20% black, 20% Hispanic and 10% Asian students.

Procedure

Surveys were administered at the beginning and end of each school year, so that each subject was surveyed four times over the seventh–eighth-grade period. Data were obtained through group administration of a questionnaire that included items on smoking and alcohol use, stress, coping, and psychosocial variables. The questionnaire was administered in science classes by project staff, who followed a standardized protocol in giving instructions to students and answering questions about particular items. Questionnaires were labeled with only a code number (used for longitudinal tracking); students were informed that all their answers were confidential and that they should not write their name on the survey. When the questionnaire was distributed, project staff collected a saliva sample, and students were informed that the sample would be analyzed confidentially to determine whether the student had smoked cigarettes (the "bogus pipeline" technique; Evans, Hansen, & Mittelmark, 1977). The questionnaire was completed in one class period. Because of a daily absentee rate of approximately 20%, there was some data loss at each administration.

Measures

Stress. The original stress measure, the Stress Reactions Scale, was a 15-item scale indexing subjective reactions to stress, such as feelings of tension and time pressure, difficulty in sleeping or relaxing, and feelings of stress or nervousness. Pretesting indicated that this scale was correlated with a measure of current negative events, $r(200) = .60$, $p < .001$. In the first survey administration the stress scale was used with a 3-point scale to index occurrence of feelings during the past week and had high internal consistency (Cronbach alpha = .85); comparable reliability was found for subsequent administrations. As an alternative approach to measurement of stress, an affect balance scale (Zevon & Tellegen, 1982) was included, based on a 20-item adjective checklist that indexed orthogonal dimensions of negative mood and positive mood. Like the Stress Reactions Scale, the affect scales were completed to describe frequency of a particular mood during the past week. Beginning in Year 2, two 12-item scales of negative and positive events occurring during the past week were included. These scales, based on checklists developed by Lewinsohn and associates (e.g., Lewinsohn & Amenson, 1978), were rated on a 3-point frequency scale.

Factorial Coping Measure. With the original cohort, coping was indexed by factorial measures of generalized coping patterns. A set of 35 items derived from the Response Profile of the Coping Assessment Battery (Bugen

& Hawkins, 1981) was given to subjects with the heading, "When I have a problem, I _____." (The nature of the problem was left unspecified except to say that it was a problem "at school or home.") Items were responded to on a 1–5 frequency scale with the anchor points "never" and "usually." This item set was then factor analyzed using the principal-factor method with iteration and varimax rotation. From a default analysis of 11 factors, a solution with 8 factors was selected and factor scores were constructed based on standardized items. In the eight-factor solution the first two factors were Decision Making and Cognitive Coping. Consistent with the conceptual framework, the first factor contained items that tap the kind of coping behavior termed *problem solving* or *direct action*. The second factor included a variety of cognitive strategies exemplifying the type of coping that has been termed *emotion-focused coping, cognitive restructuring,* or *situation redefinition*. The remaining factors included one concerning physical activity (bicycle riding, sports), and one termed Distraction, which was loaded by the items "I daydream" and "I try to put the problem out of my mind." In the third and fourth waves (beginning and end of eighth grade) the coping inventory was expanded to 54 items to clarify some ambiguous factors in the original instrument. From a 13-factor default solution an 11-factor solution, presented in Table 3.1, was selected. Some of the previous factors were replicated, and the revised instrument provided factors that separately defined social support from peers and from adults, distinguished social entertainment activity from solitary relaxation activity, and included factors titled Aggression and Prayer.[1]

Psychosocial Measures. In addition to measures of stress and coping, several psychosocial variables were included in the surveys. Two subscales from the Multidimensional Health Locus of Control Scales (MHLC, Wallston, Wallston, & DeVellis, 1978) were included to index health-specific beliefs. Also, an 18-item assertiveness inventory based on Gambrill and Richey (1975) was used in the original survey. Factor analysis indicated that this instrument comprised three factorial dimensions that were termed General Assertiveness (e.g., "ask for service when you are not getting it," "re-

---

[1] In a replication study with a new cohort, an alternative approach to the measurement of coping was used, based on the method developed by Stone and Neale (1984). The purpose was to assess the same basic dimensions of coping using a different measurement approach. Subjects were given generalized descriptors (e.g., "Something to try to solve the problem") designed to represent a particular coping pattern (e.g., Decision Making) and then were asked to rate how often they did this (with the intention of coping) when they had a problem. Eight dimensions of coping were assessed, and frequency of use of coping patterns was assessed for each of five different problem areas. Because the results were generally similar to those obtained with the previous approach to coping measurement, these results are not reported in detail. Some exceptions are noted.

Table 3.1
ELEVEN-FACTOR SOLUTION FOR 54-ITEM COPING INVENTORY: SPRING 1983 DATA[a]

Factor title/items[b]	Loadings										
	1	2	3	4	5	6	7	8	9	10	11
Factor 1: Decision Making											
Think about which information is necessary	.77	.16	.06	.07	-.06	.02	-.06	.10	.01	.00	.11
Think about choices before taking any action	.71	-.07	-.01	.07	-.03	.10	-.06	-.06	.08	-.03	.08
Get information needed to deal with problem	.70	.14	.02	.07	-.04	.09	-.01	.04	-.01	-.03	.07
Think about which of alternatives is best	.68	-.04	.08	.12	-.05	.03	-.10	-.02	.12	.13	-.05
Think about risks of different ways	.68	-.06	-.03	.11	-.08	.01	-.02	-.03	.06	-.03	.08
Think about possible consequences of alternatives	.64	.01	.11	.07	-.09	.10	-.03	-.06	.10	.06	.00
Compromise to get something positive from situation	.50	.01	.30	.08	-.15	.10	-.03	.10	.04	.14	-.06
Change an attitude which contributes to the problem	.45	.00	.18	.13	.03	.09	-.05	.04	.05	-.03	-.01
Change behavior that contributes to the problem	.45	-.14	.08	.09	-.03	.13	-.05	.04	.00	.01	-.12
Factor 2: Adult Social Support											
Talk with a doctor	.02	.68	.00	.02	.02	.02	.02	.09	.03	.03	-.02
Talk with teacher	-.01	.56	.00	.13	.08	.09	-.01	-.01	.03	.03	-.02
Talk with counselor or psychologist	-.06	.55	-.07	.09	.02	.02	-.01	.03	.05	.00	.00
Talk with a minister	.01	.53	.12	.03	.09	.13	.07	-.03	-.12	.05	.10
Practice meditation	.07	.39	-.01	-.03	.17	.13	.15	.02	.08	.03	.12
Go to a social club	-.05	.39	.01	.01	.11	.14	-.04	.20	.12	-.21	-.05
Go to an after school program	.00	.35	.07	.00	-.02	.09	-.07	.15	.13	.05	.05

(*continued*)

Table 3.1
(Continued)

Factor title/items[b]	Loadings										
	1	2	3	4	5	6	7	8	9	10	11
Factor 3: Cognitive Coping											
Tell myself it will be over in a short time	.05	.09	.65	.07	−.09	.06	−.02	−.02	.08	−.01	.04
Not worth getting upset about	.10	.06	.61	.12	−.03	.06	−.06	.08	.06	.06	−.07
Wait and hope that things will get better	.05	.00	.58	.07	−.08	.01	.03	.03	.09	−.10	.26
Try to put it out of my mind	.02	−.09	.54	−.04	.05	.03	.15	.02	−.01	.04	.02
Remind myself that things could be worse	.28	.04	.54	.17	−.10	−.05	−.04	.04	.09	.07	.07
Try to notice only the good things in life	.23	.03	.53	−.02	.03	.15	.02	.09	.05	.03	−.06
Go on as if nothing had happened	−.03	.02	.47	−.11	.13	.16	.13	.21	.09	−.03	.06
Factor 4: Peer Social Support											
Let out feelings with someone I feel close to	.17	.06	.02	.81	.00	.03	.02	.05	.12	.06	.01
Look for a person who might understand problem	.21	.08	.01	.79	−.04	.07	.02	.11	.12	.04	.09
Find someone special to share my problem with	.18	.08	.05	.78	.01	.08	−.04	.04	.05	−.07	−.01
Talk with one of my friends	.12	.01	.08	.64	.04	.03	.04	.15	.22	.02	.10
Talk with my brother or sister	.11	.18	.09	.29	−.01	.11	.06	.00	.03	.11	.12
Factor 5: Substance Use											
Drink beer or wine	−.15	.07	−.06	.06	.80	.10	.16	.12	−.09	−.03	−.03
Smoke grass	−.14	.12	−.05	−.04	.77	.03	.11	.13	−.07	.01	.03
Take pills to feel better	−.11	.33	.00	−.08	.66	−.04	.18	−.01	.00	−.05	.00
Factor 6: Physical exercise											
Work if off by physical exercise	.12	.03	.06	.13	.09	.67	.04	.03	.07	−.11	−.13
Play sports	.07	.14	.15	−.01	−.09	.63	−.05	.23	.11	.17	.07
Go to the gym and work out	.15	.25	.03	.07	.07	.57	.03	.10	.08	.01	−.03
Go jogging	.16	.17	.04	.06	.03	.56	−.01	.01	.06	−.04	.05
Go bicycle riding	.11	.09	.10	.02	−.03	.55	−.06	.15	.08	.08	.00

	F1	F2	F3	F4	F5	F6	F7	F8	F9	F10	F11
Factor 7: Aggression											
Get mad at people	−.11	.00	−.04	.04	.15	−.03	*.70*	.05	.07	.05	.12
Blame or criticize other people	−.13	.01	.21	.09	.02	−.07	*.53*	.04	−.02	.01	−.01
Do something bad or cause trouble	−.18	.18	.02	−.09	.32	.10	*.50*	.18	−.05	−.06	.10
Do something exciting or risky	−.03	−.03	.10	.01	.19	.35	.35	.35	−.04	−.03	.12
Avoid being with people	−.04	−.01	−.04	−.07	.16	−.03	.34	−.17	.21	−.13	.00
Factor 8: Social Entertainment											
Hang out with other kids	.06	.01	.11	.19	.10	.18	.07	*.65*	.08	−.03	−.04
Go to a party	.01	.22	.09	.17	.17	.18	.05	*.60*	.06	−.09	−.10
Go to the movies	.03	.19	.15	−.01	−.02	.25	.03	*.46*	.28	.12	.03
Go shopping	.00	.19	.15	.07	.04	.01	−.06	.33	.24	.11	.14
Factor 9: Individual Relaxation											
Go walking	.10	.05	.07	.19	−.14	.17	.03	.07	*.56*	−.05	.09
Read books or magazines	.09	.12	.10	.02	−.06	.07	.02	.01	*.54*	.11	.04
Get away from things for a while	.09	.07	.05	.11	.03	.16	.34	.05	*.44*	−.19	.02
Listen to music	.06	−.03	.06	.18	.02	.10	.12	.23	*.44*	.05	.00
Sit quietly and relax	.15	.09	.16	.21	−.01	−.03	−.14	.09	*.42*	.08	.05
Factor 10: Parental Support											
Talk with my mother or father	.17	.26	.02	.22	−.06	.09	−.17	−.03	.14	*.55*	−.10
Watch TV	−.08	−.07	.22	−.08	−.02	.05	.13	.17	.22	.31	.27
Factor 11: Prayer											
Pray for guidance or strength	.13	.27	.15	.13	−.09	.02	.03	.05	.07	.03	*.54*
Worry a lot about the problem	.01	−.05	.03	.19	.13	−.07	.20	−.11	.11	−.07	*.43*
Eigenvalue (nonrotated)	6.99	4.38	2.41	2.16	1.84	1.59	1.28	0.93	0.72	0.61	0.56
Eigenvalue (rotated)	4.16	2.45	2.65	2.91	2.12	2.37	1.71	1.74	1.71	0.73	0.87
Percentage of variance	18	11	11	12	9	10	7	7	7	3	4

[a] Analysis performed using principal-factor method with iteration. Tabled values are varimax-rotated loadings. Values ≥.40 are in italics. Analysis based on all subjects with complete coping data; $N = 509$.

[b] Items are responses to "When I have a problem I _____."

turn items to a store or restaurant"), Social Assertiveness (e.g., "start a conversation with a stranger," "tell someone you like them"), and Substance-Related Assertiveness (e.g., "resist pressure to smoke cigarettes," "resist pressure to drink"). In later waves, measures of self-efficacy and self-esteem were included, and these are described during presentation of results.

Substance Use. Smoking was measured by four items asking whether the subject had smoked cigarettes ever, more than four times, in the past month, in the past week; responses to these items were on a dichotomous (yes or no) scale. Comparable items were employed for alcohol use (defined as beer, wine, or liquor), and an additional item on heavy drinking asked whether there was a time in the past month when the subject had had three or more drinks on one occasion; responses for this item were "No," "Yes, it happened once," and "Yes, it happened more than once."

RESULTS

Prevalence Rates for Smoking and Alcohol Use

Data for the individual smoking and alcohol items are presented in Table 3.2. Rates of experimental and regular substance use are consistent with rates found in national surveys (Fishburne, Abelson, & Cisin, 1980; Green, 1979) and show more exposure to alcohol than to cigarettes. Data for this population indicate that most transitions from experimental to regular use occurred during the seventh-grade year; rates for regular use almost doubled during this period, from 8 to 14% for smoking and from 8 to 15% for alcohol. After the end of seventh grade there was little change in regular substance use, although there was a slight increase in rates of heavy drinking. This transition is more rapid than that observed in national samples, but it should be remembered that this was an urban population from the central areas of Manhattan, where students already enter junior high school with a considerable exposure to these substances; for example, at the beginning of seventh grade more than 25% of this sample had smoked or drunk alcohol more than four times.[2] Because Guttman scaling analyses indicated

---

[2]The validity of self-reports of smoking was checked through two methods. In the first wave, analyses for saliva cotinine (see Haley, Caryn, & Tilton, 1983) were done for all students in one junior high school ($N = 235$). This sample produced eight positive assays for cotinine indicating regular smoking; of these, 100% of the subjects indicated that they had ever smoked, and 75% reported smoking during the past week. For the second wave, saliva thiocyanate analyses (Borgers & Junge, 1979) were done for the entire population. Thiocyanate analyses were less specific but showed significant differences between students who stated they had smoked the previous day (assessed by another item not reported here) compared with students who had never smoked ($p < .01$) and students who had smoked in the past month ($p < .07$).

Table 3.2

PREVALENCE RATES, IN PERCENTAGES, FOR SUBSTANCE USE ITEMS: FIRST THROUGH FOURTH WAVES

Variable	Measurement wave			
	Fall 1981	Spring 1982	Fall 1982	Spring 1983
Smoking items				
Ever smoked	45	54	54	58
Smoked >4 times	24	38	37	42
Smoked in past month	15	21	21	20
Smoked in past week	8	14	14	14
Summary score[a]				
M	1.89	2.22	2.25	2.32
SD	1.23	1.40	1.42	1.41
Alcohol items				
Ever drank	69	73	73	79
Drank >4 times	38	46	48	55
Drank in past month	22	29	29	28
Drank in past week	8	15	14	13
Heavy drinking ≥2 times in past month	6	9	10	11
Summary score[b]				
M	2.38	2.69	2.75	2.84
SD	1.37	1.54	1.57	1.49

[a]Scored on 1–5 scale; higher score indicates more cigarette smoking.
[b]Scored on 1–6 scale; higher score indicates more alcohol use.

that the smoking and alcohol items had good scaling characteristics, summary scores were derived from the four smoking items (1–5 scale) and the five alcohol items (1–6 scale), and these continuous scores were used as criterion variables in multivariate analyses. Descriptive statistics for the summary scores of smoking and alcohol use are included in Table 3.2.

In this population, cigarette smoking and alcohol use were interrelated. For example, of students who had smoked more than four times 70% had also used alcohol more than four times; this compared with 32% of nonsmokers, $\chi^2(1, N = 499) = 60.1, p < .001$. Of students who had smoked in the past week, 34% had also used alcohol in the past week; this compared with 6% of nonweekly smokers, $\chi^2(1, N = 501) = 41.3, p < .001$. Interrelationships were strongest for heavy drinking; of those who had smoked in the past week, 57% had done heavy drinking once or more in the last month, compared with 16% for nonweekly smokers, $\chi^2(2, N = 570) = 77.1, p < .001$. Correspondingly, the summary scores for substance use were substantially intercorrelated. The correlation between smoking and alcohol summary scores was .47 in the first-wave data, and the intercorrelation increased steadily as the students grew older ($r = .51$ for second wave, $r = .59$ for third wave).

Predictors of Smoking and Alcohol Use

For analysis of these data a multiple regression approach was employed, with stress, coping factors, and psychological variables as predictors, and a summary score for smoking or alcohol use as the criterion variable.[3] Regression analyses were performed with forced entry of the full predictor set, and beta weights in the tables represent the unique contribution of each variable in the full model (Cohen & Cohen, 1983). Because some sex and race differences were found for predictor and criterion variables, all analyses were performed with controls for sex and race, and the results reported subsequently are ones that obtained with sex and race controls. Tables 3.3 and 3.4 report data from the first and fourth waves of the study, respectively. The following discussion focuses on consistencies in main-effect results over the four waves; results on interactions are presented in a subsequent section. It should be noted that the results indicated in the tables are concurrent associations between predictor variables and substance use criteria at the same point in time.[4]

Main Effects

Stress. Stress was a significant predictor of both smoking and alcohol use over all four measurement waves, although predictive patterns tended to change as students grew older. In all cases, stress was positively related to substance use. In the first-wave data, the measure of subjective stress reactions was a significant predictor of both smoking and alcohol use. This finding was replicated in the second-wave data. In data from eighth grade, where scales of both negative events and subjective stress reactions were included, negative events were a significant predictor at both measurements.

---

[3] To determine whether the summary scores met the assumptions for multiple regression, discriminant function analyses were performed with the various levels of smoking or alcohol use treated as discrete categories and the set of stress, coping, and psychological variables used as predictors. In general these analyses indicated that the data were consistent with a multiple regression model because they showed one signifcant discriminant function that indexed an overall tendency for use of a substance. With alcohol use, there was a tendency for a second function that discriminated heavy drinkers from regular but nonheavy drinkers, but this function was always secondary to the major function that indexed overall involvement in drinking.

[4] Additional analyses were performed using the stress and coping variables from Time 1 as predictors of change in smoking status from Time 1 to Time 2. Results were comparable to those from the concurrent analyses, and so the discussion in this chapter focuses on the concurrent relationships.

Table 3.3

MULTIVARIATE ANALYSIS OF PSYCHOLOGICAL PREDICTORS: FIRST WAVE DATA SET[a]

Predictor	Smoking index				Drinking index			
	Type I SS	Type II SS	β	t	Type I SS	Type II SS	β	t
Stress Reactions Scale	22.93	10.44	.12	2.70**	25.32	10.94	.12	2.55**
Decision Making	12.66	9.46	−.11	2.57**	6.45	10.43	−.12	2.49**
Cognitive Coping	4.16	7.86	−.10	2.34**	1.64	4.28	−.07	—
Social Support	1.00	0.69	.03	—	0.24	0.33	.02	—
Behavior Change	2.29	1.44	.04	—	4.75	1.24	.04	—
Physical Activity	0.77	0.71	−.03	—	5.38	6.53	.09	1.97*
Relaxation	7.50	9.66	−.11	2.60**	3.38	6.54	−.09	1.97*
Distraction	10.13	9.07	.11	2.52**	9.69	6.72	.09	2.00*
Internal Health Locus of Control	0.05	0.02	.01	—	0.84	0.86	−.03	—
Chance Health Locus of Control	0.12	0.05	.01	—	2.90	0.75	−.03	—
Social Assertiveness	3.27	2.61	.06	—	21.01	12.72	.15	2.75**
General Assertiveness	0.09	3.54	.09	—	3.16	3.25	.09	—
Substance Assertiveness	10.87	10.87	−.14	2.75**	0.29	0.29	−.02	—
	Multiple R = .31		df = 1, 508		Multiple R = .32		df = 1, 434	
	MS error = 1.43				MS error = 1.68			

[a]Substance use indices are constructed such that a higher score indicates more involvement in substance use. Predictor variables are constructed such that a higher score indicates more of the named quantity. Type I SS is for F at entry in sequential order listed; Type II SS is for partial F in full model.
*$p < .05$. **$p < .01$.

For data from the beginning of eighth grade, the negative events scale was strongly associated with both smoking and alcohol use ($p < .0001$ for both), and the subjective stress scale showed only a marginal contribution in the multivariate analyses. For data from the end of eighth grade, the negative events scale continued to show a significant, although weaker, association with smoking; for alcohol use, negative events again were a significant predictor, but the subjective stress scale now showed a significant unique contribution ($p < .01$) net of the negative events measure, largely because of its association with heavy drinking. The results suggest that stress is a factor in both smoking and alcohol use in early adolescence (from the beginning of seventh grade) and that it may be more important as a predictor of problematic alcohol use as students grow older.

Positive Events. In each measurement wave, measures of positive occurrences were included in order to investigate the possibility that positive occurrences have main effects on substance use (or buffer the impact of

Table 3.4

MULTIVARIATE ANALYSIS OF PSYCHOLOGICAL PREDICTORS: FOURTH-WAVE DATA SET[a]

Predictor	Smoking index				Drinking index			
	Type I SS	Type II SS	β	t	Type I SS	Type II SS	β	t
Negative Events	25.56	6.39	.11	1.93*	85.89	19.40	.18	3.31***
Positive Events	2.53	0.15	−.02	—	8.78	0.95	.04	—
Stress Scale	2.22	0.52	.03	—	11.93	15.14	.17	2.92**
Decision Making	3.78	2.75	−.06	—	1.48	0.40	−.02	—
Social Support (adult)	14.10	9.52	−.11	2.36**	5.86	2.81	−.05	—
Cognitive Coping	3.59	1.89	−.06	—	11.37	7.91	−.09	2.11*
Social Support (peer)	17.26	19.64	.15	3.39***	0.86	2.51	.05	—
Physical Exercise	1.88	3.20	−.06	—	2.48	1.60	.04	—
Aggression	9.26	9.88	.11	2.40**	5.77	7.38	.09	2.04*
Social Entertainment	41.98	43.29	.23	5.03****	25.37	26.93	.18	3.90****
Individual Relaxation	7.29	5.40	−.08	—	17.77	13.16	−.12	2.72**
Social Support (parental)	21.98	23.25	−.16	3.68***	7.89	8.88	−.10	2.24*
Prayer	2.93	1.59	−.04	—	16.12	11.03	−.11	2.49**
Internal Health LOC	2.95	3.92	−.07	—	4.76	6.43	−.08	1.90*
Self-esteem	1.64	0.41	.03	—	5.52	2.81	.08	—
Self-efficacy	1.16	1.16	.05	—	0.71	0.71	.04	—
	Multiple R = .41 df = 1, 470				Multiple R = .48 df = 1, 458			
	MS error = 1.71				MS error = 1.77			

[a]Substance use indices are constructed such that a higher score indicates more involvement in substance use. Predictor variables are constructed such that a higher score indicates more of the named quality. Type I SS is for F at entry in sequential order listed; Type II SS is for partial F in full model.
*$p < .05$. **$p < .01$. ***$p < .001$. ****$p < .0001$.

negative occurrences). In the first-year data, a scale of positive mood (Zevon & Tellegen, 1982) generally showed no unique contribution to substance use, with the exception of two interactive relationships discussed subsequently. In the second year, analyses of the 12-item positive events item set indicated that it consisted of two different subscales, one representing positive social events and the other representing positive nonsocial events. On a main-effect basis the nonsocial-events scale proved to be inversely related to smoking and alcohol use. In contrast, the social-events scale was always positively related to substance use. These results were qualified in some cases by Positive Events × Negative Events interactions, discussed in a subsequent section.

Decision Making. This pattern of coping was significantly related to a lower probability of smoking and alcohol use at the beginning of seventh grade. This relationship was replicated at other measurement points but grew weaker as the students grew older. In general the pattern of the findings suggests that this type of coping may be most important as a deterrent to early experimentation with substance use; after students have actively begun to experiment with smoking or drinking, other factors may become more important.[5]

Cognitive Coping. Although this type of coping was associated with a lower probability of substance use, the associations were less consistent. Cognitive Coping was a significant predictor of smoking at beginning of seventh grade. It was negatively associated with alcohol use but the main effect was statistically significant only at the end of eighth grade. The associations of Cognitive Coping with alcohol use at subsequent points are suggestive of somewhat different dynamics in the processes underlying smoking and alcohol use.

Social Support. In the first-year data a 3-item measure of general social support was not related to substance use. After the first year, the social support scale was revised to include more items and to indicate specifically the source of the support. The new measures showed strong associations between support and substance use that depended upon the type of support. A coping factor termed Adult Support, representing support from parents, teachers, or other significant adults (e.g., doctors, ministers) was significantly negatively associated with substance use; the more a student was able to talk comfortably with parents or other adults when he or she had a problem, the *less* likely the student was to be engaged in substance use. Conversely, a coping factor termed Peer Support was positively associated with smoking; the more a student tended to depend on same-age friends for talking about a problem, the *more* likely he or she was to be involved in substance use. These associations between social support and substance use occurred mainly for cigarette smoking. (For a detailed analysis of the social support variables, see Wills & Vaughan, 1985.)

Physical Exercise. One of the original coping factors indicated that when a student had a problem, he or she tended to cope through physical exercise such as running, bike riding, or sports. This measure showed a significant sex difference, with males consistently scoring higher on this coping factor. However, relationships with substance use were erratic. The

---

[5]With the subjective approach to coping measurement (see footnote 1), a significant relationship between Decision Making and smoking was found through the eighth-grade year ($p < .01$). Because of measurement and cohort differences this finding is not definitive, but it does indicate that this type of coping may show more general relationships to substance use than the initial data suggested.

factor tended to be negatively associated with smoking and positively associated with alcohol use, but in most cases the relationships were not statistically significant.

Social Entertainment. During the second year of the study, a new coping factor termed Social Entertainment reflected the use of entertaining or pleasure-seeking activities as a way of coping with problems. As Table 3.4 indicates, the final version of this measure was positively associated with both smoking and alcohol use. There is still some possible ambiguity in this measure because the items in the factor (e.g., hanging out with other kids, going to a party, going to a movie, going shopping) could be construed as involving either social activity, pleasure seeking, or distraction and entertainment. It should be noted, however, that it made a significant unique contribution net of the Peer Support coping factor, so it seems unlikely that this measure merely indexes social activity. Perhaps it is relevant that a small factor termed Distraction, loaded by items about daydreaming and trying to put the problem out of one's mind, was positively associated with substance use in both the first-wave data (see Table 3.3) and the second-wave data. There is the suggestion that some of this content, of trying to reduce stress and anxiety by distracting oneself from the problem, may be represented in the Social Entertainment factor. There is no doubt that this approach to coping is, overall, a strong positive correlate of substance use. This relationship was also replicated using the subjective coping inventory (see footnote 1).

Individual Relaxation. Throughout the course of the study an attempt was made to test the concept that a relaxation-oriented coping style would be negatively associated with substance use. This proved a difficult measurement task. In the original coping inventory used in the first and second waves, a factor termed Relaxation was found, loaded by three items about relaxation, meditation, and solitary walking. This measure was negatively associated with both smoking and alcohol use in the first wave (see Table 3.3), and this relationship was replicated for alcohol use in the second wave. During the third-and fourth-wave measurements an attempt was made to clarify the meaning of this factor through additional items. The best representation of the construct seems to be that represented by the factor termed Individual Relaxation, which reflects coping through individual activities such as walking, reading, and getting away from things in order to relax. This factor showed a significant negative association with alcohol use in the fourth-wave data (see Table 3.4); the relationship with smoking was in the same direction but was nonsignificant. Thus, there is evidence that a coping pattern based on individual activities pursued with the intent of relaxation and stress reduction may operate to decrease the probability of substance use.[6]

Aggression. On the basis of downward comparison theory (Wills, 1981), some items were included to test the proposition that an aggressive style of coping would be positively correlated with substance use. The relevant coping factor (see Table 3.1) included items about getting mad at people, blaming or criticizing others, and causing trouble. As predicted, this dimension showed a significant positive association with both smoking and alcohol use.

Religion. In order to explicitly separate religiously oriented coping from other coping dimensions such as Adult Support and Relaxation, items about coping with problems through prayer were included the second year. As indicated in Table 3.4, this coping pattern was significantly negatively associated with alcohol use. In the replication study a religious coping dimension showed similar relationships with both smoking and alcohol use.

Health Locus of Control. To index locus of control the Internal and Chance subscales from the Wallston et al. (1978) MHLC were employed. In this cohort the Internal Health Locus of Control subscale showed consistent negative associations with smoking and alcohol use but the relationships were generally nonsignificant. It was only at the end of eighth grade that a significant relationship with alcohol use was noted (see Table 3.4). Some cohort effects were also evident, because in the replication study it was found that Internal Health Locus of Control was a highly significant predictor of alcohol use from the beginning of seventh grade onwards.

Assertiveness. In the first year of the study, factor analysis of the assertiveness factor indicated that it comprised three orthogonal factors: Substance-Related Assertiveness (refusing specific offers of cigarettes or alcohol), General Assertiveness (in everyday situations), and Social Assertiveness (relevant to social or dating situations). Quite different relationships were found

---

[6]The wording of such measures is crucial, however. Items concerning meditation may index religiously oriented coping, and investigators should be careful to provide separate measures of that coping pattern. In addition, subjects may interpret subjective items about relaxation to mean achieving relaxation through substance use. This was found in the replication study, where a dimension concerning "coping with the intent of relaxation" showed a strong positive association with substance use. Apparently with this measure the subjects consistently construed the item not in terms of stress-reducing behaviors but in terms of smoking or drinking as a means of relaxing. Given the widespread perception that substance use can reduce stress (see Wills & Shiffman, Chapter 1, this volume), this is not an unreasonable interpretation, and investigators should be alert to this possible interpretation of relaxation measures.

for these three factors. Substance-Related Assertiveness was significantly negatively associated with substance use at all measurement points. In contrast, General and Social Assertiveness tended to be positively associated with smoking and alcohol use. The associations were statistically nonsignificant in the first-wave data but by the end of the seventh grade the associations were highly significant. The same measures were included in the replication study, and again the same pattern of significant relationships was observed. (For a detailed analysis of data on assertiveness and substance use, see Wills, Baker, & Botvin, 1985.)

Self-Esteem and Self-Efficacy. In Year 2, global measures of self-esteem (Rosenberg, 1965) and self-efficacy (Ilfeld, 1978) were included in the survey. Data from the third and fourth waves with the original cohort indicated that neither of these measures was significantly related to substance use. In the replication study, an attempt was made to resolve these findings by using multidimensional measures of self-esteem (Fleming & Watts, 1980) and perceived control (Paulhus, 1983) with new cohorts of students. The self-esteem measure was scored for a five-factor solution, and a factor indexing generalized self-regard proved to be negatively associated with smoking ($p < .01$). The perceived control measure produced a four-factor solution, and in these data a factor indexing general self-efficacy was negatively associated with smoking and alcohol use ($p < .01$ for both). In contrast, a factor from the self-esteem battery indexing social self-confidence was positively associated with alcohol use ($p < .01$), and a factor from the perceived control battery indexing perceived control in social situations was positively associated with both smoking and alcohol use ($p < .001$ for both).

Interactions: Coping Variables

Tests of stress buffering for the coping variables were performed by forcing a cross-product term (Stress Variable × Coping Variable) into the regression model after the main-effect terms for stress and coping (Cohen & Cohen, 1983). As the type of interaction typically found for buffering processes is a difficult one to demonstrate statistically (Cohen & Wills, in press), interactions at marginal significance levels were analyzed if they were replicated over different measurements. Two general conclusions emerged from these analyses. First, Stress × Coping interaction effects were found most often for indices of recent use (e.g., smoked in past week, heavy drinking in past month) rather than for indices of overall involvement in substance use, although some significant interactions were found for the summary scores of smoking and alcohol use. Second, it was found that the domain of coping variables measured provided several different types of interaction effects: Some coping patterns represented true buffering processes (i.e., coping reduced substance use only under high stress), some represented mixed buffers, and a few produced reverse interactions (i.e., this type of coping *increased* substance use under high stress). The following sections summarize the findings for these different types of interaction processes.

True Buffers. Consistent with the theoretical formulation of stress, coping, and substance use, it was found that several coping dimensions produced interactions that represented stress-buffering: Under higher stress there was a substantial inverse relationship between coping and substance use (i.e., the higher the level of coping, the lower the level of substance use), whereas under low stress there was little or no relationship between coping and substance use. This pattern was found for the coping dimensions of Decision Making and Cognitive Coping. The coping pattern of Physical Exercise showed consistent buffering, but there tended to be some crossing of the interactions, especially for alcohol (i.e., physical exercise coping was related to a slightly higher level of alcohol use at a low level of stress). The original coping measure termed Relaxation Coping produced some buffering interactions at early measurement points, and the social support measure termed Parental Support showed a true buffering interaction at the end of 8th grade.

Mixed Interaction. Some measures showed interactions of a type where coping increased substance use somewhat at a low level of stress but had lesser, and sometimes inverse, effects at higher levels of stress. The net effect, statistically, is that the coping variable reduces the impact of stress on substance use, so that the pattern can be classified as a mixed interaction. This pattern of interaction was found for the coping measures termed Distraction and Withdrawal, used at some points with the original cohort.

Reverse Interaction. In two cases, coping dimensions were found to have virtually no effect at a low level of stress but to markedly increase substance use at a high level of stress. This pattern was found for the dimensions representing Substance Use and Aggression as coping mechanisms. Less consistent results were found for two other measures, one termed Social Entertainment, the other a specialized support measure termed General Adult Support (as distinguished from parental support). These variables tended to produce reverse interaction effects, although results were not totally consistent and sometimes a mixed interaction was found.

Interactions: Stress Variables

In this study, measures were included that indexed both positive and negative affect (in Year 1), positive and negative recent events (in Year 2), and positive and negative major events (in Year 3). This made it possible to test for interactions of Positive × Negative Events (cf. Cohen & Hoberman, 1983). The analytic model was analogous to that used previously, with main-effect terms for positive and negative dimensions forced into the regression model first, and the cross-product term (Positive × Negative) added subsequently. These analyses showed a number of interaction effects for the stress measures.

Affect Measures. In the first wave, an interaction of Positive Affect × Negative Affect was found for the heavy drinking variable. This was a true buffering interaction, indicating a strong relationship between negative affect and drinking among subjects with low positive affect, but no such relationship among subjects with high positive affect. A similar buffering interaction was found for experimental smoking in the second wave.

Recent Events Measures. The measures of positive and negative recent events showed a number of significant interactions that varied according to the type of event analyzed. In the fourth wave, there were significant interaction effects of negative events with the positive events scales, but of quite different types for the social and nonsocial events scales. Analyses for Positive Nonsocial Events showed true buffering interactions for alcohol use: There was a strong relationship between recent negative events and alcohol use among subjects with a lower level of positive nonsocial events, but essentially no such relationship among subjects with a high level of positive nonsocial events. This represents a pure buffering process because positive events essentially eliminated the impact of negative events on alcohol use. A quite different form of interaction was found for positive social events, where significant interactions occurred for both smoking and alcohol use. These analyses indicated that positive social events increased substance use at all levels of negative events, but it was also the case that among subjects with a high level of positive events the relationship between negative events and substance use was reduced (i.e., the slope of the regression line decreased). This, then would be termed a mixed buffering interaction because there was an overall reduction of the impact of stress on substance use behavior. There were some measurement differences in these effects. In the original cohort, no interactions of positive and negative events were found at the third-wave measurement, but a number of significant interactions were found at the fourth wave. In the replication cohort, interactions for the recent events measures occurred mainly at the fourth wave, although some interaction effects were found at the third-wave measurement. The suggestion is that the finding of numerous interactions at one particular time point indicates that the subjects are undergoing a transition phase during which the balance between positive and negative dimensions of life events is particularly crucial for substance use.

Summary and Discussion

Data on the predictors of smoking and alcohol use in this cohort of urban adolescents provide considerable support for the conceptual framework advanced in Chapter 1 (Wills & Shiffman, this volume) indicating that stress and coping patterns are both related to substance use. With respect to coping, the measurement of coping by two different methods produced generally comparable results, so the findings do not appear to be method-specific. The significant negative associations between coping factors such as Decision Making, Cognitive Coping, and substance use support the basic tenet that constructive coping patterns act to increase people's resistance to internal or external pressures for substance use. A second general conclusion is that stress is related to an increased probability of substance use. Whether stress was indexed by subjective feelings of stress or by objective negative occurrences, the findings were essentially the same, so again the results do not seem to depend on a particular measurement method. The data do seem to indicate that problematic drinking (as opposed to occasional alcohol use) is more related to subjective feelings of stress, particularly toward the end of eighth grade.

In addition to the finding that some coping mechanisms showed overall main-effect relationships to substance use, the finding of buffer interactions for some of the coping variables is noteworthy. In particular, the fact that the major coping dimensions of Decision Making, Cognitive Coping, and Relaxation are most strongly related to reductions in substance use at a high level of stress is specifically supportive of a stress-coping formulation of substance use. At the same time, there was a good deal of specificity in the types of interactions found. Some coping variables showed true buffering effects, but different types of interactions with stress were found for some coping dimensions. For example, Distraction Coping produced a mixed buffer interaction, showing an overall positive correlation with substance use but serving to reduce the impact of stress. This paradoxical type of interaction may be relevant for further research on stress-buffering processes.

Two additional points about buffering are suggested by these data. One is that with substance use as a criterion variable, buffering interactions may be more easily detected for measures indexing recent use or rate of use, rather than for global classifications as user versus nonuser. The reason is that some types of substance use, such as cigarette smoking, have an inherent momentum of their own. Once begun and established as a regular habit, smoking becomes governed more by physiological, addictive processes and less by contemporaneous psychological influences. Thus coping variables, which may be quite relevant for early stages of substance use, may lose predictive power (for distinguishing users and nonusers) once a pattern of regular use has become established. It is conceivable that there is a shift in coping–substance use relationships, with some coping processes being most relevant for early stages of initiation and other processes being more related to rates of ongoing, regular use. A second proposition is that buffering processes may be particularly relevant for substance use at certain life transition points where a substantial proportion of adolescents are undergoing a challenging environmental or social change (e.g., from junior high school to high school). The finding in the present study that buffer interactions for positive and negative events measures were found at specific time points is suggestive of this more specific model of buffering.

The relationship between substance use and hedonic, pleasure-oriented activities is also noteworthy. Consistent with the formulation proposed in Chapter 1 (Wills & Shiffman), several aspects of the data suggest that smoking and alcohol use are pursued in the context of pleasure-seeking activities. In addition, measures of positive social events showed consistent associations with substance use. Together with the fact that negative events showed an independent contribution to substance use, these findings support the theoretical formulation in Chapter 1, proposing that substance use may serve the dual purpose of reducing negative affect and increasing positive affect. Whether there is a shift from a positive-affect mechanism (early in the initiation process) to a negative-affect management mechanism that subsequently maintains regular substance use as was suggested by McKennel and Thomas (1967) is a question that deserves further investigation. The present data are not inconsistent with this formulation, but a strong test of the proposition requires extensive measures of positive affect and negative affect that would be obtained systematically with a cohort of students followed from early adolescence through middle adolescence.

That substance use is pursued in social contexts is evident in these data in several respects. For one thing, the coping dimensions indexing support seeking from peers were consistently positively associated with smoking (but not with alcohol use), suggesting that initiation of cigarette smoking is facilitated by strong involvement in peer-group activities. Also, measures indexing social assertiveness were positively correlated with substance use. The exact interpretation of these results, however, is still somewhat ambiguous. Social settings may provide an opportunity for pleasure seeking and relaxation; they may represent a situation in which explicit peer pressure is exerted; or it is also possible that persons who are more socially active simply have more opportunities to be exposed to substance use. In addition, the fact that the Parental Support measure was strongly negatively associated with substance use indicates that the values of a reference group are just as important as the mere fact of involvement in a social group (see Wills & Vaughan, 1985).

The findings also support the proposition that both generalized and substance-specific coping skills are independently related to substance use. The results showed that generalized coping skills relevant for a variety of problems and stressors, such as Decision Making, Cognitive Coping, and Relaxation, were negatively associated with substance use. At the same time, the specific coping skill of substance-related assertiveness showed a unique contribution to smoking and alcohol use in the full regression models. The latter skill was not strongly related to sex or race and was not substantially correlated with any of the psychological variables, so at present the determinants of substance-specific assertiveness are not known. Further research may show that the determinants of substance-specific assertiveness lie in other domains, such as family values and training by parents, or general attitudes about the desirability of substance use.

INTERVENTION PROGRAM

Based on the psychosocial model of substance use described previously, an intervention program, the Decision Skills Curriculum (Spitzhoff, Ramirez, & Wills, 1981), was developed and implemented with a sample of seventh-grade students. The program was designed to affect mediating variables presumed relevant for deterrence of smoking initiation, specifically decision-making ability, locus of control, knowledge about negative consequences of smoking, and assertiveness skills. The primary intervention method was a psychosocial curriculum consisting of eight modules, which was taught in the first project year in consecutive sessions over a 2-week period. The curriculum was taught by project staff (two health educators) while the regular classroom teachers observed and assisted where necessary with exercises and activities. The curriculum began with a values-clarification exercise focused on leisure activities and moved next to decision-making instruction, first introduced as a systematic process for dealing with general problems of adolescence and then applied in role play exercises using prepared scenarios involving both everyday decisions and substance-related decisions. Following were modules on social influence, applying this concept both to general influences (especially media advertising about smoking) and to specific influences such as peer pressure for substance use. In these modules, instruction was given on how to counteract influence, using both cognitive and direct-action approaches. Following from the latter concept was a module on assertiveness, which began by introducing the distinction between aggressive, assertive, and passive behavior, and then applied this concept in role play exercises involving both everyday, general assertiveness situations (e.g., being served in a department store) and substance-specific situations (e.g., being offered a cigarette in a group setting).

Two concluding modules on stress management dealt with both short-term and longer term issues. The first module taught an approach for dealing with stressful situations based on the cognitive modification approach of Meichenbaum (1977, Chapter 5), which uses a four-step process of preparing for and coping constructively with stressful situations such as test taking or new social encounters. The other module presented ways of incorporating stress-management techniques into one's life-style, focusing on progressive muscle relaxation. Other activities such as meditation and physical activity (e.g., running) were discussed as positive ways of using leisure time and dealing with periods of stress. Finally, a module on the health consequences of smoking provided cognitive material on both short- and long-term physiological effects of cigarette smoking; this module included a lecture section, a biofeedback demonstration on the physiological effects of nicotine using pulse rate, blood pressure, and hand tremor, and a discussion of the psychological and economic benefits of nonsmoking.

Design

The intervention program was conducted with the entire seventh grade ($N = 800$) in three junior high schools. Two of the schools (School E1 and School E2) were assigned to the experimental condition, receiving the smoking prevention program and associated educational activities; the other school was assigned to the control condition. Baseline data indicated that the schools were closely matched on prevalence rates of regular smoking; for smoked in past month, $\chi^2(2, N = 662) = 1.73$, ns, and for smoked in past week, $\chi^2(2, N = 661) = 1.52$, ns.

The intervention program was first implemented immediately after completion of the baseline survey in Fall 1981. A follow-up program, based on the original curriculum, was implemented with the same population during their eighth-grade year. Evaluation data were obtained from the Behavior Survey, which was administered in school classrooms by project staff at the beginning and end of each school year. The survey included measures of smoking and alcohol use as well as the measures of stress, coping, and locus of control described previously in this chapter.

Results

Preliminary analyses of data on substance use and process variables indicated that the overall effect for the intervention was only marginal and was moderated by school differences. Thus further analyses were performed at the school level, contrasting data for each of the two experimental schools with those from the control school. Data on substance use are presented in Table 3.5. These data are incidence figures, based on the pool of students who were initially nonusers (as defined by a particular index) and computing the percentage of the initial pool who were users (as defined by that index) at a subsequent measurement. It is evident from the data on smoking incidence that the intervention was effective in School E1; in this school, there was a 42% reduction in smoking incidence at the end of seventh grade. By the third-wave measurement there was a 39% reduction in regular experimental smoking as well. For school E2, however, there was no significant effect on smoking, even though the identical intervention had been implemented in both of the experimental schools. Data for alcohol use (defined by the heavy drinking measure) were mixed, showing a nonsignificant reduction in School E1 and an increase in School E2.

Data on the process variables were consistent with the outcome data on

Table 3.5
CONDITIONAL PROBABILITIES FOR SMOKING AND DRINKING INITIATION VARIABLES, BY SCHOOL[a]

	Variable									
	Ever smoked		Smoked >4 times		Smoked in last month		Smoked in last week		Heavy drinking (≥once)	
School	p	z	p	z	p	z	p	z	p	z
	END OF SEVENTH GRADE (5-MONTH FOLLOW-UP)									
E1	.24	−0.80	.15	−3.48***	.15	−1.31	.12	−0.11	.12	−1.33
E2	.22	−0.33	.30	+0.79	.13	−1.65	.11	−0.45	.19	+1.02
C	.28		.26		.18		.12		.16	
	BEGINNING OF EIGHTH GRADE (10-MONTH FOLLOW-UP)									
E1	.25	−0.61	.20	−2.22**	.11	−2.22**	.10	+0.16	.15	+0.13
E2	.22	−1.10	.29	+0.14	.19	+0.41	.17	+2.53**	.22	+2.03*
C	.28		.29		.18		.09		.15	

[a]Tabled p values are the proportion of subjects indicating a "Yes" response to a substance-use item at the follow-up measurement, given that they indicated a "No" response at baseline. Tabled z values are for two-sample proportion test comparing an experimental school (E1 or E2) with the control school (C). Analysis based on cohort subjects only.
*$p < .05$. **$p < .025$. ***$p < .001$.

substance use. The process data were analyzed through analysis of covariance, and comparisons of schools were based on covariate-adjusted means (with baseline measure as the covariate). Data for the second-wave measurement indicated that in School E1 there were increases in Decision Making ($p < .10$) and Internal Health Locus of Control ($p < .05$), and significant decreases in stress and use of substances as a coping strategy. Changes for Cognitive Coping, Social Support, and Substance-Related Assertiveness were in the predicted direction but were not significant. Data from the third-wave measurement indicated that changes in the coping patterns of Decision Making ($p < .03$), Cognitive Coping ($p < .10$), and Social Support ($p < .10$), as well as for Internal Health Locus of Control ($p < .01$), were maintained over time in School E1. In contrast, no significant desired changes were noted for School E2. Indeed, some changes in a nondesirable direction (increased stress and tendency to use substances as a coping strategy) were found for this school. From these data it is evident that the intervention was effective in one experimental school, affecting the process variables in the predicted direction and achieving a significant reduction in smoking initiation, but the intervention did not have an impact in the second experimental school.

In interpreting these results, staff members thought that the variable of school atmosphere was possibly responsible for the marked differences in program impact. Staff members found that School E1 was generally well organized and that they enjoyed good relationships with the teachers and administration. In contrast, the principal of School E2 was notably uncooperative and sometimes obstructive in relation to the prevention program, and the level of discipline in School E2 was markedly lower so that it was sometimes difficult for project staff to teach the decision-making curriculum because of frequent interruptions and noisy classroom conditions. The effect of school atmosphere on the impact of intervention programs is a topic that needs further investigation. It should be emphasized that in the present study the curriculum was implemented by project staff and the schools were matched at baseline on rates of regular smoking, so the differential results cannot be attributed to implementation or base-rate variables. These results argue that process measures and indices of school atmosphere should be included in research on school-based smoking prevention (see Botvin & Eng, 1982; Luepker, Johnson, Murray, & Pechacek, 1983) so that individual- and school-level variation in outcome effects can be accounted for through direct measures.

GENERAL DISCUSSION

In summary, the results of this study provide considerable support for a formulation applying concepts of stress and coping to the study of substance use among adolescents. Notably, measures of stressful experiences were consistently significant predictors of both smoking and alcohol use across all waves of data collection. In addition, the present results show that both generalized and specific coping skills are related to the probability of substance use. As predicted, constructive generalized coping patterns of Decision Making and Cognitive Coping were negatively associated with substance use, and the specific skill of Substance-Related Assertiveness was negatively associated with both smoking and alcohol use. In the intervention program, the results suggest that teaching these skills to students early in adolescence can achieve a significant reduction in the initiation of cigarette smoking.

The present results argue that initiation of substances in early adolescence is not simply a matter of unwilling adolescents being pressured into substance use by peers. Rather, these results are consistent with other studies of smoking initiation (Friedman, Lichtenstein, & Biglan, 1983; Hirschman, Leventhal, & Glynn, 1983) in showing that some adolescents are attracted to smoking situations and enter such situations with the full knowledge that they will (and will want to) have an opportunity to smoke. To better understand why adolescents are attracted to smoking, we need further research on the perceived stress-reducing functions of substances and how social coping difficulties may affect the perceived attractiveness of smoking.

A final aspect of the data that deserves comment is the possibility of some degree of specificity in mechanisms of substance use. Cigarette smoking in adolescence seems more closely connected with social activity and social settings and less related to what might be termed psychological disturbance. Alcohol use is portrayed by these data as somewhat more of a reaction to psychological distress, heavy drinking in particular being strongly associated with subjective negative affect. Thus, although there is a clear rationale for considering the commonality in basic processes of stress reduction and addictive behavior, there is also evidence that it may be productive to investigate differential determinants in the etiological patterns for various substances.

This study suggests a number of directions for further research on stress, coping, and substance use. It seems desirable to have more basic knowledge about the determinants of stress in early adolescence, and longitudinal research to study correlations between coping and drug use across a wide age range (from sixth to tenth grade) would probably be informative. Several aspects of the present data suggest studying specific transition points, such as the transition from elementary school to junior school or the transition from junior high school to high school, as these may be crucial time points for the initiation of particular types of substance use. Attention should be given to buffering mechanisms as well as main effects, since the present data show buffering at transition points. With respect to substance abuse prevention research, there are good reasons for recommending that researchers obtain multidimensional process measures to determine the mediating variables in school-based intervention programs. These would include not only psychological variables, such as locus of control, decision making, and assertiveness, but also ecological variables such as school atmosphere and type of community (e.g., inner city vs. suburban). There is also a need for studies to determine the effective components of broad-based primary prevention programs, which currently include material on health knowledge, decision making, assertiveness, personal control, and stress reduction. Currently there is little evidence on which component(s) of the complex, multifactorial smoking prevention programs is responsible for the observed results, and more detailed studies testing particular components or combinations of components would add considerable knowledge to this area.

REFERENCES

Abrams, D. B. (1983). Psychosocial assessment of alcohol and stress interactions: Bridging the gap between laboratory and treatment outcome research. In L. A. Pohorecky & J. Brick (Eds.), *Stress and alcohol use.* New York: Elsevier.

Bentler, P. M., & Speckart, G. (1979). Models of attitude-behavior relations. *Psychological Review, 86,* 452–464.

Borgers, D. & Junge, B. (1979). Thiocyanate as an indicator of tobacco smoking. *Preventive Medicine, 8,* 351–357.

Botvin, G. J., & Eng, A. (1982). The efficacy of a multicomponent approach to the prevention of cigarette smoking. *Preventive Medicine, 11,* 199–211.

Botvin, G. J., & McAlister, A. (1981). Cigarette smoking among children and adolescents: Causes and prevention. In C. B. Arnold, L. H. Kuller, & M. R. Greenlick (Eds.), *Advances in disease prevention* (Vol. 1). New York: Springer.

Bugen, L. A., & Hawkins, R. C., III. (1981, August). *The Coping Assessment Battery: Theoretical and empirical foundations.* Paper presented at the meeting of the American Psychological Association, Los Angeles.

Coates, T. J., Perry, C., Killen, J., & Slinkard, L. A. (1981). Primary prevention of cardiovascular disease in children and adolescents. In C. K. Prokop & L. A. Bradley (Eds.), *Medical psychology: Contributions to behavioral medicine.* New York: Academic Press.

Cohen, J., & Cohen, P. (1983). *Applied multiple regression/correlation analysis for the behavioral sciences* (2nd ed.). Hillsdale, NJ: Erlbaum.

Cohen, S., & Hoberman, H. (1983). Positive events and social supports as buffers of life change stress. *Journal of Applied Social Psychology, 13,* 99–125.

Cohen, S., & Wills, T. A. (in press). Stress, social support, and the buffering hypothesis. *Psychological Bulletin.*

Evans, R. I., Hansen, W. B., & Mittelmark, M. B. (1977). Increasing the validity of self-reports of behavior in a smoking in children investigation. *Journal of Applied Psychology, 62,* 521–523.

Fishburne, P. M., Abelson, H. I., & Cisin, I. (1980). *National survey on drug abuse, 1979* (DHHS Publication No. ADM 80–976). Washington, DC: National Institute on Drug Abuse.

Fleming, J. S., & Watts, W. A. (1980). The dimensionality of self-esteem: Some results for a college sample. *Journal of Personality and Social Psychology, 39,* 921–929.
Friedman, L. S., Lichtenstein, E., & Biglan, A. (in press). Smoking onset among teens: An empirical analysis of initial situations. *Addictive Behaviors.*
Gambrill, E. D., & Richey, C. (1975). An assertion inventory for use in assessment and research. *Behavior Therapy, 6,* 550–561.
Green, D. E. (1979). *Teenage smoking: Immediate and long-term patterns.* Washington, DC: U.S. Government Printing Office.
Haley, N. J., Axelrod, C. M., & Tilton, K. A. (1983). Validation of self-reported smoking behavior: Biochemical analyses of cotinine and thiocyanate. *American Journal of Public Health, 73,* 1204–1207.
Hirschman, R. S., Leventhal, H., & Glynn, K. (1984). *The development of smoking behavior: Conceptualization and supportive cross-sectional data.* Manuscript submitted for publication.
Ilfeld, F. W., Jr. (1978). Psychologic status of community residents along major demographic dimensions. *Archives of General Psychiatry, 35,* 716–724.
Jessor, R., Chase, J. A., & Donovan, J. E. (1980). Psychosocial correlates of marijuana use and problem drinking in a national sample of adolescents. *American Journal of Public Health, 70,* 604–613.
Kandel, D. B. (Ed.). (1978). *Longitudinal research on drug use: Empirical findings and methodological issues.* New York: Wiley.
Kandel, D. B., Kessler, R. C., & Margulies, R. Z. (1978). Antecedents of adolescent initiation into stages of drug use: A developmental analysis. In D. B. Kandel (Ed.), *Longitudinal research on drug use: Empirical findings and methodological issues.* New York: Wiley.
Leventhal, H., & Cleary, P. D. (1980). The smoking problem: A review of the research and theory in behavioral risk modification. *Psychological Bulletin, 88,* 370–405.
Lewinsohn, P. M., & Amenson, C. S. (1978). Some relations between pleasant and unpleasant mood-related events and depression. *Journal of Abnormal Psychology, 87,* 644–654.
Luepker, R. V., Johnson, C. A., Murray, D. M., & Pechacek, T. F. (1983). Prevention of cigarette smoking: Three-year follow-up of an education program for youth. *Journal of Behavioral Medicine, 6,* 53–62.
McKennel, A. C., & Thomas, R. K. (1967). *Adults' and adolescents' smoking habits and attitudes.* London: British Ministry of Health.
Meichenbaum, D. (1977). *Cognitive-behavior modification: An integrative approach.* New York: Plenum Press.
Paulhus, D. (1983). Sphere-specific measures of perceived control. *Journal of Personality and Social Psychology, 44,* 1253–1265.
Rosenberg, M. (1965). *Society and the adolescent self-image.* Princeton: Princeton University Press.
Spitzhoff, D., Ramirez, S., & Wills, T. A. (1981). *The Decision Skills Curriculum: A program for primary prevention of substance abuse.* Unpublished manuscript, American Health Foundation.
Stone, A. A., & Neale, J. M. (1984). A new measure of daily coping: Development and preliminary results. *Journal of Personality and Social Psychology, 46,* 892–906.
Wallston, K. A., Wallston, B. S., & DeVellis, R. (1978). Development of the Multidimensional Health Locus of Control (MHLC) scales. *Health Education Monographs, 6,* 160–170.
Wills, T. A. (1981). Downward comparison principles in social psychology. *Psychological Bulletin, 90,* 245–271.
Wills, T. A., Baker, E., & Botvin, G. J. (1985, August). *Dimensions of assertivness: Differential*

relationships to substance use in adolescence. Paper presented at the meeting of the American Psychological Association, Los Angeles.

Wills, T. A., & Vaughan, R. (1985). *Relationship of peer and adult social support to smoking and alcohol use in middle adolescence.* Manuscript submitted for publication.

Zevon, M. A., & Tellegen, A. (1982). The structure of mood change: An idiographic/nomothetic analysis. *Journal of Personality and Social Psychology, 43,* 111–122.

Chapter 4

Coping with Social Influences to Smoke*

ANTHONY BIGLAN
WENDY WEISSMAN
HERBERT SEVERSON

INTRODUCTION

Cigarette smoking is the single most preventable cause of death due to cardiovascular disease and cancer (U.S. Department of Health and Human Services [USDHHS], 1982). Given the importance of cigarette smoking as a health risk, considerable research has been devoted to ways to assist people to stop smoking and to prevent smoking before it is established. Since most smoking begins in adolescence (Biglan, Severson, Bavry, & McConnell, 1983; Evans & Raines, 1982; Mettlin, 1976), it is imperative that the onset of smoking and continued use of cigarettes by adolescents be better understood. Based on that understanding, more effective methods of deterring smoking can be developed.

Peer social influence has emerged as one of the most important factors in the onset and maintenance of adolescent smoking. This chapter describes studies that have recently been done by our group to clarify the role of peer influences in adolescent smoking. Strategies for teaching young people skills to cope with such social influences are presented, then procedures for assessing the acquisition of those skills are described. Finally, evidence regarding the impact of refusal skills training on adolescent smoking is presented.

---

*The preparation of this paper was supported in part by two grants from the National Institute of Child Health and Human Development (# R01 HD15825–01 and #5 RO1 HD 13409–02). The authors thank Kate Marquez for invaluable assistance in the preparation of the manuscript.

SOCIAL INFLUENCES TO SMOKE AMONG ADOLESCENTS

A number of studies have shown that adolescents who report current smoking also report having friends who smoke (Botvin & McAlister, in press, Leventhal & Cleary, 1980). However, studies correlating questionnaire reports of adolescent smoking and friends' smoking do not indicate whether peers induce their friends to smoke or if those who are already smokers become friends. Moreover, most of the studies that have been done have not used multivariate procedures. This means that the importance of peer influences relative to other factors in predicting smoking have not been clarified. For example, data presented by Wills (Chapter 3, this volume) suggest that smoking initiation depends, in part, on background factors (such as stress) which predispose young people to try cigarettes. Finally, most of the earlier studies of peer influence processes rely solely on self-reports of smoking (e.g., Salber & MacMahon, 1961), which may lead to significant underreporting of smoking (Bauman & Dent, 1982).

The First Three Cigarettes

One point in the transition to regular smoking which may be particularly influenced by peers is the experimentation with the first few cigarettes. Initial experimentation may or may not be prompted directly by peers. If it is, teaching refusal skills to young people may reduce their experimentation. However, if initial experimentation is not prompted directly by the offers of cigarettes from peers, other factors such as the correction of normative beliefs about how many adolescents smoke (Evans, Rozelle, Maxwell, et al., 1981; Evans, Rozelle, Mittelmark, et al., 1978) may be more relevant than the teaching of social skills.

In order to obtain more information about initial experimentation, Friedman, Lichtenstein, and Biglan (1985) conducted a study in which a sample of 157 teen-agers were interviewed regarding their first three smoking experiences or the first three instances in which they felt pressured to smoke. The results confirmed that the overwhelming majority (89%) of initial experiences with cigarettes occurred in social settings. Of the people who were present in these incidents, 77% were friends or acquaintances and 11% were siblings. Initial smoking situations were much more likely to involve people of the same sex. In approximately half of the initial smoking incidents, another young person was trying a cigarette for the first time.

Friedman et al. also examined whether there were any variables that could distinguish between adolescents who went beyond initial experimentation to smoke more than 10 cigarettes and those who stopped experimenting before this point. Persistent experimenters were more likely to have experienced social influences to smoke in their first three experimentations. There were more smoking models present and they were more likely to have been encouraged by others to smoke. At the same time, the study contained evidence that is consistent with Wills' (Chapter 3, this volume) notion that there are factors that predispose some adolescents to try cigarettes. The persistent experimenters were more likely to have come to the initial incidents with the intention to smoke. The adolescents who were offered cigarettes but did not smoke appeared to possess more effective strategies for refusing cigarettes than did those who experimented. In sum, there appears to be ample justification for attempts to teach young people skills for coping with direct social influences to smoke, since it appears that the vast majority of initial experimentation occurs in circumstances where other adolescents are smoking. Initial experimentation with cigarettes under conditions where an adolescent is socially isolated appears to be a relatively rare phenomenon.

A Longitudinal Test of the Peer Influence Hypothesis

We have conducted a longitudinal study of the factors predicting adolescent smoking in order to test whether peer smoking predicts smoking over time or is simply a concurrent correlate of adolescent smoking (Ary & Biglan, 1985). Subjects were tested 6 months and 1 year after an initial assessment. Multivariate procedures were used to analyze the data. Physiological measures of smoking were collected at the same time that questionnaire reports were obtained (Evans, Hansen, & Mittelmark, 1977; Pechacek et al., 1983).

A total of 1181 teen-agers participated in the initial assessment. Of these subjects, 887 (75%) were available at 6-month follow-up and 801 (68%) at 1-year follow-up. Subjects were divided approximately equally between male and female. At the 6-month follow-up there were 562 students in middle schools and 325 in the ninth and tenth grades. At 1-year follow-up there were 506 students in seventh and eighth grade and 295 in ninth and tenth grade. The questionnaire asked students to indicate how many cigarettes they had smoked in the previous day and how many they had smoked in the last week. Answers to these items were combined to form a smoking index indicating the average number of cigarettes smoked in the prior week.

Preliminary analyses indicated that the predictors of smoking onset were significantly different from the predictors of change in smoking rate. In addition, it was found that the predictors of onset were significantly different depending on the grade level of the subject (seventh grade vs. ninth and tenth). For these reasons, predictors of smoking onset and of changes in rate are described in separate sections and, for the predictions of onset, results are presented separately for seventh versus ninth and tenth grades.[1]

In general, the amount of variance in smoking onset that could be accounted for was small. The largest R^2 was .19. One reason for this may be that the variables that account for onset occur much closer in time to onset than 6 months or 1 year (Collins, Graham, & Hansen, 1984). For example, over a 6-month period, groups of adolescents who were not smoking initially, may take up smoking. These subjects would be indicating that neither they nor their friends smoked at Time 1, yet they would all be smoking at the end of 6 months.

The most consistent predictor of later smoking onset was prior experience with cigarettes (for example, having puffed on a cigarette). At the same time, peer and sibling influences accounted for variance in later smoking even after the variance due to prior experience with cigarettes had been removed. The predictability was much greater at the high school level than at the middle school level. Peer and sibling influences accounted for significantly more variance in smoking onset among high schoolers at 1-year follow-up (11% of the variance) than they did among middle schoolers (2% of the variance). At least two other studies have shown that peer influences on smoking are greater among older adolescents than among younger adolescents (Chassin, Presson, & Sherman, 1984; Krosnick & Judd, 1982). The use of alcohol and marijuana at initial assessment predicted onset of smoking for middle school subjects at 6 months and 1 year and for high school subjects at 6 months. This was true even after variance due to prior experience and peer and sibling influences had been removed.

Social Influences Maintaining Smoking

There is increasing reason to believe that the factors that maintain adolescent smoking need to be investigated separately from the factors associated with onset. The results of the preliminary analysis in our longitudinal study indicated that the predictors of onset are not the same as the predictors of whether an adolescent increases or decreases his or her smoking. Moreover, as data presented later suggest, it may be possible to reduce the prevalence of adolescent smoking by getting adolescents who have already started to

---

[1] The subjects' rated intentions to smoke were entered as a predictor in all equations. In all but one analysis it was found that rated intentions to smoke did not account for variance in later smoking once the variance due to social factors and substance use variables had been removed. In predicting onset among seventh graders at 6 months, rated intentions accounted for 1.8% of the variance in later smoking after variance due to other predictors had been removed.

quit. Knowledge of factors that maintain adolescent smoking could facilitate such an effort.

We originally assumed that adolescents become dependent on cigarettes soon after they begin smoking them each day. Preventive efforts therefore had to concentrate on dissuading young people from beginning to experiment. However, there are a number of findings that suggest that such a rapid development of dependency may not occur. First, a substantial proportion of adolescents smoke at low levels (Biglan, Nautel, Ary, & Thompson, 1983) and many young people eventually give up smoking (USDHHS, 1982). Second, the typical rate of smoking among adolescents is lower than that for adults (Biglan, Severson, Hops, et al., 1983). Third, recent evidence suggests that the dose per cigarette increases over a long period of time (Pechacek et al., 1983; Biglan, Nautel, et al., 1983). This suggests that tolerance may develop slowly.

Our research thus far has indicated that social influences continue to be important in maintaining adolescent smoking. We first describe the results of our longitudinal study that involved prediction of changes in rate of smoking. Then self-monitoring and direct observation data that bear on the social influence hypothesis are reviewed.

Prediction of Changes in Smoking Rate. At both 6-month and 1-year follow-up, the best predictor of changes in the rate of smoking among those who had been smoking at Time 1 was the initial smoking rate ($r = .62$, $p < .01$ for 6 months, and $r = .47$, $p < .01$ for 12 months). A questionnaire measure of addiction accounted for additional variance at 6 months that was over and above that accounted for by smoking rate. When the variance due to initial smoking rate was controlled for, the number of friends who smoked at Time 1 significantly predicted later smoking (4.8% of the variance). No additional predictors of change in smoking rate were identified for the 12-month analysis. However for the 6-month analysis, a composite measure of parental influences to smoke accounted for significant variance (11%) in later smoking rate. In addition, even after the variance at the initial assessment that was due to smoking rate, addiction, parental influences, and peer smoking was removed, the number of offers of cigarettes in the week prior to assessment accounted for significant variance in smoking rate at 6 months. This suggests that social influences to smoke involve specific prompts to smoke at specific times, not simply an effect on the adolescents' attitudes and intentions.

The results of our longitudinal research suggest that peer influences are an important factor in maintaining an adolescent's smoking during the time that tolerance and dependence are developing. However, by themselves, longitudinal studies are an insufficient method of determining whether the smoking of peers helps to maintain adolescent smoking. It would be useful to examine more directly whether the smoking of adolescents is prompted by the smoking behavior of peers. Two studies conducted at Oregon Research Institute bear on these issues.

Self-Monitoring of Smoking Situations. In one study (Biglan, McConnell, Severson, Bavry, & Ary, 1984), 44 adolescents self-monitored their smoking for a week. They noted the situations in which they smoked during two 2-hour blocks of time each day. The subjects ranged in age from 12 to 17. We found that among adolescents who were smoking daily, the majority of cigarettes continued to be smoked in the presence of other people. Another person was present for an average of 71.8% of the cigarettes. Another adolescent was present for 35% of the cigarettes. Thus, even after smoking is occurring each day, much adolescent smoking is social. However, one cannot conclude from these results that peer smoking functions as a discriminative stimulus for the adolescent to smoke. Data on the degree to which the other people present were smoking was not obtained. Moreover, it is possible that the adolescent smokers in that study simply distributed their smoking over the day and happened to be with people 71% of the time.

Modeling Effects on Smoking. Kniskern, Biglan, Lichtenstein, Ary and Bavry (1983) experimentally evaluated the possibility that other smoking teen-agers function as discriminative stimuli for teen-age smoking. Twenty-eight female and 28 male teen-agers were exposed to the three experimental conditions: a male smoking confederate, a female smoking confederate, and no model present. The effects of these conditions on the number of cigarettes smoked and the frequency of puffing were examined. It was found that the presence of a teen-age model who was smoking increased the number of cigarettes smoked. However, subjects appeared to compensate for the increased smoking in the presence of a smoking model by taking significantly fewer puffs per cigarette in the model-present conditions. The sex of the model did not matter. Regardless of condition, male subjects tended to take more puffs than female subjects, and when there was a model present, the difference was significant. These results confirm that adolescents who are smoking regularly continue to be influenced by other adolescents who smoke. However, considering that 70% of the subjects smoked at least one cigarette in the no-model condition, it is clear that peer influences do not entirely account for the maintenance of adolescent smoking.

Summary

The results reviewed here clearly indicate that peer influences are a fundamental reason for adolescents' beginning and continuing to smoke. Examination of the details of this process indicates that it is not simply a matter of peers' affecting the attitudes and intentions of other adolescents. Rather, the typical adolescent appears to be exposed to frequent and direct prompts to experiment with cigarettes and to continue smoking. Thus, there appears to be ample empirical justification for developing programs that teach young people social skills for coping with peer influences. Strategies for teaching such skills are described in the next part of this chapter. The problem of assessing these social skills is then examined in some detail.

TEACHING TEENAGERS TO COPE WITH PRESSURES TO SMOKE

In developing our prevention program, we assumed that it is critical to teach young people ways to cope with the social influences to smoke that were just described. The prevention program described here focuses upon sensitizing students to overt and covert pressures to smoke, development of social skills to respond to such pressures and to support peers' refusals of cigarettes. The curriculum also includes a brief review of health consequences, elicitation of a public commitment not to smoke, and information on the addictive nature of nicotine. The program is taught by health or science teachers in the seventh and ninth grades, in four class periods.

Refusal Skills Training. Two types of modeling of effective refusals occurred. First, excerpts from a film created by Richard Evans entitled "Resisting Pressure to Smoke" (1978) demonstrated effective refusals in social pressure situations. Second, peers modeled refusals in practice situations in the classroom as the other students observed and critiqued their demonstration. Behavioral rehearsal occurred in two forms. Students role played refusal skills in front of the class and in small groups. Repeated rehearsals were designed to prompt both negative statements about smoking and effective refusal responses, which were reinforced by the teacher and classmates.

Public Commitment. Public commitment to a particular attitudinal position enhances a person's adherence to the position taken (Festinger, 1972). In our curriculum, teachers asked for a show of hands to indicate those students who did not intend to become smokers. Evidence of a nonsmoking commitment at the beginning of the program makes it more likely that students will identify with the curriculum's nonsmoking language and will participate more fully in classroom activities. Further, students will see their participation in the curriculum as supportive of their own goal—continuing to be a nonsmoker. A more subtle public commitment occurred whenever the students practiced refusal behavior or described negative features of smoking in the presence of their peers.

Health Facts and the Development of Addiction. Existing evidence indicates that providing information about the dangers of smoking and hazards of addiction is not by itself effective (Thompson, 1978) in deterring adolescent smoking. For this reason, detailed teaching of these facts did not occur. However, a short review of these issues provides students with information that could be used to combat prosmoking statements by others and to refuse cigarettes. The curriculum focused on a description of the immediate effects of smoking a cigarette and information about how a person can become addicted to tobacco, using a brief videotape adaptation of the film "The Feminine Mistake" (Cosgrove, 1977). In a subsequent discussion, students reviewed the major points of the film, namely, how cigarettes cause carbon monoxide elevations in the blood, blood pressure increases, heart rate increases, decreases in blood volume to the extremities and increases in respiration rate.

Booster Session. To promote generalization of refusal skills to the natural environment, students were asked to report anonymously on the occurrence of any cigarette offers and the refusal behavior they employed. This information was fed back to the class at a follow-up or "booster" session 2 weeks following the presentation of the basic curriculum. These real life situations were used as a basis for additional practice and reinforcement of the refusal skills. Student-elicited situations provided the necessary link between the classroom and real life experiences.

Additional Features of the Program. Frequently during a discussion of cigarettes in a typical health class, teachers prompt students to discuss their experiences with cigarettes. Students do this readily. However, attention to these experiences may serve to reinforce the prosmoking behavior described and thereby encourage use or experimentation. Our curriculum minimized such discussions and at the same time prompted and reinforced the expression of antismoking attitudes, intentions, and the refusal skills. The curriculum was designed to prompt all students to engage in these behaviors, whether the students were committed nonsmokers or not.

THE ASSESSMENT OF REFUSAL SKILLS

The teaching of refusal skills is a fundamental component of virtually every current smoking prevention program (Evans et al., 1981; Flay, d'Avernas, Best, Kersell, & Ryan 1981; Luepker et al., 1983; Perry, Maccoby, & McAlister, 1980). Yet despite the laudatory efforts of these studies to evaluate the effects of the programs on smoking, the assumption that these programs do indeed modify refusal skills has remained untested. Therefore we (Hops et al., in press) have developed a test of adolescents' refusal skills, called the Taped Situations Test (TST). Because the assessment of these skills has received so little attention, in this section we describe some of the considerations that went into the TST development and present a comparison of the performance of students who received the smoking prevention curriculum and students who did not.

Limitations of Self-Report Techniques

Self-report strategies are in widespread use in studies of social behavior (Eisler, 1976) as well as in the assessment of social behaviors related to smoking (Biglan, Severson, Hops, et al., 1983). Yet self-report strategies have serious limitations that need to be considered.

Questionnaires. Questionnaires are economical to administer and can be objectively scored. However, questionnaires about social skill have several important limitations. Respondents may not be able to identify or describe accurately the verbal and nonverbal behaviors included in the social interactions with peers. Further, individuals vary in their ability to assess accurately the social behavior of peers. Questionnaire items often require respondents to indicate how they would respond across different social situations (e.g. "I say 'No' to cigarette offers most of the time"). If their behavior varies across situations, this approach further obscures an accurate appraisal of their refusal skills (Eisler, 1976).

Structured Interviews. Interview formats are useful since subjects can provide detailed descriptions of social interactions and smoking behavior. Similar to a questionnaire, however, an interview requires respondents to demonstrate good discriminative skills in assessing their own and others' social behaviors and in judging their appropriate use of refusal skills.

Self-monitoring. Self-monitoring provides highly systematic data about an individual's ongoing behaviors, collected at specified intervals (Nelson, 1977). It can prompt an individual to provide details that would not be obtainable from retrospective accounts. However, detailed descriptions of interpersonal behaviors require judgments regarding complex and oftentimes subtle behavioral interactions (Nelson, 1977).

Although correlations among measures derived from these self-report methods may be high, the ability of any of these methods to predict an individual's behavior in the real world is often too low to be of value (Eisler, 1976).

Direct Observation

In contrast to the self-report strategies, direct observation of behaviors in the natural environment is the most desirable method for assessment of social skills (Bellack & Morrison, 1982). Yet it is extremely difficult to implement. Ideally, we should have direct observation of the subject's real life coping with pressures to smoke. But this is unattainable for a variety of reasons. First, the subject may not yet have experienced social pressures to smoke. Second, even if this has occurred, it may have occurred infrequently and at times and in places where we do not have direct access. It is conceivable that unobtrusive assessments might be done in the natural environment by, for example, having a confederate offer the subject a cigarette. However, this procedure could increase the likelihood that subjects would smoke and therefore seems to be inappropriate. Finally, procedures in which direct access to smoking pressure situations was achieved might be highly reactive.

The Value of Role Play Analogue Tests

One compromise between self-report instruments and direct observation is the role play analogue test. Role play analogues are designed to approximate the subjects' natural environment by recreating the important stimuli thought to be present in targeted situations (Kern, Miller, & Eggers, 1983). Role play situations typically include three steps: (1) the social situation is described, including the people present and their relationship to the subject, the activity, and the context; (2) appropriate sound effects and actors engaging in conversation create the scene, then the actor(s) deliver a prompt line (in the present case, a cigarette offer); and (3) the subject responds to the prompt as though he or she were actually in the situation. Analogue tests employing role play enactments are the most frequently used procedure for the assessment of social skills (Bellack & Morrison, 1982).

Role play analogue tests can be employed to compare treated and untreated groups on their social behavior (Bellack & Morrison, 1982). For example, Horan and Williams (1982) compared junior high school students who received one of three levels of assertiveness training that were designed to prevent drug abuse. Following training, treated students had higher levels of assertiveness on the role play test than did untreated students. They also reported less drug use at the 3-year follow-up.

We applied the same strategy in the evaluation of the effects of our refusal skills training. We compared the performance of subjects who had received refusal skills training with those who had not. By doing this we provided an initial test of the assumption that prevention programs affect refusal skills.

It should be recognized that discrimination between treated and untreated groups is not the only form of validity that could be assessed. Some studies have compared role play performance with behavior in related criterion situations (see Bellack, Hersen, & Lamparski, 1979). The prediction of behavior in these situations has proved inconsistent. Even if the TST comparison shows that trained students outperform untrained, we cannot be sure that those who will become smokers perform less well on the test than those who remain nonsmokers. Further, it is unclear whether the test is accurately predicting adolescents' behavior in a natural environment. Nevertheless, in developing our role play test, we constructed it in ways that seemed likely to maximize its ability to predict behavior in real life.

Improving the Validity of Analogue Tests

Several procedural modifications of traditional role plays tests were employed in an effort to make it more likely that the TST would be capable of predicting behavior in the natural environment (Hops et al., in press). First we selected actors or confederates of similar age to the subjects. Confederates provide background effects and/or deliver important conversational cues to which the subject responds. Especially for adolescents, peer group influence is a critical variable, and the use of same-aged confederates is important.

Second, a wide variety of relevant situations were included. For example, adolescent responses to cigarette offers may vary as a function of the source of the offer, that is, same- or opposite-sex peers, older or younger friends, or pressure exerted by a group versus a single adolescent. Hence these variations are included.

Third, we created situations that varied in the level of pressure to smoke. The role play format has generally consisted of brief presentations of situations to which subjects are required to respond with brief discrete responses (Bellack & Morrison, 1982). Yet real life situations may not end with a simple prompt or single rejoinder. For example, in situations where cigarettes are being offered to peers, a simple refusal may have the effect of increasing harassment and social pressure. For these reasons we created some situations in which very strong pressure to smoke was presented.

Development of the Taped Situations Test

In developing the Taped Situations Test (TST) we attempted to construct items which were representative of situations that young people actually encounter by drawing on the evidence from the study by Friedman, Lichtenstein, and Biglan (1985). Scene locations included outdoor neighborhood sites, friends' homes, and school. Friends, acquaintances, siblings, and parents were described as those present and offering cigarettes.

Junior and senior high drama students were recruited as actors in the audiotaped situations. A total of 26 scenes contained social situations in which an offer of a cigarette occurred. The type of offer varied across scenes. They included a single individual applying light pressure or heavy pressure. In another category, labeled group pressure, multiple offers were presented. Each scene was introduced by a female narrator describing the activity and context, whereupon appropriate sound effects and teen-age voices presented a social interaction.

DESIGN AND PROCEDURES

As a first test of criterion validity, the TST was given to a sample of treatment ($n = 63$) and control ($n = 68$) seventh graders. These students came from four middle schools that were participating in the smoking prevention program described earlier. Subjects were offered a coupon for a free hamburger in exchange for 1 hour of participation. Parental consent was required in order to participate. A large pool of students ($n = 200$) from treatment and control classrooms volunteered and roughly equivalent samples from each school were randomly selected to participate. Prior to the program's initiation, treatment and control subjects were assessed (Time 1) with a questionnaire. Follow-up assessments occurred at 6-month and 1-year intervals.

The TST was individually administered during school hours, in office space providing visual and audio privacy. Taped instructions requested that the subjects use their imaginations to place themselves in the situations described. One practice situation was presented with the experimenter present so that any questions about the procedure could be answered. The student was then left alone to complete the 50-minte task.

One tape recorder provided the taped situations. A second tape recorder recorded the subject's response for later analysis. There was a 30-second pause between scenes.

CODE DEVELOPMENT

Subjects' taped responses to the role play test were analyzed for verbal content. Code categories were based on the specific verbal skills taught in the refusal skills curriculum. Appropriate statements by students could include negative statements about cigarettes and effective refusal responses. Inappropriate statements and acceptances were also coded.

The code scheme contained nine response categories: direct–simple refusals, health facts, conciliatory remarks, excuses, withdrawal statements, aggressive comments, references to external authority figures, assertive "I" statements, and acceptances. Table 4.1 provides examples of each type of response and presents frequencies for each code for treatment and control subjects.

Each discrete phrase uttered by a student was considered a codable response. Thus a student could respond to an offer using multiple code categories in a single role play situation. Intercoder reliability was checked on a

Table 4.1
TST RESPONSE CODES

Code categories[a]	Examples of response statements	Mean number of responses over 26 situations	
		Control	Experimental
Direct–simple (+)	No thanks. No, that's OK.	17.35	20.02
Health facts (+)	It will give me cancer. I'm allergic to smoke. It makes me cough.	3.00	3.74
Conciliatory–supportive (+)	You can go ahead and smoke. I won't tell if you smoke. I'll just pass it on.	3.13	4.06
Excuses–change of subject (+)	I'm not in the mood. Maybe later. I want to go shopping	18.41	26.00
Withdrawal (+)	I have to go. Let's go back to the party.	2.34	3.23
Aggressive–sarcastic (−)	Only creeps smoke. Cigarettes are dumb. If you want to kill yourself...	8.97	7.77
External consequences (+)	We'll get into trouble. I'll smell like smoke.	2.99	4.98
Direct "I" statements (+)	I don't want to. I don't like cigarettes. I don't smoke.	13.22	13.19
Acceptance (−)	Gee... thanks. Yeah, sure.	1.41	0.68

[a]Signs indicate inappropriate (−) and appropriate (+) statements.

random basis with 15% of the audiotapes. Percentage agreement ranged from 81 to 100%, with an average of 92% agreement.

TST RESULTS

To analyze the effects of refusal training on students' social skills, a MANOVA was conducted that compared treatment and control subjects on the vector of nine content codes. That is, nine dependent variables were present in the MANOVA where the total number of responses of each of the nine code types over all 26 situations was analyzed. Treatment and control subjects were significantly different on this MANOVA (Wilks's lambda $=.85$, approximate $F[9, 120] = 2.37$, $p < .017$). Subsequently, univariate Fs were calculated to compare treatment and control subjects on each of the nine content codes. Subjects receiving refusal training responded significantly more often with direct–simple refusals, $F = 5.32, p < .023$, offered excuses–changes of subject significantly more often, $F = 12.61, p < .001$, and mentioned external consequences to smoking more often, $F = 6.30, p < .01$. All three of these responses had been taught in refusal training.

The subjects' first response to a peer's influence attempt may be particularly important since it may affect whether the peer persists in pressuring the student to smoke. For this reason, we analyzed the subject's first utterance separately. It should be noted that this analysis is redundant to some extent with the one just described. Here too a MANOVA comparing treatment and control subjects was conducted across the nine content codes. In the analysis, the subject's total number of first utterances in each code category was summed across the 26 situations. This analysis also indicated that treatment subjects differed significantly in their refusal responses from control subjects (Wilks's lambda = .82, approximate $F[9, 120] = 2.78, p < .005$). In the first utterance trained subjects gave significantly more direct–simple refusals, $F = 6.05, p < .015$, and cited health reasons for not smoking significantly more often, $F = 12.45, p < .001$. The groups did not differ at the .05 level on any of the other codes. However, trained subjects tended to mention more external consequences for smoking than did untrained subjects, $F = 3.33, p = .07$. Trained subjects actually tended to give fewer excuses for refusing the cigarette than did untrained subjects as their first utterance, $F = 3.49, p < .06$. Note that this is opposite to the result when all utterances are considered together. Overall, treated subjects were giving more excuses, but they were giving fewer excuses as their first response to the pressure to smoke.

Effects of training on response time and latency to respond were also assessed since both variables had been shown to discriminate assertive and nonassertive subjects in other studies (Dow et al., 1981; Glasgow & Arkowitz, 1975). In assessing total response time, treatment and control subjects were compared using a MANOVA in which the response time on each of the 26 situations constituted the dependent variables. There was an overall difference indicating that treatment subjects talked significantly longer (Wilks' lamda = .60, approximate $F[26, 88] = 2.20, p < .003$). Subsequent univariate analyses of variance indicated that subjects who received refusal skills training had significantly longer response times on 8 of the 26 situations.

The MANOVA comparing the latencies to respond of treatment and control subjects over all 26 situations did not indicate that the groups were significantly different (Wilks's lambda = .726, approximate $F[26, 87] = 1.26, p < .21$). It can be noted, however, that in 23 of the 26 situations the latency for trained subjects was shorter than that for control subjects. Univariate Fs comparing treatment and control subjects on each situation indicated that these differences were significant at the .05 level for only three of the situations.

EFFECTS OF THE REFUSAL SKILLS TRAINING PROGRAM ON SMOKING

We evaluated the effects of the prevention program in deterring smoking in the ninth-grade classes of three high schools and the seventh-grade classes of six middle schools (Biglan et al., 1985). In each school the classes of health and science teachers who had agreed to participate were randomly assigned to treatment or control conditions. This design probably made it less likely that deterrence would occur, since treated and untreated students who were in the same school could influence each other, thus reducing the differences between the two groups. The design, however, provides a true experimental comparison at the classroom level.

SUBJECTS

Initial questionnaire and physiological data regarding smoking were provided by 1730 participating teen-age students. Of these subjects, 1325 (76.6%) also responded to a 6-month follow-up questionnaire regarding their current smoking behavior. One year later, 1178 (68.1%) of the subjects were available for follow-up. At 6-month follow-up, 562 middle school subjects were assessed, and 509 were assessed at 1 year in seventh-grade health and science classes. There were 322 high school students at 6-month follow-up and 298 at 1-year follow-up.

MEASURES

A questionnaire regarding smoking experiences was administered to all subjects. Items explored the respondent's socioeconomic status, smoking history, attitudes toward cigarettes, and the smoking behavior of parents, siblings, and friends. Current self-reported cigarette smoking and use of alcohol, chewing tobacco, and marijuana were also probed. A composite measure of smoking was developed which was a weighted average of the reported number of cigarettes smoked in the last week and the reported number of cigarettes smoked yesterday. A measure of refusal of offered cigarettes was calculated by dividing the reported number of accepted offers of cigarettes in the last week by the reported number of cigarette offers in last week. Students also provided expired air samples and saliva samples under bogus pipeline conditions (Evans et al., 1978).

DETERRENCE AMONG REGULAR SMOKERS

Smokers were classified into the following smoking categories based on their pretest self-report: (1) never smoked—not even a puff; (2) tried smoking—not currently smoking, but had smoked at least a puff; (3) experimental smoker—smoked 1–7 cigarettes in the last week; or (4) regular smoker—smoked more than 7 cigarettes in the last week. There was a smaller proportion of experimental and regular smokers in the treatment group than in the control group at 6-month follow-up, although the differences was not significant. At 1-year follow-up there was little difference between the groups.

Analyses of the effects of the program on smoking rate indicated that Time 1 regular smokers who were exposed to refusal skills training were smoking at a significantly lower rate 1 year later than were regular smokers who did not receive the program. However, analysis of the attrition among subjects suggested that this result may have been due to more regular smokers being missing from the treatment condition than from the control condition.

These results are in contrast to most other published prevention studies. Most programs have been found to reduce the incidence of *new* experimenters. Indeed, some have not even reported the effects of their program on students who were already smoking when the prevention program began. The present results suggest that refusal skills training may help adolescents who are already smoking to resist continued social influences to smoke. The results presented earlier in this chapter on the factors associated with the maintenance of adolescent smoking suggest that such skills are needed by young people who are already smoking, since social influences appear to induce people to continue to smoke.

At the same time, there are several reasons to be cautious about these results. First, the results were analyzed using individual subjects as the unit of analysis, while the unit of random assignment was the classroom. This procedure, while frequently used in assessing the effects of prevention programs, underestimates the Type I error rate. Second, analysis of attrition suggested that the effect of the program may have been an artifact of differential attrition between the two conditions. Clearly, replication of the study is needed.

FUTURE DIRECTIONS

Our research thus far makes us cautiously optimistic that social skills training of the type we have done may contribute to the deterrence of cigarette smoking. However, the size of the effects we have achieved and our failure to replicate others' deterrences of the onset of experimentation leave ample room for modesty. We make no claim that refusal skill training is the only factor relevant to deterrence. In Chapter 3 (this volume), Wills has shown that stress may play a role in inducing young people to begin smoking. Such a factor may be independent of refusal skills, in that young people who have the skills, yet are experiencing some stress, may be disinclined to use their refusal skills.

There is still much that needs to be learned about how adolescent social skills relate to the onset and continuance of smoking. In the space remaining we discuss the directions of future research that appear most needed.

Improved Role Play Assessment Procedures

Certain methodological changes could enhance the validity of role play assessments. First, a procedure that required more extended responding on the part of the subject might provide a more valid sample of his or her refusal skill. Role play situations in which a confederate continued to insist that the subject smoke a cigarette might more accurately discriminate those who could successfully cope with such social pressures from those who could not.

A study by Kern et al. (1983) identified some instructional procedures that may further enhance the validity of role play tests. For most role play tests, the instructions have been to behave "as you typically would in such a situation." These were the instructions given for the TST described here. Kern et al. (1983) showed that validity of a role play test was increased when subjects were asked to "behave as they had" when they were in the same situation previously. Even further improvements in the validity of the role play tests were obtained when subjects were asked to produce specific behaviors at the same rate that they had produced them in the situation previously. The latter instructions improved the validity of the role play test for the specific behaviors that had been identified. Moreover, Kern et al. (1983) presented evidence suggesting that only the "typical response role play" produced criterion performance that was significantly greater than that found in the unobtrusive assessment. Thus the instructions to replicate previous behavior, particularly when certain key behaviors are specified, may produce a sample of refusal behavior that is more representative of the behavior that occurs in the natural setting.

A third factor that might improve the validity of role play tests is the use of videotapes in both the presentation and recording of responses to them of situations. The videotaping of the subject response would allow coding additional relevant behavioral responses. Audiotapes are limited to analysis of the verbal response given, yet other components of the response such as eye contact, body posture, and other nonverbal cues may be important predictors of whether the subject would use the response in a subsequent situation.

The Need for Prospective Studies

Studies are needed that examine the extent to which tests of refusal skills predict later smoking. Further research will require studies with much larger Ns, since the proportion of young people who experiment with smoking is fairly small and the onset is spread out over a long period of time. As Collins et al. (1983) have suggested, failure to assess smoking onset over the appropriate time period may greatly decrease our power to detect effects. For example, a measure of refusal skill that predicted changes in smoking status very well over 3 months may be entirely unrelated to smoking status over 6 months.

The data presented earlier in this chapter also underscored the need to study the onset of experimentation and the factors affecting the maintenance of regular smoking. In the sample that received our Taped Situations Test, there were too few smokers to assess accurately whether the refusal skills were related to a later smoking rate for those who were already smoking at Time 1. It might be fruitful to assess the refusal skills of young people who were entering a smoking cessation program in order to see if these skills predict their success in the program. The lower smoking rates among regular smokers who received our smoking prevention curriculum do suggest that the teaching of refusal skills is relevant to coping with continued social pressure to smoke. However, the results demand replication.

Relationship of Refusal Skills to Other Social Skills

It is possible that the assessment of other social skills would provide better prediction of onset and continuance of smoking than does the assessment of skill in refusing specific offers of cigarettes. Consider that assertiveness in other situations may be more predictive, especially if we ask about using the kind of instructions that Kern et al. (1983) have developed. This is because many subjects may never have had experiences in which they were offered cigarettes. Yet it is likely that they have had many instances in which peers pressured them in a variety of ways and they successfully or unsuccessfully dealt with those pressures. Asking them to behave as they have in prior pressure situations may produce a more accurate assessment of their repertoire of assertive behaviors with peers than do role play items that have to do with smoking. This should be the case for young people who have never experienced social pressures to smoke. For those who have experienced social pressures to smoke, the smoking items on the role play task should be more valid than items having to do with other social pressures.

The Nature of a Skilled Response

A critically important issue is the specification of what constitutes a skilled response in a peer pressure situation. The refusal skills that we taught were, unfortunately, not based on any evidence that they are effective with adolescents. We need to know more about the types of adolescent social behaviors that are truly effective with other adolescents. This problem goes well beyond the issue of deterring cigarette smoking. Social influence among adolescents is very important across a wide range of behaviors. At the same time, adults' influence appears to be limited. If we can find ways to teach adolescents to cope with peer influences, we may be able to prevent a number of unfortunate consequences of social pressure, such as death in auto accidents due to pressure to take risks.

We need to enumerate specific behaviors that are hypothesized to be skilled and unskilled and to test empirically their impact on adolescents. New methods appear relevant. First, adolescent subjects could be asked to rate samples of assertive and unassertive behavior in order to identify more or less acceptable responses. Dow et al. (1981) used such a method in an attempt to identify socially skilled responses for college age women. Audiotapes of a brief conversation between a man and a woman were produced. The tapes varied only in the rates of three behaviors of the woman: (1) her compliments to the man, (2) her questions about the man, and (3) her latency to respond, to him. Subjects who listened to these tapes rated the woman who gave more questions and more compliments as more socially skilled. In applying these methods to assessing the social impact of adolescent assertive behavior, it would be particularly valuable to assess the adolescents' responses to more and less aggressive refusal responses.

One advantage of the method just described is that a fairly large number of social behaviors can be evaluated with relative efficiency. However, adolescents' indication that a behavior is preferred does not necessarily indicate what the functional effect of that behavior will be when used in a social situation. For this reason a second method is needed. Specifically, studies are required in which the impact of various assertive behaviors on the behavior of naive subjects is assessed. Confederates could be trained to vary the degree and nature of their assertive responses in different experimental conditions. The impact of this on the subject's response to the confederate could be assessed, as could the effect of the confederate's behavior on the subject's ratings of the confederate.

CONCLUSION

The role of peer influences in the initiation and continuance of smoking is confirmed by our research. Yet we are just beginning to unravel the details of the process and the ways in which it can be modified. Social skills training plays a central role in attempts to modify the impact of peer influences to smoke. But we need more detailed experimental validation of the most effective methods of teaching these skills. And, we need more fine-grained methods of assessing those skills and determining precisely how they contribute to the deterrence of smoking.

REFERENCES

Allegrante, J. P., O'Rourke, T. W., & Tuncalp, S. (1977–1978). A multivariate analysis of selected psychosocial variables on the development of subsequent youth smoking behavior. *Journal of Drug Education, 1,* 237–248.

Ary, D. V., & Biglan, A. (1985). *Onset and cessation in adolescent cigarette smoking: A prospective analysis.* Manuscript submitted for publication, Oregon Research Institute, Eugene, OR.

Ary, D., Biglan, A., Nautel, C. L., Weissman, W., & Severson, H. H. (1983, July). *Longitudinal prediction of the onset and change in rate of adolescent smoking.* Paper presented at the World Conference on Smoking and Health, Winnipeg, Canada.

Ary, D., Biglan, A., & Severson, H. (1983, August). *Concurrent correlates and longitudinal predictors of adolescent cigarette smoking.* Paper presented to annual meeting of the American Psychological Association, Anaheim, CA.

Bauman, K. E., & Dent, C. W. (1982). Influence of an objective measure on self-reports of behavior. *Journal of Applied Psychology, 67,* 623–628.

Bellack, A. S., Hersen, M., & Lamparski, D. (1979). Role play tests for assessing social skills: Are they valid? Are they useful? *Journal of Consulting and Clinical Psychology, 47,* 335–342.

Bellack, A. S., & Morrison, R. L. (1982). Interpersonal Dysfunction. In A. S. Bellack, M. Hersen, & A. E. Kazdin (Eds.), *International handbook of behavior modification and therapy.* New York: Plenum Press.

Biglan, A., McConnell, S., Severson, H. H., Bavry, J., & Ary, D. V. (in press). A situational analysis of adolescent smoking. *Journal of Behavioral Medicine, 7,* 109–114.

Biglan, A., Nautel, C., Ary, D., & Thompson, R. (1983, August). *Self-reported marijuana smoking: Relationships to carbon monoxide and Thiocyanate measures.* Paper presented at the annual meeting of the American Psychological Association, Anaheim, CA.

Biglan, A., Severson, H., Ary, D., Faller, C., Gallison, C., Thompson, R., Glasgow, R., & Lichtenstein, E. (1985). *Do smoking prevention programs really work? Attrition and the internal and external validity of an evluation of a refusal skills training program.* Manuscript submitted for publication, Oregon Research Institute, Eugene, OR.

Biglan, A., Severson, H., Bavry, J., & McConnell, S. (1983). Social influence and adolescent smoking: A first look behind the barn. *Health Education,* 14–18.

Biglan, A., Severson, H. H., Hops, H., Faller, C., Ary, D. V., Friedman, L. S., Weissman, W., & Nautel, C. L. (1983, August). *Methodological considerations in studying the smoking acquisition process.* Paper presented at the annual meeting of the American Psychological Association, Anaheim, CA.

Botvin, G., & McAlister, A. (in press). Teenage cigarette smoking: Causes and prevention. In C. B. Arnold (Ed.), *Annual review of disease prevention*. New York: Springer.

Chassin, L., & Clark, C. P. (1984). Cognitive and social influence factors in adolescent smoking cessation. *Addictive Behaviors, 9*, 383–390.

Cohen, J., & Cohen, P. (1975). *Applied multiple regression/correlation analysis for the behavioral sciences*. Hillsdale, NJ: Erlbaum.

Collins, L. M., Graham, J. W., & Hansen, W. B. (1983, August). *Measuring developmental processes in health-related behavior acquisition*. Paper presented at the annual meeting of the American Psychological Association, Anaheim, CA.

Collins, L. M., Graham, J. W., & Hansen, W. B. (1984). *Testing and developing dynamic models for longitudinal data: Some considerations when a dynamic process is measured at fixed intervals*. Manuscript submitted for publication.

Cosgrove, J. (Producer). (1977). *The feminine mistake* [Film]. San Francisco: Pyramid Films.

Dow, M. G., Glaser, S. R., & Biglan, A. (1981). The relevance of specific conversational behaviors to ratings of social skill: An experimental analysis. *Journal of Behavioral Assessment, 3*, 233–242.

Eisler, R. M. (1976). The behavioral assessment of social skills. In M. Hersen & A. S. Bellack (Eds.), *Behavioral assessment*. New York: Pergamon Press.

Evans, R. I. (Producer). (1978). *Resisting pressure to smoke* [Film]. Houston: University of Houston.

Evans, R. I., Hansen, W. B., & Mittelmark, M. B. (1977). Increasing the validity of self-reports of smoking behavior in children. *Journal of Applied Psychology, 62*, 521–523.

Evans, R. I., & Raines, B. E. (1982). Control of prevention of smoking in adolescents: A psychosocial perspective. In T. J. Coates, A. C. Peterson, & C. Perry (Eds.), *Promoting adolescent health: A dialogue on research and practice*. New York: Academic Press.

Evans, R. I., Rozelle, R. M., Maxwell, S. E., Raines, B. E., Dill, C. A., Guthrie, T. J., Henderson, A. H., & Hill, P. C. (1981). Social modeling films to deter smoking in adolescents: Results of a three-year field investigation. *Journal of Applied Psychology, 66*, 399–414.

Evans, R. I., Rozelle, R. M., Mittelmark, M. B., Hansen, W. B., Bane, A. L., & Havis, J. (1978). Deterring the onset of smoking in children: Knowledge of immediate physiological effects and coping with peer pressure, media pressure, and parent modeling. *Journal of Applied Social Psychology, 8*, 126–135.

Festinger, L. (1972). An introduction to the theory of dissonance. In E. P. Hollander & R. G. Hunt (Eds.), *Classic contributions to social psychology*. New York: Oxford University Press.

Flay, B. R., d'Avernas, J. R., Best, J. A., Kersell, M. A., & Ryan, K. B. (1981). Cigarette smoking: Why young people do it and ways of preventing it. In P. Firestone & P. McGrath (Eds.), *Pediatric behavioral medicine*. New York: Springer.

Friedman, L. S., Lichtenstein, E., & Biglan, A. (1985). Smoking onset among teens: An empirical analysis of initial situations. *Addictive Behaviors, 10*, 1–13.

Glasgow, R. E., & Arkowitz, H. (1975). The behavioral assessment of male and female social competence in dyadic heterosexual interactions. *Behavior Therapy, 6*, 488–498.

Hops, H. H., Weissman, W., Biglan, A., Faller, C., Nautel, C., & Severson, H. H. (1983). *A taped situation test of cigarette refusal skill acquisition*. Paper presented at the annual meeting of the American Psychological Association at Anaheim, CA.

Horan, J. J., & Williams, J. M. (1982). Longitudinal study of assertion training as a drug abuse prevention strategy. *American Educational Research Journal, 3*, 341–351.

Kern, J. M., Miller, C., & Eggers, J. (1983). Enhancing the validity of role-play tests: A comparison of three role-play methodologies. *Behavior Therapy, 14*, 482–492.

Kniskern, J., Biglan, A., Lichtenstein, E., Ary, D., & Bavry, J. (1983). Peer modeling effects in the smoking behavior of teenagers. *Addictive Behaviors, 8,* 129–132.

Krosnick, J. A., & Judd, C. M. (1982). Transitions in social influences at adolescence: Who induces cigarette smoking? *Developmental Psychology, 18*(3), 359–368.

Leventhal, H., & Cleary, P. D. (1980). The smoking problem: A review of the research and theory in behavioral risk modification. *Psychological Review, 88,* 370–405.

Luepker, R. V., Johnson, C. A., Murray, D. M., & Pechacek, T. F. (1983). Prevention of cigarette smoking: Three year follow-up of an education program for youth. *Journal of Behavioral Medicine,* 1983, 53–62.

Mettlin, C. (1976). Peer and other influences on smoking behavior. *Journal of School Health, 46,* 529–536.

Mittelmark, M. B., Murray, D. M., Luepker, R. V., Pechacek, T. F., Pirie, P. L., & Pallenon, U. (1983, August), *Adolescent smoking transition states over two years.* Paper presented at the annual meeting of the American Psychological Association, Anaheim, CA.

Nelson, R. O. (1977). Methodological issues in assessment via self-monitoring. In J. D. Cone & R. P. Hawkins (Eds.), *Behavioral assessment: New directions in clinical psychology.* New York: Brunner/Mazel.

Pechacek, T. F., Murray, D. M., Leupker, R. V., Mittelmark, M. B., Johnson, C. A., and Schultz, J. M. (1984). Measurement of adolescent smoking behavior: Rationale and methods. *Journal of Behavioral Medicine, 7,* 123–140.

Perry, C. L., Maccoby, N., & McAlister, A. (1980). Adolescent smoking: A third year follow-up. *World Smoking and Health,* 40–45.

Salber, E. J., & MacMahon, B. (1961). Cigarette smoking among high school students related to social class and parental smoking habits. *American Journal of Public Health, 51,* 1780–1789.

Sherman, S. J., Presson, C. C., Chassin, L., & Olshavsky, R. (1983, August) *Becoming a cigarette smoker: A social psychological perspective.* Paper presented at the annual meeting of the American Psychological Association, Anaheim, CA.

Thompson, E. L. (1978). Smoking education programs, 1960–1976. *American Journal of Public Health, 68,* 250–257.

U.S. Department of Health and Human Services. (1982). *The Health Consequences of Smoking: Cancer. A report of the Surgeon General* (DHHS Publication No. PHSD 82–50179). Washington, DC: U.S. Government Printing Office.

Chapter 5

Social Competence and Self-Efficacy as Determinants of Substance Use in Adolescence

MARY ANN PENTZ

INTRODUCTION

This chapter focuses on the promotion of general social competence as an approach for preventing substance use among early adolescents. Based on social learning theory, a competence model of drug use prevention is proposed. The model is then tested by analyzing the relationship between normative social competence and drug use and by evaluating the effects of a broad-based social competence training program on enhanced competence and reduced drug use. Results support the capability of social competence for preventing drug use but suggest that this capability may be mediated by individual differences in adolescent development, behavior, and environment. The findings are discussed in terms of the relative effectiveness of general social competence and specific resistance skill approaches for prevention of drug use, and the implications of competence for generalized coping in adolescence.

Defect-to-Competence

Until recently, research and treatment on adolescent drug use espoused a medical or "defect" model which depended on the identification of pathological *intra*personal factors (e.g., delinquency and poor self-esteem) for predicting the onset and course of drug abuse (see Levine & Kozak, 1979; Quay & Quay, 1965). This model, however, failed to account for recreational drug use, for developmental shifts in proneness to drug use during early adolescence, or for specific behavioral and environmental influences on drug use (Jessor & Jessor, 1977; Perry, 1983).

In contrast, the last decade has witnessed an increase of research into the training of social or *inter*personal skills for resisting drug use and promoting healthy alternatives (Albee, 1981). The targeted skills include both the cognitions associated with confidence and perceived mastery of social skills and the observable behaviors expressing skill demonstration. Collectively, these cognitive and behavioral skills are referred to as social competence, and the shift from pathology identification to skills training is known as the defect-to-competence movement (Brickman et al., 1982; Meichenbaum, Butler, & Gruson, 1981).

In the area of drug use prevention, social competence can include either broad-based interpersonal skills that are applicable to a wide variety of life situations (e.g., the general skill of assertiveness), skills that are pertinent to a particular type of person or age group (e.g., assertiveness for peer pressure resistance in adolescence), or skills that are specific to drug use (e.g., assertiveness for resisting peer pressure to use drugs). Current research on adolescent drug use suggests a relationship between social competence and prevention of drug use, regardless of the particular skills being evaluated (see Pentz, 1983a). The research draws heavily from both social learning theory (Bandura, 1977; Rosenthal & Bandura, 1978) and problem behavior theory (Jessor & Jessor, 1977). From this perspective, drug use is attributed to direct learning or modeling influences (e.g., peer use) in conjunction with certain individual behaviors (e.g., rebelliousness) and environmental influences (e.g., availability of drugs and support for drug use). Social competence acts to lessen the impact of these direct influences. For example, a socially competent adolescent may be able to resist a friend's persistent pressure to try a cigarette by saying "no" assertively. In fact, recent programs employing social competence training have shown this to be the case, regardless of whether the training included broad-based or specific drug resistance skills (see Botvin, Eng, & Williams, 1980; Hurd, Johnson, Luepker, Pechacek, & Jacobs, 1980; Perry, Killen, Telch, Slinkard, & Danaher, 1980; Schinke & Gilchrist, 1983).

Even with a background of supportive research, however, the dynamics of the social competence–drug use relationship are still not understood. No well-designed prospective study has been published in this area. To fill the gap, evidence for a causal relationship must be inferred from other bodies of research which have addressed, at least indirectly, the question of how drug use develops in adolescence. These bodies of research encompass competence development, psychosocial correlate and retrospective studies on drug use, and coping with stress.

Competence, Drug Use, and Coping in Adolescence

Developmental research has indicated that adolescents are concerned with acquiring a broad base of social competence (Ford, 1982; Piaget & Inhelder, 1969). The concern is particularly apparent during early adolescence (Grades 6 through 9 or the middle-school years), when school, family, and peer relationships are in transition and increased pressure is exerted on adolescents by adults to accept responsibility for a variety of interpersonal behaviors (Kelly, 1980; Parkes, 1971; Perry & Murray, 1982). Some of the more commonly recognized skills that constitute general social competence during this period include assertiveness, ability to disagree and refuse, and ability to make requests and initiate conversations (Gilchrist, 1981; Goldstein, Sprafkin, Gershaw, & Klein, 1979).

During this same age period, psychosocial correlate studies have shown steady increases in the prevalence of cigarette smoking and alcohol use, the gateway substances which have been linked with illicit drug use in later adolescence (see Kandel, Kessler, & Margulies, 1978; Pentz, 1983a). These increases have been related to an inability to exert social competence skills such as refusal of cigarette offers (McAlister, Perry, & Maccoby, 1979). This relationship is further supported by retrospective research that demonstrates a history of lower social competence among drug-using adolescents (see Kellam, Brown, & Fleming, 1982; Levine & Kozak, 1979).

Finally, support for the relationship between social competence and drug use is provided by research on how persons cope with stress. Two perspectives have guided this research. One, termed the *stress coping model*, conceptualizes drug use as a compensatory or coping behavior in reaction to stress in an individual's environment. For example, an individual may engage in drug use to reduce stress arising from fear of social isolation. The use of drugs under such circumstances may temporarily alleviate stress and provide a sense of being "in" with the peer group. In fact, preliminary studies on young adults and adolescents have provided some support for this model by showing decreases in anxiety or depression following drug use, at least for drug use assessed over short-term periods of 6 months or less (see Aneshensel & Huba, 1983). The alternative view, the *stress response model*, is that drug use is a behavior that increases rather than alleviates stress over the long-term. The model assumes that if individuals are using drugs as a coping mechanism, they are inhibited from learning or practicing more adaptive, alternative coping behaviors.[1] Thus, social com-

---

[1]The stress response model is consistent with two theories of reciprocal behavior change. Wolpe's (1958) theory of reciprocal inhibition asserts that a behavioral response will decrease the strength of a simultaneous competing response. Use of drugs as a coping mechanism decreases the likelihood that an individual will seek another coping mechanism that does not

petence and adaptive behaviors would be expected to decrease as a consequence of heavy drug use (Wrubel, Benner, & Lazarus, 1981). At least one study has supported this trend in the long-term, showing an increase in depression and related behaviors following continued alcohol use (Aneshensel & Huba, 1983).

A Competence Model of Drug Use Prevention

According to social learning theory, social competence is represented as a dynamic sequence of cognitions and behaviors that modify each other over time. The cognitions represent self-efficacy, that is, "the conviction that one can successfully execute the behavior(s) to produce the desired outcomes" (Bandura, 1977, p. 193); the behaviors represent the actual overt performance of social skills. Initial perceptions of self-efficacy may prompt an individual to make an initial attempt to refuse a friend's offer of a cigarette. Successful refusal heightens subsequent self-efficacy, which in turn is likely to prompt more frequent or stronger refusals in future situations involving drug use. Thus social skills and self-efficacy are examined for their effects on each other, the outcome being mastery of social competence, that is, easily and successfully applied social skills. Self-efficacy and social skills are also assessed for their relationship to other cognitions and behaviors that are related to drug use (see Jessor & Jessor, 1977). For example, in early adolescence, the need to develop self-efficacy and social skills in prosocial ways may override an initial intention to experiment with drugs. Conversely, precocious or well-developed drug use behavior in this age group may replace or offset the need to master social competence. In this case, self-efficacy and social skills diminish as a result of lack of practice of prosocial behavior over time (see Jessor & Jessor, 1977; Jessor, 1982).

The remaining sections of this chapter describe a longitudinal study that focused on empirical validation of a bidirectional relationship between social competence and drug use. Self-efficacy and social skills, the two components of social competence, are evaluated for their ability to increase each other and decrease drug use over time. Conversely, initial drug use is evaluated for its effect on lowering subsequent social competence. Finally, a performance-based modeling program is evaluated for its effect on both increasing social competence and decreasing drug use.

---

involve drug use. Bandura's (1977) theory of reciprocal determinism suggests that behaviors and cognitions about mastery of behaviors influence each other over time. Initial drug use may increase a sense of confidence about using drugs in the future. In turn, increased confidence about the ability to handle drug use leads to more drug use rather than the practice of more adaptive behaviors for coping with stress.

SOCIAL COMPETENCE AS A PREDICTOR OF DRUG USE

Rationale

A major problem in earlier studies is the lack of a clear conceptual model of the causal relationship between drug use and social competence. Two models have dominated the literature. One posits that drug use-specific variables (primarily prior drug use, and secondarily, friends' use of drugs, sanction for drug use, and availability of drugs) are the major determinants of drug use in adolescents (Huba & Bentler, 1982). Social competence may indicate or lessen these influences by providing an adolescent with skills to resist drug use or to seek alternative activities. The other model treats current and prior drug use behavior as determinants of subsequent social competence. In this case, lower social competence is predicted to be the result of heavier drug use.

The present study compares both models of drug use. The purpose of the investigation was to test the ability of social competence measures to predict drug use in adolescents, and second, to validate previous short-term research on drug use relationships by testing the models over a longitudinal period of 2 years.

Method

PARTICIPANTS

Participants were 254 sixth- through ninth-grade students who constituted a subsample of the control group for a 2-year drug abuse prevention study having a total N of 1472 sixth- through ninth-grade students in eight public schools in Knox County, Tennessee. Participants were randomly selected from four of the eight schools (one rural middle, one suburban middle, one rural high, and one suburban high school). The sample represented respondents who provided complete data on self-report and audiotaped role play measures across four waves of assessment (every 6 months for 2 years). A high degree of correspondence was found in sociodemographics between the current study sample, the total drug abuse prevention sample, and the 1980 census for Knox County. Thus, the current study sample appears representative of the eligible population. The sample was 96.3% white and 51.3% female. Consistent with national survey data, the sample was characterized by an initially low rate of drug use, with sharp increases by grade (see Johnston, Bachman, & O'Malley, 1980). At Wave 1, the percentages of students reporting any cigarette and/or alcohol use in the past month were 4.7, 5.2, 18.5, and 37.5% for Grades 6–9, respectively.

The subsample of 254 was derived from a sequential sampling plan as follows. Twenty-five percent of students in participating schools were randomly selected by classroom within each grade. This procedure resulted in 1472 students, with school-representative proportions at each grade level. Within each grade, classrooms were randomly assigned to a drug abuse prevention training condition, a prevention instruction condition, or a no-training control condition. Two-thirds were randomly selected further for testing on an audiotaped role play measure of social skills. Over a 2-year period, 11% of the respondents dropped out of the study and 10% had missing data on one or more of the 177 items assessed in the larger drug abuse prevention project. Thus, the effective sample size was 254.

MEASURES

Three measures were administered to all subjects at each of four successive semesters, in standardized questionnaire and audiotaped role play administrations. Data were collected by three pairs of graduate students and a supervising program assistant trained in questionnaire and role play test administration. All questionnaire data were collected in two mass testing sessions per grade per school. Audiotaped role play data were collected individually. Questionnaires and role play taped were numerically coded for each subject at each wave.

Drug Use. Ninety-seven items on this measure were adopted from other standardized measures of adolescent drug use.[2] Items were repeated for each of the gateway drugs (cigarettes, beer, wine, hard liquor). These included 3-item scales which measured environmental aspects of drug use: (1) friends' use of drugs (number of friends using each substance at least once a month); (2) sanction for use by adults; and (3) availability of drugs. Three additional items measured drug use by the respondent: (1) amount of use on days used in the last month and, for alcohol, number of times drunk or abused in the last 6 months, (0 [none] to 6 [6 or more]); (2) frequency of use per month (a continuous scale of 0–30 days; responses were rescaled to 1 [none] to 5 [20 days or more] format); and (3) assessed intentions to use in the future (1 [never] to 5 [yes, for sure]).

Self-Efficacy. This 18-item scale measured the cognitive component of social competence. Nine items measured self-efficacy in familiar interpersonal situations (i.e., expected to occur on a frequent basis) requiring assertiveness, requests, or refusal with teachers, parents, and peers. Nine involved

---

[2]Content, criterion-oriented and construct validities, and test–retest and internal consistency reliabilities are reported in detail elsewhere (Huba & Bentler, 1980; Kandel, 1975; Pentz, 1983a).

the same skills, but in nonfamiliar interpersonal situations (i.e., expected to occur rarely or only occasionally, for example, with a waiter in a restaurant), with persons other than teachers, parents, or peers. Each item assessed level of self-efficacy (0 = no, could not; 1 = yes, could perform the skill) and strength of self-efficacy (certainty that the skill could be performed; 1 = not at all sure; 5 = very sure). Item ratings were summed to yield scores for level and strength of self-efficacy in familiar and unfamiliar situations.[3] An example of self-efficacy in a familiar situation was the following:

> You're trying to take notes in class, but the teacher is going so fast that you can't keep up. You raise your hand and say, "Could you stop a minute and go back to the last topic? I'm really having trouble keeping up. Could you slow down a little?"
>
> Could you do this?   Yes _____   No _____
>
> How sure are you? 1   2   3   4   5
>   Not   Somewhat   Very
>   at all   sure

Social Skills. The 12-item social skill measure assessed the behavioral component of social competence. Participants were required to respond to social situations presented by audiotape.[4] Six of the situations involved responding to teachers, parents, or peers; six involved responding to others such as a stranger pushing in a ticket line. Each response by the subject was audiotaped and later rated by two graduate student raters trained in scoring verbal interactions. Two scores were derived: type of overall response (1 [unassertive] to 3 [assertive]); and level of social competence (1 [no or off-topic response] to 5 [direct, reasonable response toward situation resolution]). Average interrater reliability was .92. An example of a social skills test in a familiar situation was the following:

> *Narrative prompt on tape.* You're sitting at the dinner table with your family. Your mother starts discussing your good friend Charlie.

---

[3]Derivation, validity, and reliability information is reported elsewhere (Bandura, 1977, 1978; Pentz & Kazdin, 1982; Pentz, 1983a, 1983b).

[4]The 12 items were those that yielded the greatest item-to-total correlations and Chronbach's alpha values from the situations used to measure self-efficacy. Validity and reliability information are reported elsewhere (Pentz & Kazdin, 1982; Pentz, 1983a, 1983b). In the present study and in a 1-year pilot study on 875 sixth- through ninth-grade students (Pentz, 1983b), the order of self-efficacy and social skills testing was counterbalanced to determine any effects of method variance or test sensitivity on participant responses. In both studies, order of test administration had no effect ($p > .09$).

Adult female dialogue prompt. Why do you hang around with Charlie? Why don't you hang around with Billy instead? He's such a nice boy.

The dialogue prompt is followed by a 30-second delay for recording the subject's response.[5]

PROCEDURE AND DESIGN

Subjects were administered the self-report measure in groups in school classrooms and the audiotape measure in individual testing sessions every 6 months (November and May) over a 2-year period. This procedure yielded four waves of data. Audiotape data were later rated by two pairs of raters. The design was a single group (control group) design with repeated measures across four waves.

Results

Causal modeling was used to determine if initial drug use led to decreases in social competence, whether the reverse was true, or whether drug use and social competence influenced each other over time. Causal modeling can estimate both unidirectional and bidirectional relationships.[6]

Several preliminary models were tested at separate and successive waves to determine the initial strength and stability of the social competence–drug use relationship.

The preliminary analyses supported the testing of a model of a bidirectional relationship of social competence and drug use over time. This model,

---

[5]The response-type rating was based on both the verbal response and three nonverbal indices (response lag in a 60-second period, hesitation or break in responding, and tone of voice). An unassertive response was defined as a response lacking expression of rights or opinions. An assertive response involved appropriate expression rights or opinions. An aggressive response involved expression without regard to the other person's rights or opinions. Response level was based on verbal content and direct address to the other person which, with expression of both persons' opinions and suggestion for situation resolution, was rated as a highly socially competent response. Details are described elsewhere (Pentz & Kazdin, 1982).

[6]The LISREL IV program was used (Jöreskog, 1979) to obtain maximum-likelihood estimates of model parameters, chi-square goodness-of-fit, and normed and nonnormed fit index values, using the covariance matrix of measured variables. Unlike the chi-square statistic, the index values estimate the extent to which the observed covariance matrix is explained by the causal model independent of sample size (see Bentler, 1980; Huba & Bentler, 1982). Thus the index values are useful with large samples or complete models, where trivial departures from the observed data may lead to rejection of the hypothesized model. The normed fit coefficient ranges from zero to unity (perfect model fit); the nonnormed coefficient assumes similar values but is corrected for the size or complexity of the model (Huba & Bentler, 1982).

as tested, is presented in Figure 5.1 (adapted from Pentz & Huba, 1984). Criterion construct refers to actual drug use behavior by an adolescent (the dependent variable). The construct was represented by four indicators: cigarette, beer, wine, and liquor use. Each indicator was developed by standardizing and summing the scores for frequency and amount of the particular substance used. The relationship between self-efficacy, social skills, and drug use was tested based on the social learning model described earlier in this chapter. Results showed that across all four waves the theoretical model was accurately and reliably represented by the data (average fit index value was .96 out of a possible 1.00). Prior drug use had the strongest influence on subsequent drug use (average beta weight was .92). Higher levels of drug use at Time 1 led to decreased levels of self-efficacy, decreased social skills (mediate through self-efficacy), and higher levels of drug use at subsequent time periods (beta weights ranging from .28 to .45). The bidirectional relationship of drug use was more stable over time than unidirectional relationships (i.e., the beta weights fluctuated less from wave to more stable wave). This pattern of influence was replicated across subsamples split by sex and grade.

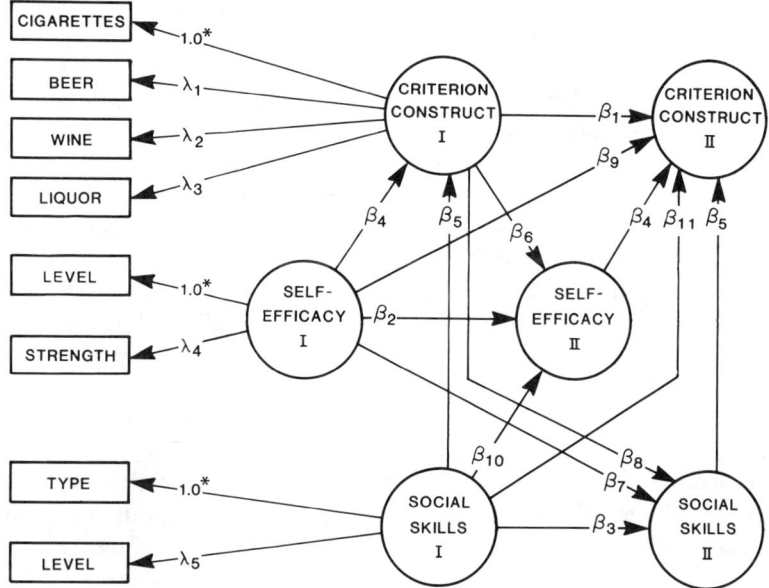

Figure 5.1 A causal model of social competence and drug use. Criterion construct refers to the dependent variable, drug use. The model was also estimated using intentions, peer use, sanction for use, and availability of drugs as criterion constructs. Roman numerals I and II refer to Waves 1 and 2, respectively; the same relationships were found through Waves 3 and 4. Boxes refer to standardized and summed scores representing each of the constructs. $N = 254$.

Supplementary analyses were also conducted on the model, replacing the dependent variable of own drug use with drug use intentions, sanction for use, availability, and friends use. These models yielded only weak relationships, indicating that social competence relates more to actual drug use by a respondent than to external drug use influences. Conversely, when drug use influences were tested along with social competence for their combined influence on respondents' own drug use, the model produced an even better fit with the data.

Conclusions

High levels of initial drug use led to decreases in social competence and increases in drug use over time. The finding that drug use decreased both self-efficacy and social skills suggests that over time, drug use may heighten rather than alleviate stress. Thus, consistent with recent findings from other longitudinal research, the results support a stress-response rather than a stress-coping model of drug use (see Aneshensel & Huba, 1983; Wrubel et al., 1983).

Several findings bear directly on the validity and reliability of the social competence–drug use relationship. First, the three major variables, respondent's drug use, self-efficacy, and social skills, were highly stable over time. Conceivably, the stability of these variables may be due to the fact that each was developed by summing and averaging across a wide variety of representative items: Drug use included cigarettes, beer, wine, and liquor; and social skills and self-efficacy involved a variety of interpersonal situations with teachers, parents, and peers. Past research supports the principle that the stability of measures of behavior is increased when summing and averaging techniques are used instead of simple repeated measures of single behaviors (e.g., monthly frequency of beer use; see Epstein, 1980).

Second, the direction of the causal relationship replicated the direction of cognitive-behavior change obtained by Bandura (1977) and others (Wandersman & Florin, 1981). Self-efficacy and social skills influenced each other, with initial levels of self-efficacy mediating changes in social skills as well as effects of drug use on skills. The positive relationship found between self-efficacy and social skills is supported by recent formulations of attitude-behavior change, which hypothesize strong effects of attitudes on attitude-consistent behaviors (Bentler & Speckhart, 1979; Kahle, Kingel & Kulka, 1981).

Third, prior drug use had a larger impact on subsequent drug use than social competence, and inclusion of external drug use influences (sanction for use, availability, friends' use) resulted in better prediction of drug use than social competence alone. These findings have two implications. One is that social competence alone may not be sufficient for accurate prediction of drug use in adolescents; other drug use influences may also have to be considered. This possibility argues for a multidimensional rather than a unidimensional approach to prediction (Huba & Bentler, 1980). The other possibility is that the strength of social competence as a predictor of drug use may depend on whether social competence skills are measured in situations directly related or proximal to drug use (e.g., resisting a drug offer), or in situations that are only indirectly related, or distal, to drug use (e.g., resisting an opportunity to cheat on an exam). Both of these possibilities have been raised elsewhere (Jessor & Jessor, 1977). Unfortunately, even in longitudinal studies of drug use, the period of assessment of drug use development rarely exceeds 1 and 2 years. In such a short time frame, it is logical to expect that variables directly related to drug use would have the larger impact. Future research should focus on causal models that are tested over a period of several years, with particular attention to shifts in proximal and distal influences.

SOCIAL COMPETENCE TRAINING FOR PREVENTION OF DRUG USE

Rationale

Social competence is regarded increasingly as a plausible intervention target for promoting stress coping ability and enhancing health (Masterpasqua, 1981; Sanchez-Craig, 1976). Currently, the major method of enhancing social competence is social competence training, defined as the set of techniques used to improve self-efficacy and social skills (Pentz & Tolan, 1984; Rosenthal & Bandura, 1978). The emphasis is on mutual benefit and maintenance of personal integrity in interpersonal situations (Gilchrist, 1981). The most commonly employed techniques include modeling (overt or covert, live or taped, with or without instruction); rehearsal (covert or overt, with or without an interactor); feedback with social reinforcement (self or other-initiated); and extended practice (intra- or extratraining, assigned as homework or spontaneous). If used together in sequence, these techniques are referred to in social learning theory as "performance-based modeling" (Rosenthal & Bandura, 1978). Whether these techniques are used singly or in combination, the theory asserts that to be maximally effective, training should address both the cognitive (self-efficacy) and behavioral (social skills) aspects of social competence. Without self-efficacy or confidence, an individual's attempts at behaving in a socially skilled manner may be tentative, sporadic, or may not occur at all, regardless of any amount of training. Conversely, if an individual is confident about behaving skillfully but has little opportunity to practice, subsequent behavioral attempts are likely to be faulty.

A few studies have assessed the effects of social competence training as an approach to drug use prevention in adolescents (e.g., Botvin et al., 1980; Pentz, 1983a; Schinke & Gilchrist, 1983). In these training programs, generic interpersonal communication skills are emphasized as means for coping with a wide variety of life situations and for selecting prosocial and health-promoting healthy behaviors. An adolescent is expected to generalize these skills for application to situations where drug use might occur. Common skills include assertiveness, making requests, and expressing disagreement. These programs are differentiated from other skill training programs that focus exclusively on skills for refusing offers of drugs (see Biglan, Weissman, & Severson, Chapter 4, this volume).

Previous smoking prevention programs have demonstrated decreases in drug use onset among adolescents, sometimes for a period of several years (see, e.g., Luepker, Johnson, Murray, & Pechacek, 1983). Few however have utilized strategies that attempt to tailor programmatic components to individual adolescent needs (see Goldstein et al., 1979; Goldstein & Pentz, 1984; Johnson, 1983). Research in areas other than drug abuse prevention has shown that individual behavior and environmental characteristics can strongly affect the results of epidemiological and intervention studies. For example, SES and individual differences in behavioral style affect attrition rates and outcome of certain types of psychotherapy (Heller, Price, & Sher, 1983). These factors and population density (SMSA-defined rural, suburban, and urban areas) also affect the incidence and prevalence of stress-related disorders (Lazarus, Averill, & Option, 1974; Radius, Dillman, Becker, Rosenstock & Horvath, 1980).

In the area of adolescent drug use, prevention programs appear to be affected by individual characteristics such as age–grade status (Jessor, 1982) and assertive behavioral style prior to training (Pentz, 1983b). Certain environmental characteristics may also contribute to program success, including the cluster and feeder patterns of students through schools in which programs are implemented (e.g., whether program students stay together as a class through successive school years; Kim, 1981) and whether the community in which program schools operate is rural, suburban, or urban (see Dunnette, 1978; Levine & Kozak, 1979; Winfree, Theis, & Griffiths, 1981). However, none of these characteristics has been systematically evaluated for their relative effects on drug use or on program outcome.

This phase of the present study evaluates a generic social competence training approach to drug use prevention in early adolescence. Two individual characteristics, age–grade status and unassertive–assertive–aggressive behavioral style, were systematically compared for their influence on drug use and training effectiveness. Type of environment (suburban vs. rural) was also assessed. The purpose was to confirm the competence model of drug use prevention tested earlier with causal modeling analysis and to identify areas where prevention strategies might be tailored to meet the individual and environmental needs of adolescents. The major hypotheses were (1) social competence training increases social competence and other prosocial behaviors and decreases drug use, and (2) age–grade status, behavioral style prior to training, and type of environment in which training is implemented, contribute to drug use levels and training outcome.

Method

PARTICIPANTS

Participants were 1193 sixth- through ninth-grade students from eight schools (four rural, four suburban).

The sample represented the full sample of 1472 students in the NIDA study described earlier, minus attrition over a 2-year period (9% in Year 1; 11% in Year 2). As part of the measurement design, two-thirds of the students received the audiotaped role play measure of social skills; thus the effective sample size for social skills analyses was 799.

MEASURES

The drug use, self-efficacy, and social skills measures were the same as described and used earlier for causal modeling analyses. The following measures were also used.

Behavioral Style. The Syracuse Scales of Social Relations (see Gardner & Thompson, 1958; Pentz, 1980, 1981; Pentz & Kazdin, 1982) were used to measure interpersonal behavior displayed in classroom situations. Teachers independently observed and rated their students relative to classmates for unassertive, assertive, or aggressive behavior (1, very unassertive; 5, appropriately assertive; 10, very aggressive). Each student was rated by four or five teachers from major curriculum areas. Students were subsequently classified as unassertive, assertive, or aggressive if more than half of their teachers' ratings were consistent within one point of agreement in the 1–3, 4–7, or 8–10 range of the scales. Only 2% of students had inconsistent ratings, and were excluded from further analyses.[7]

---

[7]Prior research has shown the scales to be valid and reliable for differentiating unassertive, assertive, and aggressive behaviors in self-report, role play, and *in vivo* tests administered to

Social Attitudes. This 50-item measure was adopted from the McLeod High Risk and Student Attitudinal Inventories for drug use (Archer & Arundell, 1983). Five scales were adopted for their significant predictive validity and test–retest reliability, and their relationship to preventive drug use intervention in school: Positive Social Attitude; Rebelliousness; School Value; Student–Teacher Relationship; and Family Cohesiveness (parent–child relationship;). Items are counterbalanced for negative and positive response choices (1, most; 5, none; or 1, very much; 5, not at all).

School Behavior Measures. Fifteen self-report items were used to measure school achievement (semester grade point average), truancy (times truant per semester), and absence (days absent per semester). Items were validated by school archival records. A 10% random sample of students' records indicated a high correlation with self-reported school behavior (average $r = .97$). Research has suggested that achievement, truancy, and absence may be related to drug use and prevention outcome (see, e.g., Bry & George, 1980; Quay & Quay, 1965).

PROCEDURE

The assessment procedure was the same as that described earlier for causal modeling. Social competence training was conducted over a 10-week period in the Spring semester between assessment Waves 1 and 2 in Year 1. The following procedure was used.

Following screening on the Syracuse scales, students were randomly assigned by classroom teams to one of three conditions varying training (active social competence training, instructions only, no-training control).[8] This procedure yielded a 3 × 3 factorial design for major analysis of prevention effects, with pretraining behavior (unassertive, assertive, aggressive as rated on the scales) nested within each classroom and training condition, and with four repeated measures across 2 years.

Training was referred to in schools as the SASS program (Socializing And Social Skills). Training groups consisted of whole classrooms, each of which

---

adolescents at 4-week intervals, and to differentiate adolescents who have received social skills training from those who have not ($p < .01$ to $p < .0001$; Pentz, 1980, 1982; Pentz & Kazdin, 1982). In addition, the scales have demonstrated predictive validity and test–retest reliability for assessing social recognition and achievement needs ($r = .71$ and $r = .79$ respectively; Gardner & Thompson, 1958).

[8]The participating schools were structured so that students and teachers were randomly assigned to self-contained class teams each school year. A team consisted of four to five classrooms and as many teachers clustered in a school wing. The number of wings in a school varied from three to eight, depending on school size. This type of structure reduced the possibility of program "leakage" across experimental conditions within each school.

received seven 55-minute sessions of sequenced modeling (live and audiotape), rehearsal, feedback with social reinforcement, and between-session practice of self-efficacy and social skills in a variety of everyday situations with teachers, parents, and peers, rather than specific drug use situations. An introductory session, the seven training sessions, and a final discussion session were conducted over a 10-week period by a trained teacher paired with a program assistant. Modeling, rehearsal, and generation of practice situations were facilitated by peers working in subgroups of four in the classroom. Peer facilitators were those students nominated by their subgroups to initiate and prompt skill practice in the subgroup during a particular training session. The program assistant demonstrated the facilitator role to the entire class just prior to peer nomination at the beginning of each training session. Students, including the nominated peer facilitators, then alternately served in active and passive roles for modeling, rehearsal, and feedback so that each student experienced each role during a classroom period. Skill sessions, sample situations, and step-by-step procedures are detailed elsewhere (Goldstein et al., 1979; Goldstein & Pentz, 1984; Pentz, 1980).

In contrast to the training group, the instruction-only group received only an introduction and two didactic sessions on the content and use of social competence. The control group completed the assessment measures but did not receive any training or instruction.

Results

Preliminary one-way analyses of variance were conducted to determine whether dropouts or students with missing data differed from students with complete data. No significant differences were obtained on a drug use composite variable that was created by standardizing and summing the frequency, amount, and abuse items for cigarettes, beer, wine, and liquor. However, there were significant differences in the use of specific substances. Specifically, by Wave 4, dropouts showed greater amounts of alcohol use in all three categories (beer, wine, and liquor) when compared to students having complete data ($p < .05$ to $< .001$; see Pentz, Leong, & Pentz, 1984).

Multivariate and univariate analyses of variance with listwise deletion were used for the major research design. Results indicated that training improved level and strength of self-efficacy, type and level ratings of social skills (e.g., unassertive responses changed to assertive responses and level of social competence increased), and grade point average increased relative to the instruction-only and control groups (p ranged from $< .05$ to $< .001$). Also, training interacted with pretraining behavior. Assertive and aggressive students in the training group showed greater increases in social competence and greater improvements in student–teacher relationships, family cohesiveness, and rebelliousness ($p < .05$ for all); and effects were maintained through Wave 4. Training also interacted with pretraining behavior to affect drug use. Relative to all other groups, assertive and aggressive students in the training group showed the lowest onset rates and the largest decreases in frequency, amount of drug use, and intentions to use drugs. In contrast, control group students showed greater onset rates and increases in drug use, with unassertive and aggressive students in this group displaying the highest levels of drug use (p ranged from $<.05$ to $<.001$).

Despite the training interaction, effects decreased somewhat over time. By Wave 4, training and instructions groups did not differ significantly from each other on levels of drug use, although both experimental groups continued to maintain lower drug use than the control group on the same variables that had produced significant differences at Wave 2 (see Table 5.1 for continued results from Wave 1 through Wave 2).

Across all four waves, significant interaction effects were limited mainly to the alcohol use variables. However, cigarette use showed similar nonsignificant trends. Assertive and aggressive students is the training group showed the lowest levels of cigarette use, whereas unassertive and aggressive students in the control group showed the highest. The nonsignificant effects for cigarette use are understandable in light of the low initial cigarette use by subjects relative to alcohol (see Pentz, 1983a for use of each substance by each grade at Wave 1).

Additional multivariate and univariate analyses were conducted to assess the contribution of grade to training effectiveness. As expected, grade alone produced linear increases in social competence and curvilinear increases in drug use (see Pentz, 1983a, for discussion of these results and the relationship of high within-grade levels of social competence to low drug use). However, results also indicated that grade interacted with training in affecting self-efficacy and social skills, with training group students in Grade 9 showing the greatest increases in social competence (p ranged from $<.05$ to $<.001$). Grade also interacted with training to produce differences in drug use and intention to use drugs. Training group students in sixth and ninth grade demonstrated the greatest decline in drug use and intention (e.g., the changes in drug use from Wave 1 to Wave 2 shown in Figure 5.2). These grades represent school transition periods from elementary to middle school and from middle to high school. Grade × Training interaction effects were maintained through Wave 4.

Finally, effects of environment were evaluated on a matched subsample of seventh- and eighth-grade students, selected for their approximately equal numerical representation in suburban and rural schools. Analyses included multiple regression analysis with variables entered by sets (e.g., sex and age

Table 5.1
TRAINING AND PRETRAINING BEHAVIOR EFFECTS ON ACTUAL DRUG USE[a]

Source	df	Mult F	Amount per day				Actual drug use Frequency in last month				Got drunk in past 6 months		
			Cig.	Beer	Wine	Liq.	Cig.	Beer	Wine	Liq.	Beer	Wine	Liq.
Between													
Training (A)	1	1.60	0.88	3.34	1.27	0.06	1.22	3.09	0.02	2.53	0.13	0.19	0.14
Pretraining behavior (B)	2	2.34***	2.70	3.56*	3.49*	0.13	2.09	4.11*	1.94	4.15*	1.42	1.06	0.90
A × B	2	3.00***	1.57	5.18**	.75	1.38	1.09	6.83***	1.45	5.02**	2.98	1.59	4.02*
Within													
Time (T)	1	2.55**	3.12	1.02	5.84*	1.07	1.21	0.07	10.66***	0.01	3.94*	3.12	3.38
A × T	1	0.33	0.17	0.35	1.93	0.03	0.00	0.67	0.08	0.02	0.00	0.45	0.16
B × T	2	1.15	0.33	2.03	1.07	0.09	2.26	1.16	0.65	0.34	0.70	2.01	1.65
A × B × T	2	1.18	0.66	3.74*	0.39	1.51	1.60	0.49	1.69	0.82	1.63	1.17	2.82

[a]Based on repeated measures over Waves 1 and 2, waves showing the greatest differences. Based on $N = 694$, with listwise deletion of cases with any missing data at any of the four waves.
*$p < .05$. **$p < .01$. ***$p < .001$.

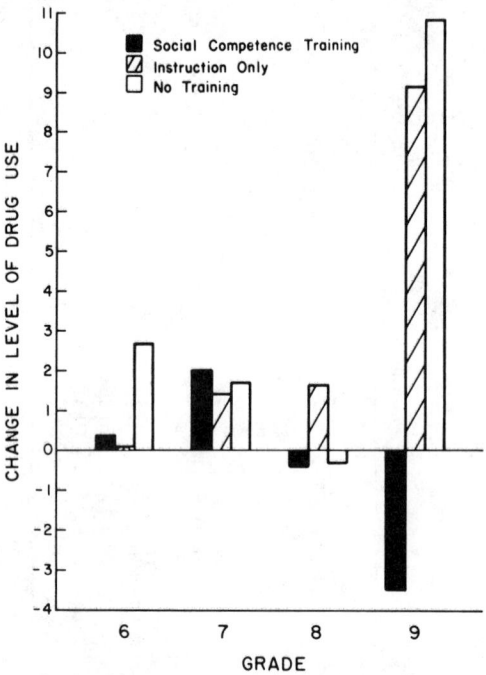

Figure 5.2 Changes in total drug use from pre- to posttraining as a function of grade. Drug use represents a standardized and summed index of frequency and amount of cigarette, beer, wine, and liquor use from Wave 1 and Wave 2. $N = 692$.

as a set of demographic variables; see Kerlinger & Pedhauzer, 1973) and multivariate and univariate analysis of variance. Results of the regression analyses conducted on Wave 1 data indicated that demographic characteristics (male sex and higher age), social competence (lack of self-efficacy and social skills), social attitude (negative scores on the five scales), and drug use influence (peer use, parent use, sanction for use, availability of drugs) contributed significantly to actual drug use and intention to use drugs (from 37 to 70% of the variance; see Table 5.2). This pattern was repeated across subsequent waves.

Despite the similarities, several differences were found. Analyses of variance showed that suburban students reported greater adult sanction of alcohol use than rural students ($p < .001$). In multiple regression analyses on the rural sample, the main contribution to drug use was low social competence, and to a lesser extent, demographic characteristics of students. In the suburban sample, drug use was affected by a broader range of variables, including to a great degree, peer and parent uses, sanction for use and

Table 5.2
ACTUAL DRUG USE: F CHANGE VALUES[a]

Variable	Suburban				Rural			
	Cig.	Beer	Wine	Liquor	Cig.	Beer	Wine	Liquor
Demographic characteristics	0.62	2.68	3.10*	2.69	4.43**	4.76**	2.03	1.60
Social competence	2.97*	1.74	2.45*	1.10	9.09****	10.76****	21.74****	25.25****
Social attitude	3.62**	8.20****	4.93****	7.96****	3.24**	0.40	1.72	2.06
Drug use influence	25.82****	29.57****	13.58****	11.00****	0.49	0.27	0.34	0.34
Overall F	11.00****	15.90****	7.95****	7.79	4.65****	3.72***	6.97****	8.20****
Multiple R	.79	.84	.74	.73	.65	.61	.72	.75
Total R^2	.62	.70	.54	.54	.42	.37	.52	.56
Cross-sample R	.42****	.51****	.46****	.41****	.39****	.67****	.50****	.41****

[a]Based on matched subsample of seventh- and eighth-grade students (147 suburban, 134 rural). Cross-sample R refers to the application of beta weights generated on one sample to the regression model for the other sample. Significance means that the variables account for a similar good fit, regardless of the sample used.
*$p < .05$. **$p < .01$. ***$p < .001$. ****$p < .0001$.

availability. Analyses of training effects also produced these differences, showing an Environment × Training interaction. Before training, suburban students reported higher peer and parent drug use and more negative social attitudes than rural students (p ranged from $<.01$ to $<.0001$); after training, suburban students in training groups reported lower peer use than rural students in training groups, but rural students reported greater increases in grade point average ($p < .05$). Differences were maintained over four waves. There were no interactive effects on actual drug use behavior.

Conclusions

Results of this phase of the study confirm a relationship between social competence and drug use prevention. Social competence training, in interaction with individual behavior and grade, produced increases in social competence and academic achievement, and decreases in drug use and intention. To a lesser extent, environment characteristics also had an effect. Social competence training had a greater effect on drug use in rural versus suburban students.

The interactive effects obtained argue strongly for the development of training strategies tailored to meet the individual and environmental characteristics of adolescents. For example, the fact that aggressive and assertive students benefited most from training suggests that they might be more actively involved in modeling and rehearsal activities than unassertive students. Given this finding, future research should investigate methods for increasing participation of unassertive and other reluctant students, perhaps by providing incentives or prompts for active participation in role playing. In addition, the fact that training effectiveness decreased over time relative to instructions suggests that booster sessions focused on active role playing might be required to maintain program effects with this age group.

In terms of Grade × Training interactions, results suggest that early adolescents who are experiencing multiple transitions (in this case, school as well as trade transitions) may be particularly receptive to drug abuse prevention efforts. This view is consistent with Jessor's notion of "transition proneness" (1982). To test this hypothesis, further research is needed to unconfound grade from school changes. For example, training effectiveness could be compared for sixth-grade students in 6–7–8 middle-school structures versus sixth-grade students in K–6 elementary school structures. A subsequent confirmation of heightened training receptiveness during periods of transition would help focus future prevention efforts and improve the cost effectiveness of prevention programming.

Finally, the rural and suburban differences obtained suggest that future prevention programs be tailored to communities by type and breadth of content. Specifically, students in suburban communities may need more training sessions devoted to changing rebelliousness and resisting drug use influences. Students in rural communities, on the other hand, may require a broader introduction to types of drug use influences they may encounter in the future.

IMPLICATIONS FOR FUTURE RESEARCH

Results of this study offer support for a competence–prevention rather than a defect–remediation model of drug use. The causal modeling analyses indicated that greater drug use led to decreases in self-efficacy, and through self-efficacy, to decreases in social skills. The multivariate analyses conducted on experimental groups supported both hypotheses: (1) that social competence training would increase social competence, improve school behavior, and decrease drug use; and (2) that training effects would interact with individual behavior style, grade and with environment (type of community). These findings argue strongly for the inclusion of social competence training in formative educational curricula for our youth, and for tailoring curricula to the individual needs of youthful populations to be served. However, the findings also point to several issues that should be addressed in future research. These include the extent of bidirectional relationships in drug use, the balance between individualizing and generalizing of training for drug abuse prevention, developmental stability of drug use levels and prevention effects, and the testing of alternative models of prevention.

The issue of bidirectional relationships bears directly on two specific findings from the present study. One finding is that drug use is negatively and causally related to subsequent self-efficacy and social skills and that social competence training decreases subsequent drug use. The sequence suggests that drug use may increase rather than alleviate stress: that is, early drug use lowers social competence and thus perhaps the ability to cope with subsequent interpersonal stressors like peer pressure to use drugs; social competence training increases social competence (by implication, coping ability) and lowers subsequent drug use. However, further research is needed to confirm a sequential bidirectional relationship. Such research should include concurrent measures of coping, physiological measures of stress, and comparison of social competence training with prevention programs that are focused directly on drug use.

The other finding is that drug use behavior, but not intention to use drugs, is related to social competence. This appears to conflict with research that has already demonstrated a strong causal relationship between intention and subsequent drug use (e.g., Chassin, Corty, Presson, & Olshavsky,

1981). To resolve this issue, future research should focus on directly comparing intentions and behavior for their relationship to social competence and as targets for social competence training. In addition, information-processing research is needed as it relates to drug use. Specifically, epidemiological and prevention studies should evaluate the developmental sequencing of decision making at different stages of drug use (see Froman & Hubert, 1980).

A second issue is the balance to be achieved in drug abuse prevention programming between tailoring program components to specific characteristics of adolescents (for maximizing program effects) and generalizability (for minimizing program costs). Currently, little is known about individual characteristics other than behavior and grade that could influence program outcome (e.g., personalities of trainers, support of parents) and other environment characteristics that could jeopardize replication of program effects (e.g., changing feeder patterns, communities that support treatment more than prevention). Furthermore, the effects of individual and environment characteristics on how drug use is conceptualized (i.e., whether it is a problem warranting intervention) is also open to question (see Kim, 1982; Levine & Kozak, 1979; Winfree et al., 1981). These questions need to be addressed before limits of program tailoring and generalizability can be tested.

Another issue that warrants further research is the developmental stability of social competence and drug use constructs and, consequently, prevention effectiveness. Whether or not the meaning and importance of social competence changes for an adolescent over time, and whether its effects on subsequent behaviors like drug use change in immediacy or strength, can be examined by several means. For example, factor structures can be examined for qualitative and quantitative invariance over time (Cunningham, 1982). Multiple measures of drug use and social competence can be administered over different behavioral domains and settings; the resultant data are then summed and weighted to yield cognitive and behavioral stability scores (see Bentler & Speckhart, 1979; Epstein, 1980). Social competence and drug use might be evaluated across several experimental laboratories as well as areas of adolescent functioning (Levenson & Gottman, 1978). This may be particularly important in determining agreement of what is meant by social competence (vs. aggression and extraversion, for example) and drug use (vs. abuse), assessing replicability of training effects, and evaluating generalizability across geographic and demographic areas. Finally, fine-grained developmental changes, such as weekly changes in social competence that may occur as an adolescent begins dating, can be evaluated by time series analyses (see Froman & Hubert, 1980).

A final issue that is relatively unexplored is the relative efficacy of drug abuse prevention programs that are based on different models of drug use. For example, it is not known whether a generic social competence program is more effective than a drug use resistance skills program or one that empirically tests and combines both approaches. It may be that a dual focus on drug use-specific variables (e.g., changing normative expectations about friends' use of drugs) *and* social competence might maximize the benefits to be derived from a drug abuse prevention program. To date, prevention programs have tended to focus on either inoculation and resistance to drugs (e.g., McAlister, Perry, & Maccoby, 1979), social competence in nondrug use situations (e.g., Pentz, 1983a), or a content—rather than empirically—determined combination of both (e.g., Botvin et al., 1980). An additional consideration is the relative effectiveness of programs that are based on a life-span view of drug use development rather than a critical periods perspective. For example, is long-term program effectivenss increased with training that includes an adolescent's family members or with training that is reported at early and mid-adulthood (see Grinder, 1982)? Finally, further pursuit of drug abuse prevention research requires basic assessment of the validity and reliability of programs that are based on different models of helping and coping, for example, teaching students how to compensate for friends' drug use and pressure to use drugs versus enlightening students about how they can influence each other positively (Brickman et al., 1982).

REFERENCES

Albee, G. (1981). Preventing prevention in the community mental health centers. In H. Resnik, C. Ashton, & C. Palley (Eds.), *The health care system and drug abuse prevention: Toward cooperation and health promotion*. Rockville, MD: National Institute on Drug Abuse.

Aneshensel, C. S., & Huba, G. J. (1983). Depression, alcohol use, and smoking over one year: A four-wave longitudinal causal model. *Journal of Abnormal Psychology, 92*, 134–150.

Archer, E., & Arundell, R. (1983). A measuring instrument for use in drug education programs: Development of the McLeod High Risk Inventory. *Journal of Drug Education, 8*, 313–326.

Bandura, A. (1977). Self-efficacy: Toward a unifying theory of behavioral change. *Psychological Review, 84*, 191–215.

Bentler, P. M. (1980). Multivariate analysis with latent variables: Causal modeling. In M. R. Rosenzweig & L. W. Porter (Eds.), *Annual Review of Psychology*. Palo Alto, CA.: Annual Reviews, Inc.

Bentler, P. M., & Speckhart, G. (1979). Models of attitude-behavior relations. *Psychological Review, 86*, 452–464.

Botvin, G., Eng, A., & Williams, C. (1980). Preventing the onset of cigarette smoking through life skills training. *Preventive Medicine, 9*, 135–143.

Brickman, P., Rabinowitz, V. C., Karuza, J., Coates, D., Cohn, E., & Kidder, L. (1982). Models of helping and coping. *American Psychologist, 37*, 368–384.

Bry, B., & George, F. E. (1980). The preventive effects of early intervention on the attendance and grades of urban adolescents. *Professional Psychology, 11*, 250–260.

Chassin, L., Corty, E., Presson, C. C., Olshavsky, R. W., Bensenberg, M., Sherman, S. J. (1981). Predicting adolescents' intentions to smoke cigarettes. *Journal of Health and Social Behavior, 22,* 445–455.

Cunningham, W. R. (1982). Factorial invariance: A methodological issue in the study of psychological development. *Experimental Aging Research, 8,* 61–65.

Dunnette, M. (1978). Individual prediction as a strategy for discovering demographic and interpersonal/psychosocial correlates of drug resistance and abuse. In D. Kandel (Ed.), *Longitudinal research on drug use.* Washington: DC: Hemisphere.

Epstein, S. (1980). The stability of behavior: II. Implications for psychological research. *American Psychologist, 35,* 790–806.

Ford, M. E. (1982). Social cognition and social competence in adolescence. *Developmental Psychology, 3,* 323–340.

Froman, T., & Hubert, L. J. (1980). Application of prediction analysis to developmental priority. *Psychological Bulletin, 87,* 136–146.

Gardner, E., & Thompson, G. (1958). *The Syracuse scales of social relations.* New York: World Books.

Gilchrist, L. O. (1981). Social competence in adolescence. In S. P. Schinke (Ed.), *Behavioral methods in social welfare.* New York: Aldine.

Goldstein, A. P., & Pentz, M. A. (1984). Psychological skill training and the aggressive adolescent: *School Psychological Review, 13,* 311–323.

Goldstein, A. P. (1979). Sprafkin, R. P., Gershaw, N. J., & Klein, P. *Skill-streaming the adolescent: A structured learned approach to teaching prosocial behavior.* Champaign, IL: Research Press.

Grinder, R. E. (1982). Isolationism in adolescent research. *Human Development, 25,* 223–232.

Heller, K., Price, R. H., & Sher, K. J. (1983). Research and evaluation in primary prevention: Issues and guidelines. In R. H. Price, R. F. Ketterer, B. C. Bader, & J. Monahan (Eds.), *Prevention in mental health: Research, policy, and practice.* Beverly Hills: Sage.

Huba, G. J., & Bentler, P. M. (1980). *Questionnaire from the UCLA Longitudinal Growth Study, Wave IV-Year V.* Unpublished manuscript.

Huba, G. J., & Bentler, P. M. (1982). A developmental theory of drug use: Derivation and assessment of a causal modeling approach. In P. B. Baltes & O. G. Brim, Jr. (Eds.), *Lifespan development and behavior* (Vol. 4). New York: Academic Press.

Hurd, P. D., Johnson, C. A., Leupker, R. V., Pechacek, T. F., & Jacobs, D. R. (1980). Prevention of cigarette smoking in seventh grade students. *Journal of Behavioral Medicine, 3,* 15–28.

Jessor, R. (1982). Problem behavior and developmental transition in adolescence. *Journal of School Health, 52,* 295–300.

Jessor, R., & Jessor, S. L. (1977). *Problem behavior and psychosocial development: A longitudinal study.* New York: Academic Press.

Johnson, C. A. (1983). Untested and erroneous assumptions underlying anti-smoking programs. In T. Coates, A. Petersen, & C. Perry (Eds.), *Promoting adolescent health.* New York: Academic Press.

Johnston, L. D., Bachman, J. G., & O'Malley, P. M. (1980). *Highlights from student drug use in America, 1975–1980.* Rockville, MD: National Institute on Drug Abuse.

Jöreskog, K. G. (1979). Statistical estimation of structural models in longitudinal developmental investigations. In J. R. Nesselroade & P. B. Baltes (Eds.), *Longitudinal research in the study of behavior and development.* New York: Academic Press.

Kahle, L. R., Klingel, D. M., & Kulka, R. A. (1981). A longitudinal study of adolescents' attitude-behavior consistency. *Public Opinion Quarterly, 45,* 402–414.

Kandel, D. (1975). The measurement of "ever use" and "frequency-quality" (in drug use surveys). In J. Elinson & D. Nurco (Eds.), *Operational definitions in socio-behavioral drug use research*. Rockville, MD: National Institute on Drug Abuse.

Kandel, D. B., Kessler, R. C., & Margulies, R. Z. (1978). Antecedents of adolescent initiation into stages of drug use: A developmental analysis. In D. B. Kandel (Ed.), *Longitudinal research on drug use*. Washington, DC: Hemisphere.

Kellam, S. G., Brown, C. H., & Fleming, J. P. (1982). Social adaptation to first grade and teenage drug, alcohol, and cigarette use. *Journal of School Health, 52,* 301–306.

Kelly, J. G. (Ed.). (1980). *Adolescent boys in high school: A psychological study of coping and adaptation*. New York: Wiley.

Kerlinger, F. N., & Pedhazur, E. J. (1973). *Multiple regression in behavioral research*. New York: Holt, Rinehart.

Kim, S. (1981). Feeder area approach: An impact evaluation of a prevention project on student drug abuse. *International Journal of the Addictions, 17,* 305–313.

Lazarus, R. S., Averill, J. R., & Option, E. M., Jr. (1974). The psychology of coping: Issues of research and assessment. In G. V. Coelho, D. A. Hamburg, & J. E. Adams (Eds.), *Coping and adaptation*. New York: Basic Books.

Levenson, R. W., & Gottman, J. M. (1978). Toward the assessment of social competence. *Journal of Consulting and Clinical Psychology, 46,* 453–462.

Levine, E., & Kozak, C. (1979). Drug and alcohol use, delinquency and vandalism among upper middle class pre- and post-adolescents. *Journal of Youth and Adolescence, 8,* 91–102.

Luepker, R. V., Johnson, C. A., Murray, D. M., & Pechacek, T. F. (1983). Prevention of cigarette smoking: Three year follow-up of an educational program for youth. *Journal of Behavioral Medicine, 6,* 53–62.

Masterpasqua, F. (1981). Toward a synergism of developmental and community psychology. *American Psychologist, 36,* 782–786.

McAlister, A. L., Perry, C., & Maccoby, N. (1979). Adolescent smoking: Onset and prevention. *Pediatrics, 63,* 650–658.

Meichenbaum, D., Butler, L., & Gruson, L. (1981). Toward a conceptual model of social competence. In J. D. Wine & M. D. Smye (Eds.), *Social competence*. New York: Guilford Press.

Parkes, C. M. (1971). Psycho-social transitions: A field for study. *Journal of Social Science Medicine, 5,* 101–115.

Pentz, M. A. (1980). Assertion training and trainer effects on unassertive and aggressive adolescents. *Journal of Counseling Psychology, 27,* 76–83.

Pentz, M. A. (1981). The contribution of individual differences to assertion training outcome in adolescents. *Journal of Counseling Psychology, 28,* 529–532.

Pentz, M. A. (1982, August). *Adolescent drug use prevention training: Hard knocks and other lessons*. Paper presented at the annual meeting of the American Psychological Association, Washington, DC.

Pentz, M. A. (1983a, August). *Preventive intervention for aggression and drug use in adolescents*. Paper presented at the annual meeting of the American Psychological Association, Los Angeles.

Pentz, M. A. (1983b). Prevention of adolescent substance abuse through social skill development. In C. Leukefeld & T. Glynn (Eds.), *Preventing adolescent drug abuse: Intervention strategies* (Research Monograph Series). Rockville, MD: National Institute on Drug Abuse.

Pentz, M. A., & Huba, G. J. (1984). *Adolescent drug use, social skills, and self-efficacy over two years: A four-wave longitudinal causal model*. Unpublished manuscript.

Pentz, M. A., & Kazdin, A. E. (1982). Assertion modeling and stimuli effects on assertive behavior and self-efficacy in adolescents. *Behaviour Research and Therapy, 20,* 1–7.

Pentz, M. A., Leong, C., & Pentz, C. A. (1984). *Predicting attrition in prevention research.* Unpublished manuscript.

Pentz, M. A., & Tolan, P. (1984). *Social skills training with adolescents: A review of time trends, dimensions, and outcome, 1974–1984.* Unpublished manuscript.

Perry, C. L. (1983). Tobacco use among adolescents: Promising trends in prevention and cessation strategies. In T. C. Coates (Ed.), *Behavioral medicine: A practical handbook.* Champaign, IL: Research Press.

Perry, C., Killen, J., Telch, M., Slinkard, L., & Danaher, B. (1980). Modifying smoking behavior of teenagers: A school-based intervention. *American Journal of Public Health, 70,* 722–725.

Perry, C. L., & Murray, D. M. (1982). Enhancing the transition years: The challenge of adolescent health promotion. *Journal of School Health, 52,* 307–311.

Piaget, J., & Inhelder, B. (1969). *The psychology of the child.* New York: Basic Books.

Quay, H. C., & Quay, L. C. (1965). Behavior problems in early adolescence. *Child Development, 36,* 215–220.

Radius, S. M., Dillman, T. E., Becker, M. H., Rosenstock, I. M., & Horvath, W. J. (1980). Adolescent perspectives on health and illness. *Adolescence, 58,* 375–384.

Rosenthal, T., & Bandura, A. (1978). Psychological modeling: Theory and practice. In S. L. Garfield & A. E. Bergin (Eds.), *Handbook of psychotherapy and behavior change.* New York: Wiley.

Sanchez-Craig, B. M. (1976). Cognitive and behavioral coping strategies in the reappraisal of stressful social situations. *Journal of Counseling Psychology, 23,* 7–12.

Schinke, S. P., & Gilchrist, L. D. (1983). Primary prevention of tobacco smoking. *Journal of School Health, 53,* 416–419.

Wandersman, A., & Florin, P. (1981). A cognitive social learning approach to the crossroads of cognition, social behavior and the environment. In J. Karvey (Ed.), *Cognition, social behavior and the environment.* Hillsdale NJ: Erlbaum.

Winfree, L. T., Theis, H. E., & Griffiths, C. T. (1981). Drug use in rural America: A cross-cultural examination of complementary social deviance theories. *Youth and Society, 12,* 465–489.

Wolpe, J. (1958). *Psychotherapy by reciprocal inhibition.* Stanford, CA: Stanford University Press.

Wrubel, J., Benner, P., & Lazarus, R. S. (1981). Social competence from the perspective of stress and coping. In J. D. Wine & M. D. Smye (Eds.), *Social competence.* New York: Guilford Press.

Part III

COPING AND ONGOING SUBSTANCE USE IN ADULT SAMPLES

The following part presents reports from three pioneering investigations that employed measures of stress and coping and related these to alcohol, tranquilizer, and opiate use in samples of community-residing adults. The intent of these studies is to use the approach of social epidemiology (Dohrenwend & Dohrenwend, 1969; Leighton, Harding, & Macklin, 1963; Srole, Langner, Michael, Opler, & Rennie, 1961), obtaining data from representative samples to examine the relationship between coping and substance use as it occurs in the natural environment of the respondents. The populations of respondents for the studies vary from a representative national sample of normal adults interviewed in their homes, to a national sample of opiate addicts surveyed in treatment, to a small sample of middle-aged community adults who provided daily data on coping over a 3-month period. The types of coping measured in these studies are what would generally be termed stress-coping skills: ways of dealing with anger or depression, social support, direct action and problem solving, and passive or avoidance coping strategies.

Tucker, in Chapter 6, reports findings from a study of male and female opiate addicts in treatment. This research examined the relationship of coping variables both to current rates of drug use and to particularly adverse outcomes such as drug overdose. In this research program, the basic focus was on social versus nonsocial coping strategies; the results showed a clear distinction, with coping through social support generally related to more favorable outcomes, whereas coping through withdrawal was generally related to adverse outcomes. Tucker's research is noteworthy because she examined both target and source differences, finding that the correlations between coping and drug use are different for males and females, and also noting that different sources of social support (e.g., mate support vs. family and/or relative support) have quite different effects in this population.

Timmer, Veroff, and Colten, in Chapter 7, report analyses of data from a major social epidemiology study: a national survey of a representative sample of 2,264 adults conducted in 1976. These researchers investigated coping mechanisms identified through research with community samples, including social support, passive coping, and prayer. They also collected data on current stressors experienced by the respondents in three different life domains: finances, marital relationship, and job situation. In this study, the focus was on alcohol or tranquilizer use that was explicitly construed by respondents as a means of relieving tension, that is, substance use as a coping mechanism. The results of these analyses provide a number of interesting suggestions about the determinants of substance use. The data consistently show perceived stress to be related to the use of alcohol and tranquilizers to cope, and indicate that some alternative coping mechanisms such as social support and religion-based coping may reduce the tendency to cope through substance use. At the same time, results obtained with these measures show considerable complexity, suggesting substantial differences in the dynamics of alcohol and tranquilizer use, sex differences in patterns of coping, and interactions between different stressors and coping mechanisms.

Stone and Neale (Chapter 8) obtained large amounts of data through daily observations with a small sample of community-residing adults. These investigators employed a comprehensive inventory of coping mechanisms to examine the relationship between coping with daily problems and alcohol use status as determined through a retrospective interview. This study found that some coping mechanisms, such as social support and emotional catharsis, were used less often by the persons classified as heavy drinkers. Also, the researchers coded subjects' reports of coping episodes and found that when alcohol was employed as a means of coping, it was most often construed as either relaxation or distraction.

The results of this research may be useful from a number of perspectives. Findings from large, representative samples have an inherent validity and must be considered carefully when evaluating theoretical propositions about substance use. The methodologies used in these studies can be applied with other samples or types of substances, and some patterns of results may suggest alternative approaches to the study of coping and substance use. Also, the demonstrated value of epidemiological approaches in both medical, psychological, and substance-related research may encourage other researchers to obtain new knowledge about substance use through further research in this area.

REFERENCES

Dohrenwend, B. P., & Dohrenwend, B. S. (1969). *Social status and psychological disorder.* New York: Wiley.

Leighton, D. C., Harding, J. S., & Macklin, D. B. (1963). *The character of danger: The Stirling County Study.* New York: Basic Books.

Srole, L., Langner, T. S., Michael, S. T., Opler, M. K., & Rennie, T. A. C. (1961). *Mental health in the metropolis: The Midtown Manhattan Study.* New York: McGraw-Hill.

Chapter 6

Coping and Drug Use among Heroin-Addicted Women and Men*

M. BELINDA TUCKER

INTRODUCTION

An understanding of the relationship between coping and substance abuse must take into account the larger social distinctions among the population of substance users. It is widely recognized by substance abuse researchers that drug use patterns differ substantially on the basis of gender, ethnicity, socioeconomic status, and age (Austin, Johnson, Carroll, & Lettieri, 1977; Gomberg, 1982; Johnson & Nishi, 1976; Kalant, 1980). Although empirical evidence is scant, there is reason to believe that coping patterns are similarly distinctive. Despite early theoretical recognition of demographic differences in drug use patterns, discussion of the relationship between demographic characteristics and coping has been virtually nonexistent. (For a review of drug theories see Lettieri, Sayers, & Pearson, 1980.) As a beginning in what must become a more comprehensive analysis of this neglected issue, this chapter focuses on the role of gender in the relation between coping behavior and drug use patterns.

For a number of reasons, the issue of coping is particularly germane to an understanding of women's drug use and abuse. The history of substance use by women, as distinct from that of men, has been characterized by use for therapeutic purposes (Gomberg, 1982). Drug use by women is accompanied by more self-perceived problems than that of male use (Tucker, 1979). Female drug abusers are held in much lower societal esteem (Colten, 1982) and are often found to be more psychologically disturbed than male abusers

*This work was supported by grants from the National Institute on Drug Abuse (# H81–DA–01496 and # H81–DA–01939) and an Institute of American Cultures Award through the UCLA Center for Afro-American Studies. The author gratefully acknowledges the comments of the editors on a draft of this chapter.

(Burt, Glynn, & Sowder, 1979; Prather & Fidell, 1978). Finally, some evidence suggests that women's coping styles in general are less effective than those used by men (Moos & Billings, 1982; Pearlin & Schooler, 1978). In the discussion that follows, these points are placed within the context of a model of stress and coping relevant to female addiction (Tucker, 1982). Data on coping and drug use from a study of women and men heroin addicts are used to illustrate the utility of the model for understanding general coping patterns in the context of addiction to drugs.

WOMEN'S USE OF DRUGS: PREVALENCE AND RESEARCH

Despite a surge of interest evident in the mid-1970s, substance abuse by women is still poorly understood and insufficiently addressed. The scientific and popular literatures, so heavily focused on male addicts, convey the image that drug use, particularly abuse of the so-called hard drugs, is primarily the domain of men. (The single exception is women's use of psychotropic, or mood modifying, drugs, which far exceeds that of men [Cooperstock, 1978; Prather & Fidell, 1978; Verbrugge, 1982]). One widely used indicator of drug abuse in the United States, statistics on admissions to federally funded drug abuse treatment programs, demonstrates that serious drug involvement by women is not inconsequential. In 1981, 28% of all clients admitted to such programs were women (National Institute of Drug Abuse [NIDA], 1982). Although the percentage has remained fairly stable over recent years, the total number of women in treatment has increased steadily, from 56,000 clients in 1977 (NIDA, 1980) to 70,000 in 1981 (NIDA, 1982). However, the rate of opiate addiction among women has increased over the past 20 years at a faster rate than that of men (Burt et al., 1979; Prather & Fidell, 1978). Contemporary opiate addicts tend to be largely urban, poor, and disproportionately ethnic minorities (Tucker, in press).

Clearly, these statistics represent the problem only partially, as they include only individuals seeking help from public agencies and exclude private treatment efforts. Professionals, such as nurses or physicians, and the more well-to-do are simply not likely to seek treatment at public facilities. Such statistics probably underestimate women's heroin addiction to an even greater extent, since women are less likely than men to come to the attention of the criminal justice system (a major source of opiate treatment referrals), may be more protected by families, and are often not attracted to the traditional drug treatment approaches that may neglect the special needs of women (Cuskey, Berger, & Densen-Gerber, 1977; Prather & Fidell, 1978).

In response to recognized limitations of research on women's substance use, the Women's Drug Research Project (WDR) was initiated in 1975, through funding by the National Institute on Drug Abuse, to coordinate research efforts underway at drug abuse demonstration programs designed to attend to the special needs of female clients. Eventually the project was broadened to include the assessment of very detailed psychosocial data on attitudes, psychological states, family and personal history, personal relationships, parenting, and problem resolution techniques. The research was also expanded to include the collection of the entire battery of questions on women and men entering traditional drug treatment centers. The present study is based on these latter data.

PSYCHOLOGICAL PERSPECTIVES ON FEMALE ADDICTION

The theoretical core of this study draws upon research and thought from several areas relevant to the coping behavior of female drug abusers: psychological perspectives on female addiction, gender differences in drug use behavior, and gender differences in coping. Previous psychological perspectives on female heroin addiction have emphasized its "pathological" nature (Marsh, Colten, & Tucker, 1982). Although a focus on individual pathology is evident in reports on both male and female substance abuse, views on female addicts have been more extreme. One review demonstrated that not one study has shown that female addicts function better than male addicts; either differences were minimal or women were found to be "worse off" than men (Burt et al., 1979). Research in this area has been criticized, however, on methodological grounds and for viewing deviations from stereotyped feminine roles as pathological indicators (Burt et al., 1979; Prather & Fidell, 1978).

Other hypothesized psychological determinants of heroin abuse among both women and men include sensation seeking and the desire to feel good. The latter is strongly suggestive of a coping function, or what Alexander and Hadaway (1982) refer to as the adaptive function of drug use. Although research has not addressed the question of gender differences in the use of heroin as a coping mechanism, case histories suggest that when the motivation for use is coping, the functional properties are the same for both sexes. For example, a representative description of subjective heroin effects by female addicts in the Bahna and Gordon (1978) study of rehabilitation experiences was, "While you're high you have only good thoughts because you can select your own thoughts and push away any bad feelings" (p. 652). Similarly, Khantzian, Mack, and Schatzberg (1974) noted clinical reports of male subjective reactions to heroin that include, "[I felt] relaxed—mellow—and didn't think about bad things on dope" (p. 160). One patient said heroin helped him deal with feelings of loneliness, noting that "things don't penetrate when you're on heroin" (p. 162). Another noted that heroin helped him feel better when he was angry, nervous, or depressed.

Although there may be little difference in motivations for the use of heroin as a coping mechanism by men and women, other evidence suggests that at least the extent of use for such purposes should differ. Previous research indicates that women on drugs are subjected to more stress than are men; they experience more problems, particularly those of a medical nature (Tucker, 1979), and more disruptive life events (Verbrugge, 1982). Women addicts have also been found to be more socially isolated and lonelier than either addicted men or socioeconomically similar nonaddicted women (Rhoads, 1983; Tucker, 1979). Furthermore, it seems plausible that some of these observed adverse psychological states could be consequences (rather than causes) of the experience of being an addicted women (Colten, 1979).

Although there have been few empirical studies of gender differences in substance use, some trends can be noted in the available evidence. Although the rate of illicit drug use by women is lower than that of men, the difference is minimal in younger populations; women are usually initiated into illicit drug use by men; and women are more likely to use psychotherapeutic drugs such as tranquilizers (Suffet & Brotman, 1976; Prather & Fidell, 1978). A study by Ryser (1983), based on the Drug Abuse Early Warning Network data set drawn from hospital emergency room cases and coroners' reports, found a similarity in the drugs most frequently used over a 4-year period, although sex differences existed in the rank orderings within each year. Among persons who reported using drugs because of their psychological effects, some changes over time were noted for men (a shift from opiates toward PCP), but a female preference for diazepam (Valium) remained constant. The findings, interpreted in the context of the available literature on gender differences in drug use, suggest that women who abuse drugs may be attempting to achieve psychic effects that are qualitatively different from those desired by men. Although this study was based on a crisis sample, the results suggest a sex difference in coping patterns, since preferences for different drugs suggest different coping needs.

Although the evidence of gender differences in coping is scant, as noted in the work on the psychology of female drug abuse, existing research suggests that women's coping preferences are deficient relative to those used by men. Pearlin and Schooler (1978), in their analysis of the structure of coping, found that women were more likely than men to use coping strategies that might exacerbate stress (e.g., selective ignoring). The researchers also suggest that the general finding that women are more psychologically disturbed than men may actually be the result of women's failure (due to socialization differences) to use more effective coping patterns. This latter point is especially significant in light of the findings described earlier on the psychological characteristics of female drug abusers.

Other theoretical statements suggest similar deficits. Moos and Billings (1982) emphasize the difference in the coping behaviors of people who are field dependent versus those who are field independent. The former, while more attuned to the social environment, tend to use global defenses, such as turning against the self, whereas a field-independent person would turn against the object. Field-dependent people may turn to the environment for readily available solutions, as evidenced by the fact that alcoholics are more field dependent than nonalcoholics. Moos and Billings state that the literature shows that women tend to be more field dependent than men. Interestingly, an earlier study by Arnon, Kleinman, and Kissin (1974) found that while both male and female heroin addicts were significantly more field dependent than "normal" subjects, female addicts were significantly more field dependent than either female controls or male addicts. In view of Moos and Billings' assertions, these findings suggest that heroin-addicted women are particularly prone to using dysfunctional coping strategies.

There is evidence, however, that the relationship between gender and coping behavior is more complex that the above findings imply. Folkman and Lazarus (1980) found that men used more problem-focused rather than emotion-focused coping than women when at work, in situations that required additional information, and in situations that had to be accepted. However, the researchers found that different situations favored different strategies, for example, work contexts favored problem-focused coping, whereas health problems and situations that must be accepted (rather than changed) favored emotion-focused coping, and certain situations were more often encountered by one sex than the other. It appears, then, that greater refinement of research strategies in this area is needed to ascertain whether men and women do use different coping behaviors and what the situational determinants of such differences might be.

A MODEL OF STRESS AND COPING RELEVANT TO FEMALE ADDICTION

The model is based on the assumption of an interplay between psychological tendencies and environmental demands and explores the relationship between coping, stress, and social support in heroin-addicted women and men (Tucker, 1982). The theoretical paradigm uses general conceptions of the role of social support as a stress buffer or mediator but incorporates a central focus on the coping response used to confront stress (see Figure 6.1). For example, the usefulness of available social support may be contingent upon the individual's ability and willingness to utilize such aid in order to cope. As previous conceptualizations of social support and stress were limited by the failure to consider individual coping behaviors, this feature of the model is presented as an enhancement of the traditional explication of the social support–stress paradigm. The model operates as follows: Individual strain is caused by stressful events and or conditions, thus necessitating a coping response. The psychological or physical outcome is a function of the adequacy of the coping response. Social support is viewed as one of a number of resources that can significantly affect the process of coping with individual strain in a number of ways: by influencing the occurrence of a stressful event or condition (e.g., support systems can actually prevent certain negative situations); by influencing the individual's perception of strain (e.g., when several people share a problem, it may not seem as onerous); and by influencing the individual's psychological and/or physical outcome (e.g., the system may tend directly to the individual's resultant physical or mental needs). Social support may also mediate the relation between stressful events or conditions and individual strain (e.g., by altering appraisal of negative events) and may mediate the relation between individual strain and choice of coping response (e.g., by encouraging selection of a particular coping strategy). The system is also bidirectional at points: Individual strain as well as individual outcome can influence the ability of the social support system to act (e.g., an extreme outcome may discourage involvement by some members of the system).

The social support–stress–coping model was partially tested by research (Tucker, 1982) which examined (1) the extent to which the availability of social relationships is related to the use of social coping mechanisms, (2) the extent to which the unavailability of social relationships is related to the use

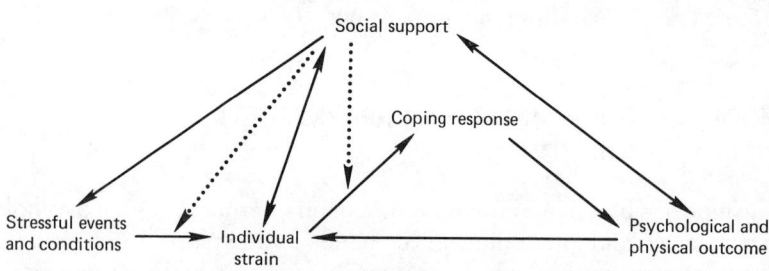

Figure 6.1 Social support–stress–coping paradigm.

Table 6.1
COPING QUESTIONNAIRE ITEMS AND DRUG USE MEASURES

QUESTIONNAIRE ITEMS

When you really get (upset or angry/depressed or feel down), what do you do about it? Do you (answer yes or no):
  a. lose your temper and yell (angry)/go to bed (depressed)?
  b. talk over things with your mother or some other female relative?
  c. talk over things with your father or some other male relative?
  d. get away from where you are or go off by yourself?
  e. talk over things with your partner or husband/wife?
  f. talk over things with a friend or neighbor?
  g. just stick it out?
  h. take it out on your children (like by punishing or yelling at them)?
  i. drink alcohol?
  j. take drugs?
  k. do something else? (What is that?)

DRUG USE MEASURES (instructions to intake worker)

Using the following drug descriptor(s), . . . describe the first drug the client used, the client's preferred drug, and all the drugs used by the client in the last two years in order of (frequency of) abuse.
  a. type drug (13 broad categories, 61 subcategories)
  b. current frequency: less than once a week, once a week, several times a week, daily
  c. time when last used: within last 3 months, 3–12 months ago, over 12 months ago
  d. current situation: in private, with other people, no current use
  e. number of overdoses: actual number, from 1–7

of nonsocial and potentially dysfunctional coping strategies (including substance use), and (3) the patterns of relations between coping strategies and support availability as differentiated by gender. Social support was measured by a series of items referring to relationships in general and specific dyadic ties (i.e., number of good friends, friends in neighborhood, availability of aid for everyday problems, romantic involvements, best friends). The coping measures are the same as those used in the present work and are listed in Table 6.1. The findings generally supported the model and showed the following results:

1. Lack of support was especially related to the use of dysfunctional coping strategies for women (e.g., withdrawal, substance use, taking it out on the kids).

This finding suggests that persons without support tend to engage in activities that either do not add to problem resolution or that may create other stresses. It provides support for Gore's (1978) assertion about the critical role in individual well-being played by the absence rather than presence of social support.

2. Although the patterns were distinctive, alcohol use was related to specific social conditions among both men and women. Among both sexes, the use of drinking to cope occurred when relations with one's mate were not optimal. Men also drank when support in general was lacking.

An increased rate of alcoholism among heroin addicts who undergo treatment has been noted before (Belenko, 1979). Research has also indicated that the support of a critical tie in the form of a spouse or opposite-sex partner is an important factor in successful treatment (Farkas, 1976; Gerstein, Judd, & Rovner, 1979). The linkage between alcohol use and the quality of a relationship known to be significant in treatment must be further explored.

3. The pattern of coping by using drugs also differed for women and men. Among women, the greatest use of drugs to cope was associated with less support and the desire for more friends, whereas men's drug use was not related to social support.

While these findings indicate that the social support variables tapped were not as relevant to men as they were to women, they also suggest that women are more driven by social considerations than are men.

These findings have several implications for the specific questions of coping at hand. First, the existence of a supportive relationship did not guarantee its use under situations of emotional distress, which suggests that the social support system must be activated in order to be effective. This activation is probably dependent upon a number of factors, but one very likely determinant is individual coping preference. Second, the fact that dysfunctional coping strategies were related to the absence of support suggests that coping repertoires are also influenced by environmental factors (i.e., no social support). (Although the reverse is a possibility, as individuals with such coping styles may discourage the establishment of social ties.) Thus the framework for an interplay between individual characteristics and environmental demands is established. A third implication is that specific coping behaviors may have different meanings and functions for women and men. That is, the fact that dysfunctional coping strategies are related to specific social conditions for women but not for men suggests that such strategies may have different meanings for each sex. Last, the drug and alcohol use findings demonstrate that addicts' use of substances to cope is condition-specific—not indiscriminate as many believe. For both women and men, substance use for coping occurred primarily under specific social conditions (e.g., lack of a romantic involvement).

Having established a relationship between certain indicators of social support and coping, the development of appropriate service delivery strategies demands a more specific determination of focal behaviors for intervention activities. This chapter, then, examines the coping element of the model in Figure 6.1 more closely by specifying the characteristics of drug use behavior (as coping) that are associated with the adoption of a particular coping style.

METHODS

SAMPLE

The sample consisted of 170 women and 202 men entering selected publicly funded heroin addiction treatment programs in Miami, Detroit, and Los Angeles in 1975–1976. Mean ages of female and male participants were 25.8 and 27.5 years, respectively. Ethnic distributions were 56% black, 35% white, and 9% other (e.g., Asian, Latino) for women and 55% black, 33% white, and 12% other for men. These figures approximate the most recent national distribution statistics: In 1981, heroin addicts admitted to federally funded treatment centers were 44% black, 36% white, and 20% Hispanic (NIDA, 1982). Latinos are somewhat underrepresented, probably because of their virtual absence in the Detroit sample and the failure to enlist program participation in the Latino communities of the other two cities.

PROCEDURE

Each respondent was interviewed by research staff upon entry to treatment. Although all entering clients were requested to participate in the study, individuals were free to refuse without jeopardizing their entry status. Interviews lasted an average of 2½ hours, and all participants were paid $4.50 per hour upon completion. Results to be presented here are based on three sets of questions: (1) ways of coping with anger, (2) ways of coping with depression, and (3) selected drug use experience and behavior items. Table 6.1 lists all the items used in the analyses to be discussed.

Coping with Anger and Depression. Respondents were asked to indicate how they usually acted under situations of commonplace emotional distress. It is recognized that these situations represent only one particular kind of stress, but the specific focus on anger and depression was based on two considerations. (1) It appeared that depression was especially critical in the study of female addiction, since drug-abusing women characteristically evidence a greater than normal number of depressive symptoms (Colten, 1979). (2) Focusing on depression as well as anger would permit an assessment of the differential use of coping mechanisms for active as opposed to passive states.

Measurement of coping through these items was somewhat limited in that verbally based interpersonal strategies are emphasized and only a few nonsocial behavioral items are included (although additional strategies were solicited through the use of an open-ended follow-up question). Nevertheless, the items used resemble factors found in certain other studies of coping structure and drug use (Moos & Billings, 1982; Wills, Chapter 3, this volume).

Drug Use Behavior. Questions regarding drug use behavior were asked for three categories of drugs: the first drug ever used by the respondent, the respondent's preferred drug, and the drug most frequently used by the respondent. The rationale behind these divisions is the recognition that use of a given drug at a particular time results from a complex set of psychological, social, economic, environmental, and political factors. Except for general agreement that the first drug used is generally milder than later drugs used by addicts, the relative importance of each category of drugs, in terms of the addiction process, is unknown. The items (as shown in Table 6.1) address severity of use for each category of drug by examining frequency and recency of use and overdose experiences. Style of use was ascertained for each drug use category by asking whether use was usually in private or with other persons.

Data Analysis. Chi-square tests of association between the drug use behaviors and the coping behaviors were the primary data analysis techniques used.[1] Due to few responses in a number of categories, combined versions of two of the drug use variables were used: heroin versus non-heroin drug type; heroin versus marijuana versus non-heroin drug type; none versus one or more overdoses. In addition, analyses of current drug use situation omitted cases of "no current use."[2] Examinations of the coping variable "take it out on your children" were limited to parents only and analyses of "talk over things with your partner or husband or wife" were

---

[1] It is recognized that this analytical approach is not capable of directly testing for gender effects in the data. Furthermore, interactions between gender and the coping and drug use variables are not assessed. A more appropriate complete determination of effects would be obtained through log-linear modeling. However, due to the exploratory nature of the present investigation and the substantial cost of conducting log-linear analyses for each of the 110 tables of interest, in addition to their derivatives (e.g., collapsed variable versions), more refined analysis awaits a more refined research paradigm.

[2] Abstainers were omitted from this item only. Analysis of the variable in the trilevel form (i.e., drug use alone, drug use in private, no current use) did not seem to make conceptual sense, since those not currently using may normally fall into one of the other two categories. This limitation excludes 35% of the women and 24% of the men but is the only way that a clear indication of the relationship between private versus social use and coping could be obtained.

limited to respondents who were either married or declared that they currently had a romantic involvement.

RESULTS

COPING PREFERENCES

A previous report examined differences between coping preferences of the men and women in this sample (Tucker, 1979). Significant differences were evident only in the tendency to lose one's temper and yell when angry and to go to bed when depressed; women endorsed both more frequently. However, when addicted women who participated through treatment centers in Detroit were compared with socioeconomically similar nonaddicted women from the same neighborhoods, differences on three preferences were obtained: When coping with either depression or anger, drug-abusing women were more likely than the comparison women to "get away . . . or go off alone," to "just stick it out," and to take drugs—all nonsocial strategies. While these latter findings may be related to the fact that addicted women have fewer social relations than nonaddicted women, notably, the same absence of social ties among addicted men did not evidence a similar coping pattern.

GENDER COMPARISONS OF DRUG USE BEHAVIOR

The male and female addicts were compared on the three sets of selected drug use measures indicated in Table 6.1. (Significant associations are indicated in Table 6.2.) Differences in the pattern of relationships among the sets indicate that the respondents did indeed differentiate between them. There were no significant differences between women and men on the type of drug first used, type of drug preferred, and the type most frequently used. However, a trichotomized version of the same variable (comparing heroin, marijuana, and other types of drugs) did reach significance for first drug of abuse only, with a greater heroin preference among women and a greater marijuana preference among men. Men and women also differed in the frequency with which they used their preferred and most frequently used drugs. In both cases, men were significantly more likely than women to be daily users, whereas women were more likely than men to use drugs less than once per week.

For first drug used, women were more likely than men to report having had one or more overdoses. There was a clear difference, however, in the number of overdoses attributed to the various categories of drugs. While more women than men had overdosed on the first drug used, more men

Table 6.2

GENDER COMPARISONS ON DRUG USE ITEMS: PERCENTAGES AND CHI-SQUARE TESTS OF ASSOCIATION[a]

	First drug		Most preferred drug		Most frequent drug	
	Males	Females	Males	Females	Males	Females
Type of drug						
Heroin	7.5	14.1*	—	—	—	—
Marijuana	69.2	55.3	ns	—	ns	—
Nonheroin	23.4	30.6	—	—	—	—
n	201	170	—	—	—	—
Frequency of use						
None	ns	—	40.3	35.3***	37.9	41.4***
Less than once per week	—	—	6.6	17.4	6.8	12.7
Once per week	—	—	2.0	6.0	1.1	5.1
Several times per week	—	—	7.7	14.4	6.3	14.0
Daily	—	—	43.4	26.9	47.9	26.8
n	—	—	196	167	190	157
Number of overdoses						
None	94.5	85.3**	ns	—	57.4	70.8*
More than one	5.5	14.7	—	—	42.6	29.2
n	201	170	—	—	188	154

[a]ns, not significant.
*$p < .05$. **$p < .01$. ***$p < .001$.

than women overdosed on their most frequently used drug. The percentage figures also suggest that men's overdose tendencies are far more a function of drug category than women's tendencies. This is probably a dual function of the fact that these women were more likely to start out with a more dangerous drug and that men reported greater daily use of preferred and most frequently used drugs (which implies a higher risk of overdose).

Overall, then, for a third of the drug use behavior items examined, indications of a gender difference were evident. The differences seem to be in line with current knowledge of women's socialization into drug use. The fact that women are more likely that men to begin drug use with heroin is probably a function of their greater likelihood of being introduced to heroin use by male partners and their greater tendency to be paired with a fellow heroin addict (Eldred & Washington, 1976). Are there implications for coping behavior here? What do gender differences in patterns of drug use indicate about coping? The fact that women are not as likely as men to use drugs on a daily basis may suggest that women's use is not indiscriminate and may be more directly tied to particular wants, needs, and situations. The lesser tendency of women relative to men to overdose is also likely related to less frequent use but may suggest more careful, discriminating use as well.

COPING PREFERENCES RELATED TO FIRST DRUG USE

Overall, compared to other drug categories, the association between coping preferences and current use of the first drug ever used was relatively weak. However, talking things over with one's mate when angry as well as when depressed was more consistently related to drug use for both sexes. Among women, those who talked with mates, compared to those who did not, reported less frequent current use of the first drug used: $\chi^2(4, n = 113) = 13.74, p < .01$ (for coping with anger); $\chi^2(4, n = 113) = 19.10, p < .001$ (for coping with depression). Since the first drug used is unlikely to be a hard drug, this finding may signal an association between talking with mates to cope and the use of more serious drugs, possibly a dysfunctional outcome.

Among men, talking with mates was associated with greater use of marijuana as the initiating drug: $\chi^2(2, n = 171) = 10.27, p < .01$ (for coping with anger); $\chi^2(2, n = 171) = 9.91, p < .01$ (for coping with depression) and with more recent use of the initiating drug, $\chi^2(2, n = 169) = 7.29, p < .05$ (for anger); $\chi^2(2, n = 169) = 8.46, p < .05$ (for depression). This finding is nearly the opposite of that observed with women. Since the first drug used by men is also likely to be a less serious drug, mate association linked with more recent use of that drug may mean a steering away from harder substances. The direct link with initial marijuana usage lends support to this view.

Also significant was the finding that men who "stick it out" when angry were more likely to report one or more overdoses from the drug first used; $\chi^2(1, n = 198) = 3.88, p < .05$. Sticking it out when depressed for men was related to no use of the drug in the last 3 months; $\chi^2(2, n = 197) = 6.25, p < .05)$. If not simply the results of chance, these seemingly contradictory findings may reflect two aspects of perseverence: continuing to take drugs despite the overdoses when committed to drug use and persisting at withdrawal once one has decided to stop using drugs.

For women, "going to bed" when depressed was associated with a history of no overdoses due to the first drug used; $\chi^2(1, n = 154) = 4.28, p < .05$. Such withdrawal behavior, which eliminates further immediate action, may effectively prevent overuse of a given substance.

COPING RELATED TO DRUG USED MOST FREQUENTLY AND PREFERRED DRUG

Relationships between coping and reported drug use behavior for most frequently used drug and for preferred drug were often similar. This was probably because the two categories elicited the same drug type for many (although clearly not all) respondents. Therefore, findings for both categories are described in one section. A few coping preferences and certain drug use behaviors accounted for most of the significant relationships. Those findings are highlighted below and displayed in Tables 6.3 and 6.4. However, due to the volume of data under discussion, the remaining findings are described only in general terms. (More specific information may be obtained directly from the author.) Overall, the association between coping and drug use behavior was much more pervasive for women than for men.

Use of Male Relatives to Cope. Talking to male relatives when both angry and depressed was the coping behavior most consistently related to drug use, but among women only. As demonstrated in Table 6.3, significant associations were found primarily for women's coping with anger rather than depression. In sum, women who talked to male relatives to cope with anger, as compared to those who did not, reported using drugs with other persons (rather than in private) and having no overdoses for the drug they used most frequently or for the drug they preferred. In addition, such copers also preferred to use drugs other than heroin. For coping with depression, the same relationships held for drug preferred and number of overdoses for both categories of drugs. Among men, talking with male relatives was related only to a greater marijuana preference in the depression coping situation; $\chi^2(4, n = 201) = 10.23, p < .05$. Among men, talking with female relatives did not play a role similar to that observed for male relative coping among women.

These results could be interpreted as indicating that female use of male relatives to cope is related to more positive drug use outcomes: Having no overdoses is clearly more functional than its opposite. Using drugs with others rather than in private could be viewed as analogous to social drinking versus drinking alone (the latter is generally viewed as the more pathological). And a preference for drugs other than heroin is a positive step from the perspective of a heroin addict.

Type of Drug Used. The significant relationships between coping and reported drug behavior were observed almost exclusively among women. As shown in Table 6.4, women who coped with anger by going off alone and sticking it out tended to have heroin as the most frequently used drug. Most frequent use of drugs other than heroin was related to drinking alcohol

Table 6.3

PERCENTAGE OF WOMEN WHO COPE BY TALKING TO MALE RELATIVE, FOR EACH DRUG USE BEHAVIOR: CHI-SQUARE TEST RESULTS[a]

	Anger				Depression			
	Most frequent drug		Preferred drug		Most frequent drug		Preferred drug	
	%	n	%	n	%	n	%	n
Type of drug	ns				ns			
Heroin			32.2***	118			24.6****	118
Nonheroin			63.3	49			63.3	49
Current situation					ns		ns	
Private	24.2**	33	29.3*	41				
With others	55.1	69	54.3	81				
Overdose occurrences								
None	47.7*	109	47.9*	117	43.1*	109	43.6**	117
1 or more	26.7	45	25.5	47	24.4	45	17.0	47

[a]ns, not significant.
*$p < .05$. **$p < .01$. ***$p < .001$. ****$p < .0001$.

when angry. For depression coping, the same variable was associated with alcohol use and with talking to female relatives. A preference for drugs other than heroin was related to taking it out on the kids and talking with male relatives when both angry and depressed. The sole significant male finding, the association between marijuana preference and use of male relatives to cope, was noted earlier.

These results suggest that frequent heroin use is associated with nonsocial (and perhaps noninstrumental) coping strategies. An increase in alcohol use during heroin withdrawal has been observed repeatedly and thought by some to be the addict's attempt to substitute alcohol for the heroin high (e.g., Belenko, 1979). However, the relationship of nonheroin use to both alcohol coping and taking out emotional discontent on the kids may be indicative of both the frustrations associated with heroin withdrawal and the calming effects of heroin during its use.

Overdose Occurrence. The associations between coping and drug use behavior were most strongly observed among women. As indicated in Table 6.4, not losing your temper and not talking with a male relative when angry were associated with a history of at least one overdose due to both the most frequently used drug and the preferred drug. Not talking with a male relative when depressed was associated with a history of at least one overdose due to the most frequently used drug as well as the preferred drug. Not

Table 6.4

PERCENTAGE OF WOMEN REPORTING LISTED DRUG USE BEHAVIOR WHO REPORTED USING LISTED COPING STRATEGIES[a]

	Loses temper		Goes to bed		Talks to female relative				Talks to male relative			
	Anger		Depression		Anger		Depression		Anger		Depression	
	%	n	%	n	%	n	%	n	%	n	%	n
									MOST FREQUENT			
Type of drug	ns		ns		ns				ns		ns	
Heroin							49.2*	122				
Nonheroin							57.6	33				
Number of overdoses					ns		ns					
None	67.0*	109	53.2**	109					47.7*	109	43.1*	109
1 or more	46.7	45	33.2	45					26.7	45	56.9	45
									PREFERRED			
Type of drug	ns		ns		ns		ns					
Heroin									32.2***	118	24.6***	118
Nonheroin									63.3	49	63.3	49
Number of overdoses			ns		ns		ns					
None	78.6*	117							47.9*	117	43.6*	117
1 or more	44.7	47							25.5	47	17.0	47

[a]ns, not significant.
*$p < .05$. **$p < .01$. ***$p < .0001$.

going to bed when depressed related to at least one overdose for preferred drug only. The first three findings taken together may signify an association between overdosing and nonexpression of strain (i.e., not "letting it out"). Going to bed may prevent excessive drug use or it may act as a substitute for the escapist effect of drugs.

OTHER TRENDS

Other trends are evident in the findings. Whether drug use occurs in private or with others was significantly related to coping strategy among both men and women. For men, talking to mate when angry was related to a greater tendency to use both the most frequently used and the preferred drug alone: $\chi^2(1, n = 125) = 4.25, p < .05$; $\chi^2(1, n = 126) = 5.46, p < .05$. Among women, talking to male relatives when angry (see Table 6.2) and taking drugs to cope was related to a greater tendency to use both

Table 6.4 (*Continued*)

	Go off alone				Sticks it out				Takes out on kids				Drinks alcohol			
	Anger		Depression		Anger		Depression		Anger		Depression		Anger		Depression	
	%	n	%	n	%	n	%	n	%	n	%	n	%	n	%	n
DRUG																
			ns				ns		ns		ns					
	86.0**	121	NS		72.1*	122							19.7**	122	21.3*	122
	67.6	34			52.9	34										
	ns		ns		ns		ns		ns		ns		ns		ns	
DRUG																
	ns		ns		ns		ns						ns		ns	
									13.4*	82	13.4*	82				
									37.1	35	31.4	35				
	ns		ns		ns		ns		ns		ns		ns		ns	

categories of drugs with others: $\chi^2(2, n = 157) = 6.90, p < .05$ (taking drugs, most frequent drug); $\chi^2(2, n = 167) = 7.96, p < .05$ (taking drugs, preferred drug).

As one of the few significant findings for men, the meaning (if any) of the association between men's talking to mate when angry and drug use as an overall pattern is unclear. It may be that mates of heroin-addicted men attempt to steer their husbands away from the bad influence of the drug-abusing peer group. If the spouse is considered a significant source of coping support, this could lead to more use in private. In contrast, however, the most supportive relationship for women (male relatives) is associated with drug use with others. Perhaps the meaning of drug use in private is different for men and women. Private use by men, in this instance, is keeping away from a negative social environment, whereas private use by women conveys the sense of a deeper, more serious drug problem. Considered in the context of the other two related coping strategies—taking drugs to cope and not going off alone—an alternative interpretation of the findings is that women who take drugs with others have more socially oriented coping styles generally.

Nonuse within the last 3 months of the most frequently used drug was related to women's use of alcohol to cope with both anger and depression: $\chi^2(2, n = 157) = 7.77, p < .05$ (anger); $\chi^2(2, n = 157) = 6.32, p < .05$ (depression). The same trend, although not significant, was observed for men. These findings seem to support the previously stated notion that the frustration of drug withdrawal can lead to the use of dysfunctional coping strategies, and they may also indicate that alcohol simply becomes a substitute for drug use during withdrawal.

Summary

The present study is an exploratory inquiry, but in this context some general trends are evident:

1. A fairly consistent pattern of associations between coping and drug use emerged for women but not for men.
2. The form of associations between drug use and coping was a function of the category of drug use considered (i.e., whether initial drug, preferred drug, or most frequently used drug).
3. Coping by talking with male relatives was a significant determinant of less severe drug use behavior among females only. Conversely, a mate-dependent coping strategy was related to more negative consequences for women but more positive consequences for men.
4. Among women, the drug use behaviors most consistently associated with coping patterns were overdose occurrence and type of drug used or preferred.
5. The use of certain dysfunctional coping strategies (i.e., alcohol use, "taking it out on the kids") was related to conditions associated with withdrawal from drug use (i.e., use of drugs other than heroin, less recent drug use).

DISCUSSION

Interpretation and Rationale

The absence of consistent associations for the male addicts in the sample could be indicative of a number of possibilities. It could represent a conceptual failure in which the coping and/or drug behavior constructs most relevant for men were omitted. Alternatively, there may be less of a relationship between coping and drug behavior for men. The fact that male drug use was observed to be more constant (therefore perhaps less discriminating) suggests that male use may be tied to more general environmental indicators than female use. A "macho" imperative that demands drug use in particular male cultures may be a more central determinant of drug use than coping. (This view is supported by the finding of a relationship between mate-coping for men and a tendency to use in private.) It is doubtful that similar heroin-using imperatives exist for women. In any event, this absence of a relationship for men parallels earlier findings from this sample: The data on men's drug use showed few significant associations between coping and social support (Tucker, 1982).

The fact that the observed associations differed as a function of the category of drug considered is one indication of the study's conceptual validity. The categories were apparently distinct in the minds of the respondents. The differences in the patterns of association observed are critical. For both males and females, mate-dependent coping was significantly related to use of the initial drug used only. The critical role of peer supports for initial drug use has been amply demonstrated (Lettieri, 1975). This is different, however, for the concern here is with *current* use of that initial drug (after the onset of addiction to what is usually a different drug) and how that relates to current coping patterns. Why are mates not similarly instrumental in the use of the preferred and most frequently used drug? Does the initial drug of abuse represent an area of shared experience (where few exist)? Since the initial drug for most is not heroin and since many (particularly men) are partnered with persons who are not heroin addicts, use of the initial drug together may be an area of common meeting. To make the association even more complex, the relationship for men and women is conceptually reversed. This may be a reflection of the fact the women addicts are more inclined than men to have drug-abusing partners (Eldred & Washington, 1976). Women's mates on that basis alone are more likely to be bad influences than the mates of male addicts.

The importance of talking with male relatives for women is particularly noteworthy. Its association with more positive drug behaviors and its functions as distinct from those associated with mates can be explained on several grounds. First, it is important that these relationships are not romantically based. These particular male relatives (i.e., those cited as coping supports) are men who apparently can be trusted to act in the interests of the woman (an uncommon situation for a woman who is a heroin addict). They are men in whom these women can have faith. Notably, the use of females as coping supports was never related to drug use, although a previous study of these same addicted women demonstrates that they do depend on other women, especially mothers, for instrumental support (Tucker, 1979). It appears then that brothers, fathers, uncles, etc., may be seen as more legitimate authorities on the issues affecting the emotional lives of these women than mothers, sisters, grandmothers, aunts, etc. Other research with these women has also indicated that they hold very traditional sex role conceptions (Colten, 1979) and may therefore consider the input of such men in general as more important.

The salience of the drug use indicators of type of drug most frequently used or preferred and overdose occurrence could imply several different things. It may signal the inefficacy of the other measures of drug use. Variables such as frequency and recency of use for primary heroin addicts may not provide sufficient variability to detect relationships. On the other hand, overdose and drug type are suggestive of very basic individual differences—the kind most subject to individual distinctions in coping patterns. It is noteworthy that the type of drug most frequently used and the drug preferred (for women at least) reflect different components of one's coping style.

The overdose findings are difficult to interpret. Although there appears to be a relationship between nonexpression as a coping style and overdose, the causes of a particular overdose must be considered. Was it due to inexperience, was it a cry for help, or was it an attempt to commit suicide? One important aspect of the observed association is that women who depend on male relatives to cope are significantly less likely to have overdosed. Whether this is a measure of the power of social support or the despair of lack of support, it represents a clear area of focus for intervention.

The fact that dysfunctional coping strategies (i.e., taking it out on the kids and the use of alcohol) appear to be related to conditions associated with drug use withdrawal is a critical observation. Perhaps the process of withdrawal removes a partially effective coping strategy (e.g., heroin use permits one to tolerate children's outbursts) without replacing it with more functional alternatives. Admittedly, however, these interviews were taken at a very early point in the treatment process. Perhaps many of the clients eventually went on to develop more effective coping strategies.

Theoretical Significance

The findings relate in important ways to recent formulations concerning the nature of drug use generally and opiate addiction specifically. The use of chemical substances to cope has long been recognized by drug abuse researchers and coping theorists alike. Recently, Alexander and Hadaway (1982) presented considerable evidence for a view of opiate addiction as an adaptive strategy (i.e., an "attempt to adapt to chronic distress") rather than the result of mere exposure. Compatible with this perspective, and as an extension of the formulation, the present data suggest a relationship between specific coping strategies and specific drug use patterns—at least among women.

In many ways, the prevailing perspectives on drug use as a coping strategy remain rather simplistic. There is a need to apply recent findings and formulations from the general coping literature (see Moos & Billings, 1982). Clearly, the use of drugs to cope with distress is a function of many factors, including the nature of the problems faced (Pearlin & Schooler, 1978), the availability of coping alternatives, the availability of resistance resources (Antonovsky, 1979), and individual characteristics (Moos & Billings, 1982). The present study illustrates the complex nature of just one aspect of such a model.

These data also provide further evidence of the utility of a person-specific approach to the study of social support. That is, as argued previously (Tucker, 1982), different persons or categories of persons in a given social network are likely to have differential influence on the support recipient. The fact that in this study relationships between drug use and coping styles using male relatives versus those using mates were so strikingly different (while female relationships were not related at all) underscores a need for more specific social support indicators.

Implications for Service Delivery

If reliable, the findings presented here have a number of direct implications for drug prevention and treatment efforts. First, service delivery attempts must recognize that the very nature of drug abuse may differ substantially for women and men. The aspects of drug abuse assessed here were related to the coping strategies examined for women but not for men. It raises the possibility that drug use means something very different for men. Prevention and treatment efforts that fail to recognize gender differences may be ineffective for one sex.

Second, recognition of the individuals to whom drug abusers and potential substance users turn for help is essential. A determination of the likely effect of such individuals on the drug using behavior of the individual must be noted. For the women in this sample, male relatives and mates are critical, but in very different ways. If these findings represent a more pervasive trend in female addiction patterns, it seems likely that male relatives have been insufficiently utilized in prevention and treatment efforts. In addition, if it appears that a mate cannot be counted on to be a positive influence on the treatment process, this fact must be directly addressed, not ignored.

Third, these data suggest that other dysfunctional coping strategies may be substituted for heroin abuse during withdrawal, a particularly stressful period. Treatment, as well as prevention, must address the coping needs of the addict. Alternative coping skills must be provided. If there is a likelihood that alcohol use will increase during withdrawal (as has been demonstrated frequently), an alternative to substance abuse in general must be developed. Obviously, drug abuse has become a way of life for those involved. Changing one aspect of their behavior (e.g., heroin use) is simply insufficient. This notion in and of itself is not new to drug abuse (e.g., Alexander & Hadaway, 1982). Mechanisms for addressing this difficulty seem to be sorely lacking, however.

Fourth, the strong association between coping behavior and overdose occurrence is informative. It suggests that overdose and other dysfunctional outcomes may be prevented if certain features of an individual's coping repertoire, such as social support and anger expression, are modified. In the present sample, several variables were found to be important determinants. Addressing the woman's tendency toward nonexpression in stressful times, as well as enlisting the aid in treatment of key responsible men in a drug-abusing woman's family, may help to prevent a tragic occurrence.

Admittedly, these recommendations are ambitious and not easily implemented. They are directions, nevertheless, that seem to be missing from the thrust of service delivery generally. In view of this society's enormously pervasive substance abuse problem, new approaches should be welcomed and tried.

REFERENCES

Alexander, B. K., & Hadaway, P. F. (1982). Opiate addiction: The case for an adaptive orientation. *Psychological Bulletin, 92,* 367–381.

Antonovsky, A. (1979). *Health, stress, and coping.* San Francisco: Jossey-Bass.

Arnon, D., Kleinman, M., & Kissin, B. (1974). Psychological differentiation in heroin addicts. *International Journal of the Addictions. 9,* 151–159.

Austin, G. A., Johnson, B. D., Carroll, E. E., & Lettieri, D. J. (Eds.). (1977). *Drugs and minorities* (Research Issues No. 21). Rockville, MD: National Institute on Drug Abuse.

Bahna, G., & Gordon, N. B. (1978). Rehabilitation experiences of women ex-addicts in methadone treatment. *International Journal of the Addictions, 13,* 639–655.

Belenko, S. (1979). Alcohol abuse by heroin addicts: Review of research findings and issues. *International Journal of the Addictions, 14,* 965–975.

Burt, M., Glynn, T. J., & Sowder, B. (1979). *Psychosocial characteristics of drug-abusing women* (Services Research Monograph Series) (DHEW Publication No. ADM 80–917). Washington, DC: U.S. Government Printing Office.

Colten, M. E. (1979). A descriptive and comparative analysis of self-perceptions and attitudes of heroin-addicted women. In *Addicted women: Family dynamics, self-perceptions, and support systems* (Services Research Monograph Series, DHEW Publication No. ADM–80–762). Rockville, MD: National Institute on Drug Abuse.

Colten, M. E. (1982). Attitudes, experiences and self-perceptions of heroin addicted mothers. *Journal of Social Issues, 39*(2), 77–92.

Cooperstock, R. (1978). Sex differences in psychotropic drug use. *Social Science and Medicine, 12b,* 179–186.
Cuskey, W. R., Berger, L. H., & Densen-Gerber, J. (1977). Issues in the treatment of female addiction: A review and critique of the literature. *Contemporary Drug Problems, 6,* 307–371.
Eldred, A. E., & Washington, M. N. (1976). Interpersonal relationships in heroin use by men and women and their role in treatment outcome. *International Journal of the Addictions, 11,* 117–130.
Farkas, M. I. (1976). The addicted couple. *Drug Forum, 5,* 81–87.
Folkman, S., & Lazarus, R. S. (1980). An analysis of coping in a middle-aged community sample. *Journal of Health and Social Behavior, 21,* 219–239.
Gerstein, D. R., Judd, L. L., & Rovner, S. A. (1979). Career dynamics of female heroin addicts. *American Journal of Drug and Alcohol Abuse, 6,* 1–23.
Gomberg, E. S. L. (1982). Historical and political perspective: Women and drug use. *Journal of Social Issues, 39*(2), 9–24.
Gore, S. (1978). The effect of social support in moderating the health consequences of unemployment. *Journal of Health and Social Behavior, 19,* 157–165.
Johnson, B., & Nishi, S. M. (1976). Myths and realities of drug use by minorities. In P. Iiyama, S. Matsunaga, & B. Johnson (Eds.), *Drug use and abuse among U.S. minorities.* New York: Praeger.
Kalant, O. J. (1980). Sex differences in alcohol and drug problems—Some highlights. In O. J. Kalant (Ed.), *Alcohol and drug problems in women: Research advances in alcohol and drug problems* (Vol. 5). New York: Plenum Press.
Khantzian, E. J., Mack, J. F., & Schatzberg, A. F. (1974). Heroin use as an attempt to cope: Clinical observations. *American Journal of Psychiatry, 131,* 160–164.
Lettieri, D. J. (Ed.). (1975). *Predicting adolescent drug abuse: A review of issues, methods and correlates* (Research Issues No. 11, DHEW Publication No. ADM 77–299). Rockville, MD: National Institute on Drug Abuse.
Lettieri, D. J., Sayers, M., & Pearson, H. W. (Eds.). (1980). *Theories on drug abuse: Selected contemporary perspectives* (NIDA Research Monograph No. 30, DHHS Publication No. ADM 80–967). Rockville, MD: National Institute on Drug Abuse.
Marsh, J. C., Colten, M. E., & Tucker, M. B. (1982). Women's use of drugs and alcohol: New perspectives. *Journal of Social Issues, 38*(2), 1–8.
Moos, R. H., & Billings, A. G. (1982). Conceptualizing and measuring coping resources and processes. In L. Goldenberger & S. Breznitz (Eds.). *Handbook of stress: Theoretical and clinical aspects.* New York: Free Press.
National Institute on Drug Abuse. (1980). *Statistical series—Women in drug abuse treatment 1979: Topical data from the Client Oriented Data Acquisition Process (CODAP)* (Series C, No. 1, DHHS Publication No. ADM 81-1049). Washington, DC: U.S. Government Printing Office.
National Institute on Drug Abuse. (1982). *Statistical series—Annual data 1981: Data from the Client Oriented Data Acquisition Process (CODAP)* (Series E, No. 25, DHHS Publication No. ADM 82–1223). Washington, DC: U.S. Government Printing Office.
Pearlin, L. I., & Schooler, C. (1978). The structure of coping. *Journal of Health and Social Behavior, 19,* 2–21.
Prather, J. E., & Fidell, L. S. (1978). Drug use and abuse among women: An overview. *International Journal of the Addictions, 13,* 863–885.
Rhoads, D. L. (1983). A longitudinal study of life stress and social support among drug abusers. *International Journal of the Addictions, 18,* 195–222.

Ryser, P. E. (1983). Sex differences in substance abuse: 1976–1979. *International Journal of the Addictions, 18,* 71–87.

Suffett, F., & Brotman, R. (1976). Female drug use: Some observations. *International Journal of the Addictions, 11,* 19–33.

Tucker, M. B. (1979). A descriptive and comparative analysis of the social support structure of heroin addicted women. In *Addicted women: Family dynamics, self perceptions, and support systems* (Services Research Monograph Series, DHEW Publication No. ADM–80–762). Rockville, MD: National Institute on Drug Abuse.

Tucker, M. B. (1982). Social support and coping: Applications for the study of female drug abuse. *Journal of Social Issues, 39*(2), 117–137.

Tucker, M. B. (in press). U.S. Ethnic minorities and drug abuse: An assessment of the science and practice. *International Journal of the Addictions.*

Verbrugge, L. M. (1982). Sex differences in legal drug use. *Journal of Social Issues, 39*(2), 59–76.

Chapter 7

Life Stress, Helplessness, and the Use of Alcohol and Drugs to Cope: An Analysis of National Survey Data

SUSAN GOFF TIMMER
JOSEPH VEROFF
MARY ELLEN COLTEN

INTRODUCTION

In this chapter, survey data from a national representative sample are used to explore the links between life stress, feelings of helplessness, and the use of alcohol and drugs to cope. This survey contained information not only about individuals' reported substance use in times of stress but also about factors that, according to a cognitive-behavioral framework suggested by Marlatt (1979), may contribute to such use. This framework encompasses the contributions to substance use from the environment made by the stressor itself and those from individuals' internal resources, attitudes toward alcohol and drugs, and the availability of alternative coping strategies. We use this model to guide our exploration of life circumstances surrounding the use of alcohol and drugs as methods of coping with stress from economic difficulties, marital dissatisfaction, and job strain. We focus on the hypothesis that individuals' internal resources and alternative coping strategies moderate the relationship between life stress and substance use as a response to that stress.

THEORY OF MODERATING EFFECTS

Why do people use substances like alcohol or drugs to cope with stressful situations? The cognitive-behavioral model proposed by Marlatt (1979) provides a framework for considering the links between role stressors and the use of drugs or alcohol to cope. The model hypothesizes that drinking (or taking drugs) will vary according to (1) the perceived stressfulness of the situation, (2) the degree of perceived personal control, (3) the availability of alcohol (or drugs), (4) the availability of an adequate coping response to the perceived stress, and (5) the person's expectations about the effects of alcohol (or drugs).

Implicit in the model is that internal psychological variables, external factors, and coping resources can affect the relationship between life stresses and the use of alcohol or drugs to cope. Demographic characteristics which describe an individual's life condition or role status within the social order (e.g., marital status, age, family income, education, employment status, and gender) can be seen as external contextual factors in this process. They play a role in determining the perceived stressfulness of a situation, the sense of personal control, and the availability and perceived efficacy of alternative coping strategies. They may also influence general access to and global attitudes toward the use of alcohol or drugs (e.g., expectancies about costs and benefits of substances). In the following sections we briefly discuss each of the four elements of the model that theoretically affect the likelihood that a person will use alcohol or drugs to cope with stress. In addition, we discuss external life conditions or demographic factors that may also influence such behavior.

Perceived Stressfulness of the Situation

The perceived stressfulness of the situation is defined here as the severity of the stressor as felt by the individual. This perspective conforms to Lazarus' cognitive appraisal model (see Coyne & Lazarus, 1980). This model proposes that stress is a direct function of evaluations of the degree to which an event has harmed or threatens to harm the self and the degree to which a person feels able to successfully cope with the event. Some stressors, like the death of a loved one, are universally felt as severe. Other stressors may vary in felt intensity according to a person's current status or history, especially with regard to available coping resources. For instance, a person with limited income or raised in a family that was continually on the brink of financial disaster might feel very stressed by economic worries that would not concern many other people. The point is that if a potentially stressful event is not perceived to be particularly stressful because the person feels he or she can adequately deal with that event, then the event is not likely to evoke much stress reaction for that person.

Internal Resources: Personal Control

The sense that one can successfully cope using available strategies conveys a sense of personal control over stress. Conversely, a lack of perceived control over stress conveys the impression that one is being swept by a tide of ill fate and that implementation of any available coping strategies would be futile. In this context, a lack of personal control over stress may be likened to learned helplessness, a syndrome that also involves an internalization of failure, feelings of dysphoria, low self-esteem, and a decreased attempt to try to change things in the future (Garber & Seligman, 1980). People generally believe that alcohol (and in some cases, drugs) will either reduce negative affect or induce positive affect (Brown, Goldman, Inn, & Anderson, 1980; Wilson & Abrams, 1977; Deardorff, Melges, Hout, & Savage, 1975). Those who feel they lack personal control may drink or take drugs to increase perceived control and relieve the negative affect associated with the failure to cope successfully.

One aspect of personal control which should be considered is the need for power, since some theoretical and empirical work has noted its importance in determining men's drinking behavior. According to McClelland, Davis, Kalin, and Warner (1972), alcohol provides men with the illusion of power, and so men who have exaggerated needs for personal power are more likely to drink heavily to enhance their need satisfaction. If a stressful event highlights a man's lack of personal power, then, according to the power motive theory, the man with the highest need should be most likely to drink to cope with the perceived loss of power. The relationship of the power motive to women's drinking behavior is less clear. Some argue that, unlike men, women are not socialized to desire high levels of personal power and, therefore, may not experience a sense of discord between their need levels and their attained levels of power. Consequently, they might not need to drink to compensate. But we suggest that the argument for compensatory drinking in response to unsatisfied power needs lies not in the absolute level of the need but in the gap between the real and ideal level of personal power. Therefore, even though women's power needs may not be as great as men's, if an event occurred which evoked feelings of low personal power, we would still expect women with a higher need for power to drink more heavily in response.

Availability of Adequate Coping Alternatives

Personal control encompasses the belief that one can effectively use alternative coping mechanisms. This is distinct from the availability of these alternatives to the person. We focus mainly on two such alternatives: social support and prayer, both of which were assessed in the national survey.

The access people have to social support from relatives, friends, and neighbors may greatly influence response to a stressful situation. Other people provide information, new ways of viewing problems and solutions, and access to other helpful people (Antonucci & Depner, 1982; Gourash, 1978; Kahn & Antonucci, 1980; Warren, 1981). Furthermore, if a person feels that there is someone to depend upon for help through a difficult time, or to talk to, then the stress may not be experienced as potentially destructive.

The use of prayer to cope with stress may also influence the consequent behavioral response. Prayer may help build faith that whatever one does to cope actively with a negative event will result in ultimate good. The use of prayer as a coping strategy may be linked to a belief that drinking alcohol shows a lack of faith and is a bad way to cope with stress, and studies of adolescent drug use show negative relationships between religiosity and drug use (e.g., Jessor & Jessor, 1977; Wills & Warshawsky, 1983). Use of prescription medications by adults to cope with tension and anxiety may be a more acceptable alternative for the religious believer, as such drugs are most likely to be prescribed by a doctor.

When there are no discernible alternatives to coping with stress, people often remain passive. We also assess in our survey those people who say they do nothing when they are unhappy or "just wait for it to pass." We call this passive coping and identify it as a response indicating an impoverished coping repertoire. We would expect, according to Marlatt's (1979) formulation, that such people would be more prone to turn to substance use as a means of coping.

Expectations for Alcohol and Drugs

Drinking alcohol or taking drugs are not necessarily effective methods for coping with many life problems. Substance use does not remove environmentally induced stress, it does not dispel conflict in marriage, and it does not find an unemployed worker a job. However, although substance use does not alter circumstances, people believe that alcohol will ease negative affect associated with stressful events and stressful life conditions (Deardorff et al., 1975; Wilson & Abrams, 1977). These expectancies about alcohol are likely to influence subsequent behavior (e.g., Marlatt, 1979). A similar pattern should be observed for drugs. Commercials, doctors, and friends may suggest that certain drugs aid in relaxation or improve mood. People who believe this would be expected to be more likely to take the drug to help them cope with those maladies.

Contextual Factors

A model of responses to potentially stressful circumstances must take into account the more general contexts determined by social roles and external conditions of life. Let us consider a few examples. Marital status may be crucial. Married people may perceive a given stressor as less severe than unmarried persons because the burden is shared. A person's age may greatly influence perception of stress. Older people, for instance, may feel that being ill is very stressful because it signals mortality. Family income may influence the degree to which job dissatisfaction is perceived as stressful. Basic needs of people with low family incomes would be more endangered by job disruption and they might, therefore, feel more stressed.

Gender may be a particularly important factor. Males and females are likely to be exposed to different stresses, as well as to conditions that cause them to experience the nature of a given stress differentially. For instance, the influence of working or not working on individuals' perceptions of stress may vary according to gender. For men, not working may increase the stressfulness of certain events, perhaps because unemployment induces low sense of self-worth and a sense of being unable to meet a fundamental criterion of adequacy for adult males. For women, working may relate to feeling more stressed by certain events because women bear major responsibilities in their familial role, and so working women may feel overloaded by any additional stress. In general, the strength of socialization to gender roles makes it very likely that there are numerous instances in which a stressor felt by men is not experienced equally as a stressor by women, and vice versa. Gender also affects the sense of personal control and the perceived availability of alternative coping strategies. Women may have more access to social supports (Antonucci & Depner, 1982). Furthermore, research has shown repeatedly that different norms govern the use of substances for men and women. For example, Parry, Cisin, Balter, Mellinger, and Manheimer (1974) suggest that men are more likely to drink in response to anxiety and depression, while women are more likely to use psychotropic drugs. They attribute the sex difference largely to social norms, possibly reinforced by other social patterns such as the greater likelihood for physicians to prescribe psychotropic drugs to women.

Implications of Marlatt's Model for Predicting Substance Use in Response to Stress

At first glance, Marlatt's (1979) model appears to imply that alcohol or drug use in response to stress arises from a failure of resources and is activated only when an individual's alternatives are so inadequate that any stress precipitates substance use, or when a stressor is of such magnitude as to overwhelm even the most robust personality and array of coping alternatives. However, we do not believe that drinking and drug use are always behaviors representing extreme dysfunction. This model can accommodate our belief. The model is additive, so that drinking or drug use behavior may be evoked by a shift in any one of the four elements: internal psychological variables, external factors, coping resources, and demographic characteristics. Internal psychological variables include reference to the perceived magnitude of the stressor and to beliefs about the utility of drugs or alcohol. Substance use as a coping strategy may reflect not only a belief that it would reduce negative affect to manageable proportions but also a belief that it can induce positive affect. The different expectations are probably influenced by different personal and situational factors.

In this paper we explore the differential influence of personal resources on the likelihood of drinking or taking drugs to handle feelings of worry, tension, or nervousness in the presence of economic worries, marital stress, or job stress. Our approach predicts that resources such as personal control and alternative coping mechanisms are inversely related to drinking to cope in the face of stressful life conditions. We are not attempting to validate fully the model developed by Marlatt (1979) in that we do not measure availability of alcohol or drugs or expectancies about the efficacy of using alcohol or drugs for coping. We assume that reported use of drugs or alcohol for coping is predicated on access to the substances and on the belief that use will have a positive effect, either a reduction of negative affect or an induction of positive affect. Also, although Marlatt does not detail the possibility of differential reactions according to the nature of the stressor, we suspect that the dynamics may differ across types of stressors and also that they may differ for men and women. We further expect, as mentioned earlier, personal characteristics of individuals, such as education, income, sex, marital status, and employment status, to function as resources and affect the extent to which a particular stressor is actually perceived as stressful as well as the availability of alternative resources to cope with that stress. Thus, these personal characteristics affect the relationship between the presence of that stressor and the use of drugs or alcohol to cope. Our analyses, therefore, focus on both the main effects of stress on substance use and on the moderating effects of personal and social resources on the use of substances to cope.

METHODS

Selected by area probability sampling, a representative national cross-section of 960 men and 1304 women living in households were interviewed in a 1976 study of subjective mental health and patterns of help seeking. (For an extensive description, see Veroff, Douvan & Kulka, 1981; Veroff, Kulka, & Douvan, 1981.) Trained interviewers made contact with a household and selected a specified respondent. The response rate was 71% of the original set of designated respondents; the demographic distributions of the resulting sample did not differ significantly from the census current population survey for 1978 (see Veroff, Douvan, & Kulka, 1981, p. 30).

The Substance Use Assessment

The interview covered a wide range of topics relevant to mental health and patterns of coping. Of special interest are two questions which asked whether and how much the respondents drank and took drugs and medicines to relieve tensions. The actual questions were:

1. When you feel worried, tense, or nervous, do you ever drink alcoholic beverages to help you handle things?
2. When you feel worried, tense, or nervous, do you ever take medicines or drugs to help you handle things? (The word *drugs* was left up to individual interpretation.)

The possible responses to these questions were: never, 1; hardly ever, 2; sometimes, 3; many times, 4. These two items were embedded in a series of similar questions asked about physical and psychological symptoms. Our study focuses on factors in the person and the situation that affect the response to these two questions that ask directly about the person's perception of substance use for stress reduction. We emphasize that these measures assess the conscious recognition of substance use as a coping strategy. Furthermore, the questions do not specify the nature of the stressor(s), so the respondent is answering with respect to general tensions. As such, the measures undoubtedly get at substance use as a general coping tendency rather than as a situationally specific one.

The Assessment of Specific Stresses

In addition, we wanted to assess specific stresses that might reflect important circumstances for substance use coping. Of the many kinds of stresses measured in the survey, three types were selected for consideration in this chapter: economic stress, marital stress, and job stress. These stresses were selected on two accounts. First, unlike others, they appeared frequently enough in the respondents' evaluations of their lives to warrant a detailed analysis. And second, they are diverse stresses—ones that can have different impacts on coping strategies. These assessments came from the following questions asked in the study:

1. *Economic stress.* Everybody has some things he worries about more or less. What kinds of things do you worry about most? (Economic stress was coded whenever a respondent mentioned a financial problem that he or she was worried about; 0, no mention of economic stress; 1, mentions economic stress.)
2. *Marital stress.* A 6-item scale used to measure marital stress included the following items:
    a. Every marriage has its good and bad points. What things about your marriage are not quite as nice as you would like them to be? (If nothing was mentioned, coded 2; if respondent mentions bad points, coded 4. This method was adopted to give this item equal weighting with the other items on the scale.)
    b. How often have you:
        i. been irritated with or resentful towards what your spouse did or didn't do.
        ii. been upset about how you and your spouse were getting along in the sexual part of your lives.
        iii. wished your spouse talked more about how he/she feels or thinks.
        iv. felt tense from fighting, arguing, or disagreeing with your spouse.
        v. wished that your spouse understood you better.
    (For each of the last five items, the response alternatives were never, rarely, sometimes, often, coded 1, 2, 3, and 4, respectively.) The scores were summed across the six items to obtain a total marital stress score. This scale had emerged from a factor-analytic study of the variety of measures of marital well-being that appear in *The Inner American* (Veroff, Douvan, & Kulka, 1981). The items in this scale cluster similarly for both men and women (Timmer, Bryant, & Veroff, in preparation).
3. *Job stress.* Taking everything into consideration, how likely is it you will make a genuine effort to find a new job within the next year? (The response alternatives were not at all likely, somewhat likely, or very likely, coded 1, 2, and 3, respectively.)

The Assessment of Personal and Social Resources

From the various measures available in the survey, we selected certain kinds of characteristics of people and their lives that we thought would affect substance use strategies of coping under stress. Each represents a resource that could affect factors specified in Marlatt's formulation, especially personal efficacy, and the availability of other coping strategies as alternatives to substance use. These are discussed below.

PERSONAL RESOURCES

Two assessments were selected because they reflect generalized personal capacities to cope. These were derived from composites of measures about self-evaluation. The interview contained many questions about self-evaluations, ranging from the assessment of general happiness to questions about physical symptoms. Bryant and Veroff (1984) have simplified many of the assessments of general subjective mental health by deriving six factor scores based on the dimensions emerging from a factor analysis of the separate questions. These factors are termed: Unhappiness, Lack of Gratification, Lack of Self-confidence, Feelings of Vulnerability, Strain, and Uncertainty.[1] In our analyses we focus on only two of these factors, Self-confidence and Vulnerability, because these come closest to assessing perceived personal resources. Lack of self-confidence is defined by endorsing items reflecting low self-esteem (e.g., saying it is rarely or never true that "on the whole, I feel good about myself"), depression (e.g., saying only some of the time or little or none of the time that "my life is interesting"), feelings of anomie (e.g., saying it is pretty true or very true that "no one cares much what happens to me"), the perception of problems and outcomes as uncontrollable, and a general lack of self-acceptance. This is not unlike what Dohrenwend, Shrout, Egri, and Mendelsohn (1980) identified as poor self-esteem in their assessment of the syndrome termed *demoralization* derived from the Psychiatric Epidemiology Research Interview (PERI). Feelings of vulnerability is characterized by endorsing such items as frequent feelings of being overwhelmed, feelings of nervous breakdown, and perceptions that bad things frequently occur. This is not unlike a dimension that Dohrenwend et al. (1980) identified as helplessness–hopelessness in the PERI.

Somewhat related to these evaluations of personal capacities to cope is a person's assessment of his or her physical health. Factor analysis of symptoms revealed a consistent cluster that concerned direct questions about physical health (see Veroff, Douvan, & Kulka, 1981, Chap. 7). These are listed below and were embedded in the same set as the drinking and drug-taking questions:

1. Has any ill health affected the amount of work you do?
2. Have you ever been bothered by shortness of breath?

---

[1]Although all of these factors deal with a general distress, each has its own configuration, and Bryant and Veroff (1984) demonstrate their divergent validity.

3. Have you ever been bothered by your heart beating hard?
4. Do you feel you are bothered by all sorts of pains and ailments in different parts of your body?
5. For the most part, do you feel healthy enough to carry out the things you would like to do?

Possible responses to the first three items were: never, 1; hardly ever, 2; sometimes 3; many times, 4. Possible responses to the last two were: yes, 4; no, 2; and yes, 2; no, 4, respectively. (Items were summed to form a scale.)

Another resource assessed was even more internal to the person's own characteristics: the strength of his or her power motive, a disposition to find gratification from having impact on the environment (see McClelland, 1975; Winter, 1973). As we discussed earlier, being concerned about power might promote alcohol use. One might view being low in this kind of motive as a resource for not using substances to create the illusion of control. Veroff, Depner, Kulka, and Douvan (1980) described the techniques used in this survey to measure power motives through thematic apperception. Stories were told in response to pictures in a standardized way by a random two-thirds of the total sample; the coding was systematic and reliable, and scores were corrected for individual differences in verbal fluency (see Veroff et al., 1980, for details).

More specific personal resources are various coping styles that the respondent says he or she uses for dealing with problems. Although we also assessed how people cope with periods of mild anxiety, we selected their reports about dealing with periods of unhappiness because the latter typically referred to more long-term and personal stresses. Worries were often about world or community problems or about very specific personal situations that clearly dictated a specific coping response (e.g., seeing a doctor about a physical problem). Respondents were asked: "One of the things we would like to know is how people face the unhappy periods in their lives. Thinking of the unhappiness you've had to face, what are some of the things that have helped you in those times?" We should note that this question calls for reports of successful coping (things that have helped). We should also note that although a person could report more than one coping strategy, this was not common and so we confined our analyses to the first-mentioned response. Furthermore, although the coding scheme for this question contained other kinds of responses (e.g., doing something about the problem) we confined ourselves to those coping responses with sufficient frequency to warrant analysis: passive coping, talking to someone, and praying. Passive coping was coded only when the respondent explicitly indicated that he or she did nothing to handle a difficult period (not when the respondent said he or she tried to forget the problem); talking to someone was coded whenever the respondent said he talked with a person (either an informal or formal resource) when difficulties emerged; praying was coded whenever the response indicated a religious form of coping. As discussed in the section, "Introduction," these coping styles should be related to substance use in times of stress.

EXTERNAL AND SOCIAL RESOURCES

External resources for coping were assessed in a number of ways. First, the person's access to a social network was coded by reports of the number of people that he or she customarily sees and the number of persons who are available to talk over problems when they arise. This measure was obtained from two questions:

1. About how often do you get together with friends and relatives—I mean things like going out together or visiting in each other's home? Would you say more than once a week, once a week, a few times a month, once a month, or less than once a month? (Coded 5, 4, 3, 2, 1, respectively.)

2. Now think of the friends and relatives you feel free to talk with about your worries and problems or can count on for advice or help—would you say you have many, several, a few, or no such friends or relatives? (Coded 4, 3, 2, 1, respectively.)

The measure of social support was based on the sum of these two items. Higher scores indicated greater access to social networks. The two items are highly correlated although the first reflects more general social activity and the second reflects more explicit availability of psychological support. Additional resources from the outside were assessed through marital status (whether a person was married or not), employment status (whether or not the person had a job), education, and family income. We assumed that each of these represented a resource that was relevant to how a person was able to cope with the social world and, hence, provided the context for a sense of personal efficacy and/or ways of dealing with stress that were alternatives to substance use.

Analysis Strategy

We are primarily interested in the moderating effects (see Cleary & Kessler, 1982) of personal resources—internal psychological, external, and coping resources—on the relationship between major life stresses and the use of alcohol and drugs to cope.[2] Therefore, we employ ordinary least

---

[2]When a variable is a modifier between stress and the use of substances to cope, then there is a different effect of stress on the use of substances to cope depending on the presence, absence, or level of the moderator.

squares regression. Predictors of the use of drugs and alcohol in the context of coping are variables measuring personal and social resources, and three different types of stress. We check specifically for interactions between the measure of life stress and each measure of the different personal and social resources, looking for evidence of variation of the effect of the life stress by levels of the measure of resource. We perform separate analyses for each stressor because they involve different populations: Economic worries are measured for the entire sample, the measure of job stress is only available for employed people, and the measure of marital stress only includes those currently married. Additionally, analyses are performed separately for men and women because there is evidence (e.g., Parry et al., 1974) that the dynamics underlying men's and women's decisions to use alcohol or drugs when they are under stress are different.

Interpreting Interactions

When a significant interaction term is included in the regression equation, this means that the effect of stress on the use of alcohol or drugs to cope varies according to the level of a particular personal resource. The measure of stress can thus be said to have a marginal effect on the use of substances to cope. For example, to estimate the marginal effect of stress on the use of alcohol to cope with tension, moderated by one particular personal resource (e.g., lack of self-confidence), the beta weight for the main effect of stress is added to the beta weights for each of the interaction terms including the stressor times the value of its respective measure of personal resources. In a standardized regression equation these values are, for example, -1, 0, and $+1$ (1 standard deviation below the mean, the mean, and 1 standard deviation above the mean of the personal resource measure). Because we are interested in the moderating effect of a lack of self-confidence, the mean value, 0, is inserted for all other measures of personal resources, and the values -1 and $+1$ are alternately inserted for the measure of self-confidence. In this way, the interaction terms including all other measures of personal resources drop out of the equation, and we can estimate the effects of a stressor on drinking alcohol to cope at low and high levels of self-confidence.

To further illustrate, the total effect of marital stress on the likelihood of drinking to cope among married men (see Table 7.2) is equal to:

$$.09 + .31 \times \text{(level of self-confidence)}$$

If standardized values of $(-1, +1)$ are substituted for the variable (level of self-confidence), the nature of the interaction becomes clear. Among men whose self-confidence is high (1 standard deviation below the mean), marital stress and drinking are negatively related ($M = -.22$). Men lacking self-confidence (1 standard deviation above the mean level of lack of self-confidence) show a strong positive relationship between marital stress and drinking equal to $+.40$. Therefore we can say that the relationship between marital stress and drinking to cope among men is moderated by self-confidence.

RESULTS

Before discussing the results of the regression analyses, we briefly discuss the nature of the dependent variables (see Veroff, Douvan, Kulka, 1981, for a more detailed discussion of these variables). More men than women report using alcohol to relieve tension: 29% of men in contrast to 16% of women. Veroff, Douvan, and Kulka (1981) note that this result runs counter to their general finding that men find it less socially desirable to admit to the presence of negative states. These authors reason that men more than women may believe that drinking is an appropriate way to relieve tension. The use of drugs to relieve tension was reported more frequently by women than by men: 34% of women and 24% of men stated that they used drugs to relieve tension. Veroff, Douvan, and Kulka (1981) concluded that drugs and medicines are a more acceptable route for substance abuse for women than for men.

On the whole, the majority of respondents do not report using either drugs or alcohol to reduce tension, and particularly alcohol. The skewed distribution of these variables (i.e., their lack of variability) does have an impact on the strength with which independent variables can predict outcomes. Because of the distributions, we expect that for women there will be fewer significant predictors of alcohol use than of drug use in times of stress.

Tables 7.1 through 7.3 show the results of regressions of respondents' use of drugs and alcohol to cope on each of the three stressors (economic worries, marital stress, and job stress) and specified measures of internal and external resources, and statistically significant interactions between the stressor and resources.

In the tables the numerical coding of the variables is indicated after each variable name. This coding will help the reader interpret the direction of significant effects. For example, in Table 7.1, in the analysis of women's use of alcohol, we can see that betas for four predictor variables (Marital Status, Employment Status, Feelings of Vulnerability, and Prayer) and two interac-

Table 7.1

REGRESSIONS OF USING ALCOHOL OR DRUGS TO HANDLE TENSION ON STRESS OF ECONOMIC WORRIES: SELECTED SOCIAL AND PERSONAL CHARACTERISTICS AND ALTERNATIVE COPING STYLES, BY SEX[a]

Predictor[b]	Use of alcohol (low–high)		Use of drugs (low–high)	
	Men (N = 366) beta	Women (N = 974) beta	Men (N = 682) beta	Women (N = 970) beta
Stress				
Economic Worries (no–yes)	.03	−.02	−.01	.01
Social characteristics				
Age (young–old)	−.05	.13	.04	.06+
Education (low–high)	.03	.05	−.02	.01
Family income (low–high)	.07	.03	.04	.03
Access to social network (little–lot)	−.09+	−.05	−.16	.03
Marital status (married–not)	.09+	−.22*	.00	.00
Employment status (yes–no)	.04	−.09**	.01	.00
Personal characteristics				
Need for power (low–high)	.43**	—	—	—
Lack of confidence (low–high)	.08	.04	.05	.06+
Feelings of vulnerability (low–high)	.17**	.17***	.15***	.21***
Physical health (good–bad)	−.04	.02	.34***	.30***
Coping styles for unhappiness				
Passive coping (yes–no)	.03	−.05	.03	−.01
Prayer (yes–no)	.07	.10*	−.21+	.02
Talk to friend (yes–no)	.06	.02	−.16	.01
Interactions				
Economic Worries × Marital Status	—	.28*	—	—
Economic Worries × Age of Respondent	—	−.23*	—	—
Economic Worries × Need for Power	−.42**	—	—	—
Economic Worries × Prayer	—	—	.22*	—
Economic Worries × Talk to Friend	—	—	.18+	—
Economic Worries × Access to Social Network	—	—	.17+	—
R^2	.13	.11	.20	.20

[a] A dash indicates that the interaction was not included in the regrssion equation because it lacked significance or that the need for power term being insignificant was excluded because it was available on only two-thirds of the sample.
[b] For all variables, numerical coding is in the order indicated.
+$p < .10$. *$p < .05$. **$p < .01$. ***$p < .001$.

tions (Economic Worries × Marital Status and Economic Worries × Age of Respondent) attained significance. The beta of −.09 for Employment Status, for example, can be interpreted to mean that use of alcohol (coded from low to high) is greater in the employed group (since employment status is coded yes or no). As another example, the beta of .10 for Prayer would be interpreted as meaning that use of alcohol is higher in those who do *not* pray as a coping style (since the prayer variable is coded yes or no). The interaction betas must be interpreted according to the method discussed in the section, "Interpreting Interactions."

In selecting regression models we used the following procedure: We included all predictor variables and included interaction terms only if they added significant predictive power to the model. We also omitted the Need for Power variable as a predictor if it did not attain significance. This was because Need for Power was available only on a random two-thirds of the sample. We emphasize that these results should not be confounded by social class, because both education of the respondent and the person's family income are included in all regression models. Thus any variability deriving from socioeconomic status per se is partialled out of the other effects reported in this paper.

For each of the three stressors, analyses were performed separately for men and women and for drug use and alcohol use. The following discussion addresses each stressor and, within that stressor, the coping use of alcohol and drugs, respectively.

The most intriguing question is about the moderating effects of personal characteristics and resources on the likelihood of using substances to cope with stress. This question is best addressed by assessing interactions between a stressor (financial, marital, and job) and personal characteristics or resources. Before we discuss the significant interactions predicting the use of drugs and alcohol to cope, we report the main effects of these resources, indicating variables that operate irrespective of the presence or absence of a particular stressor.

Relationship between Resources and General Use of Alcohol and Drugs to Cope

The analyses concerning economic worries include all men and women in the sample, whereas the analyses for marital stress include only married respondents and those for job stress include only employed respondents. Therefore, the main effects of personal characteristics, which relate to the use of alcohol and drugs to cope, vary somewhat between the analyses for each of the stressors. The variations among the different groups are discussed as they arise.

Table 7.2

REGRESSIONS OF USING DRUGS OR ALCOHOL TO HANDLE TENSION ON MARITAL STRESS: SELECTED SOCIAL AND PERSONAL CHARACTERISTICS AND ALTERNATIVE COPING STYLES, BY SEX[a]

	Use of alcohol (low–high)		Use of drugs (low–high)	
	Men (N = 482)	Women (N = 560)	Men (N = 481)	Women (N = 560)
Predictor[b]	beta	beta	beta	beta
Stress				
Marital stress (low–high)	.09+	.18***	−.05	.07
Social characteristics				
Age (young–old)	−.11*	−.21	.06	.02
Education (low–high)	.02	.04	−.22+	−.05
Family income (low–high)	.06	.11*	.02	.07
Access to social network (little–lot)	−.09+	−.02	−.21	.05
Employment status (yes–no)	.08	−.08+	−.07	.03
Personal characteristics				
Lack of confidence (high–low)	−.18	.00	.06	.02
Feelings of vulnerability (low–high)	.13**	−.24	.21***	.18***
Physical health (good–bad)	.02	.41**	.35***	.03
Coping styles for unhappiness				
Passive coping (yes–no)	−.01	−.16**	−.01	.01
Prayer (yes–no)	.02	.01	.02	.02
Talk to friend (yes–no)	.06	−.06	−.01	.03
Interactions				
Marital Stress × Lack of Confidence	.31*	—	—	—
Marital Stress × Age of Respondent	—	.27+	—	—
Marital Stress × Feelings of Vulnerability	—	.38*	—	—
Marital Stress × Education	—	—	.24+	—
Marital Stress × Access to Social Networks	—	—	.25+	—
Marital Stress × Physical Health	—	−.37*	—	.31*
R^2	.10	.12	.24	.23

[a] A dash indicates that the interaction was not included in the regression equation because it lacked significance.
[b] For all variables, numerical coding is in the order indicated.
+$p < .10$. *$p < .05$. **$p < .01$. ***$p < .001$.

In Tables 7.1, 7.2, and 7.3, we can see that persons who feel more vulnerable (or overwhelmed by life circumstances) are more likely to drink and use drugs to cope with stress. This strong result appears in each of the analyses; it is true of married men and women and of employed men and women (only for married women with respect to drinking is the result not highly significant). The strong consistent relationship between feelings of vulnerability and substance use for coping portrays an image of people imprisoned by their own feelings of helplessness. They feel unable to control

Table 7.3

REGRESSIONS OF USING ALCOHOL OR DRUGS TO HANDLE TENSION ON JOB STRESS: SELECTED SOCIAL AND PERSONAL CHARACTERISTICS AND ALTERNATIVE COPING STYLES, BY SEX[a]

Predictor[b]	Use of alcohol (low–high)		Use of drugs (low–high)	
	Men (N = 366) beta	Women (N = 974) beta	Men (N = 682) beta	Women (N = 970) beta
Stress				
Job stress, looking for another job (likely–not likely)	−.06	.07	.00	−.02
Social characteristics				
Age (young–old)	−.03	−.65***	.05	.05
Education (low–high)	.00	−.01	−.04	.01
Family income (low–high)	.06	.05	.29*	.00
Access to social network (little–lot)	−.13**	−.10*	−.02	.03
Marital status (married–not)	.03	.02	.00	.00
Personal characteristics				
Lack of confidence (high–low)	−.12**	.04	−.02	.11*
Feelings of vulnerability (low–high)	.16***	.19***	.15***	.25***
Physical health (good–bad)	.01	.00	.26***	.20***
Coping Styles for Unhappiness				
Passive coping (yes–no)	.02	−.02	−.01	−.07
Prayer (yes–no)	.11*	.11+	−.03	−.05
Talk to friend (yes–no)	.11*	−.28*	.00	−.03
Interactions				
Job Stress × Age of Respondent	—	.57**	—	—
Job Stress × Talk to Friend	—	.27**	—	—
Job Stress × Family Income	—	—	−.26*	—
R^2	.10	.14	.13	.17

[a]A dash indicates that the interaction was not included in the regression equation because it lacked significance.
[b]For all variables, numerical coding is in the order indicated.
+$p < .10$. *$p < .05$. **$p < .01$. ***$p < .001$.

their world, so they take substances that may control them, thus further perpetuating their helplessness. This conveys the sense that alcohol or drug use for coping is a response of learned helplessness resulting from the feeling that the individual does not have control over the environment and that efforts made to change are essentially futile. These results directly confirm Marlatt's (1979) formulation that a person's sense of personal efficacy is critical to whether or not he or she will cope with stress by turning to substance use.

In all but one instance across Tables 7.1, 7.2, and 7.3 there is a strong relationship between poor physical health and the use of drugs to cope among both men and women. The relationship between physical ill health and drug use is not surprising. Ill people are much more likely to use drugs in general, often in conjunction with pain relief, and therefore, they might be more likely to use drugs to cope with stress. But one could also argue that ill health might reduce coping strategies in general. This, combined with the fact that psychological vulnerability also contributes to drug taking as a coping strategy, conveys the impression that people who use drugs to cope with stress do not have many coping alternatives. It is interesting to note that ill health is largely unrelated to the use of alcohol to cope. One exception is that married women under marital stress and in poor health are less likely to drink.

As we hypothesized earlier, people who pray to cope with unhappiness do not, in general, drink to cope with stress. The effect is consistently apparent in the analysis of the women's data. All things being equal, women who use prayer as a coping strategy do not use drinking as a coping strategy. This relationship could be a reflection of the moral sanctions against using alcohol to cope (or against a failure to use prayer to cope) amongst many people who actively practice their faith. People who use prayer as a coping strategy are probably more likely to be involved with organized religion than those who do not use prayer for solace. The organizational and participatory aspects of formal religion provide yet another mechanism for reducing stress.

Other main effects discovered in Tables 7.1, 7.2, and 7.3 point indirectly to the same phenomenon about vulnerability and substance use. Among men the variables youth, bachelorhood, little access to social networks, and low self-confidence are all clearly associated with substance use to handle stress. Thus, variables that suggest life patterns of vulnerability and a lack of personal, social, and organizational commitment are likely to relate to coping with stress by substance use in men.

For women, such proxy variables for vulnerability do not appear to have the same effect as they do for men. The most important main effect for women is that being employed relates to drinking to relieve tension (see Table 7.1 and 7.2). Johnson (1982) also found that employed women drink more than nonemployed women. Our results suggest that their drinking is not solely confined to social drinking but is used for coping as well. Table 7.2 also suggests that among married women, high family income is associated with drinking as a coping strategy. Women apparently need to live in a somewhat affluent milieu in order to resort to drinking. This is evidently not an issue for men, who employ drinking as a coping strategy regardless of their economic resources.

Economic Worries and the Use of Alcohol to Cope

We turn now to findings on the interaction between stress and coping, some examples of which are diagrammed in Figure 7.1. With regard to economic stress, the results in Table 7.1 show that men with a higher need for power drink less as economic stress increases. The strong positive relationship between the need for interpersonal power and drinking exists only among those men who do not mention worrying about economic matters. This finding counters our original hypothesis that economic worries would heighten an individual's need to control the environment and other people. But perhaps the external quality of the stressor draws the focus from the self and ego-needs, triggers the performance of basic survival skills and renders the need to create the illusion of power through drinking alcohol less important. In other words, the need for power may give rise to ego-connected defense mechanisms like drinking only when the stress being experienced is more internal, or at least not easily attributed to outside forces.

There is no relationship between a need for power and drinking to cope among women. We can conjecture that either women do not find stress-related events connected to the adequacy of their egos to control their interpersonal world or that they do not experience any heightened control under the influence of alcohol. We favor the latter interpretation. We suggest that the social meaning of intoxication permits men to feel more masculine and in control but may cause women to feel unfeminine and less in control. For instance, intoxicated women have been vulnerable targets for unwelcome sexual overtures and sexual assaults.

There is a rather different pattern of factors associated with drinking in women in response to economic stress. There are interactive effects with both marital status and age. The presence of economic worries interacts with marital status in its relationship to drinking to cope so that unmarried women are more likely to report drinking to cope under conditions of financial worries, but married women are less likely to make such reports under the same conditions (Figure 1a). This interaction suggests two different explanations. The first focuses on unmarried women. The burden of their financial support falls mostly on themselves, so when they worry about finances, the stress may be quite severe. Under these conditions they may be less likely to see ways to solve their problems and drink to reduce stress because there are few coping alternatives. For unmarried women, using alcohol to cope may forestall the implementation of other coping strategies. The second explanation focuses on the married women, who are more likely to report drinking to handle tension when they are not suffering any financial stress. These women may not experience a great deal of stress in general and may simply drink to relax after a trying day.

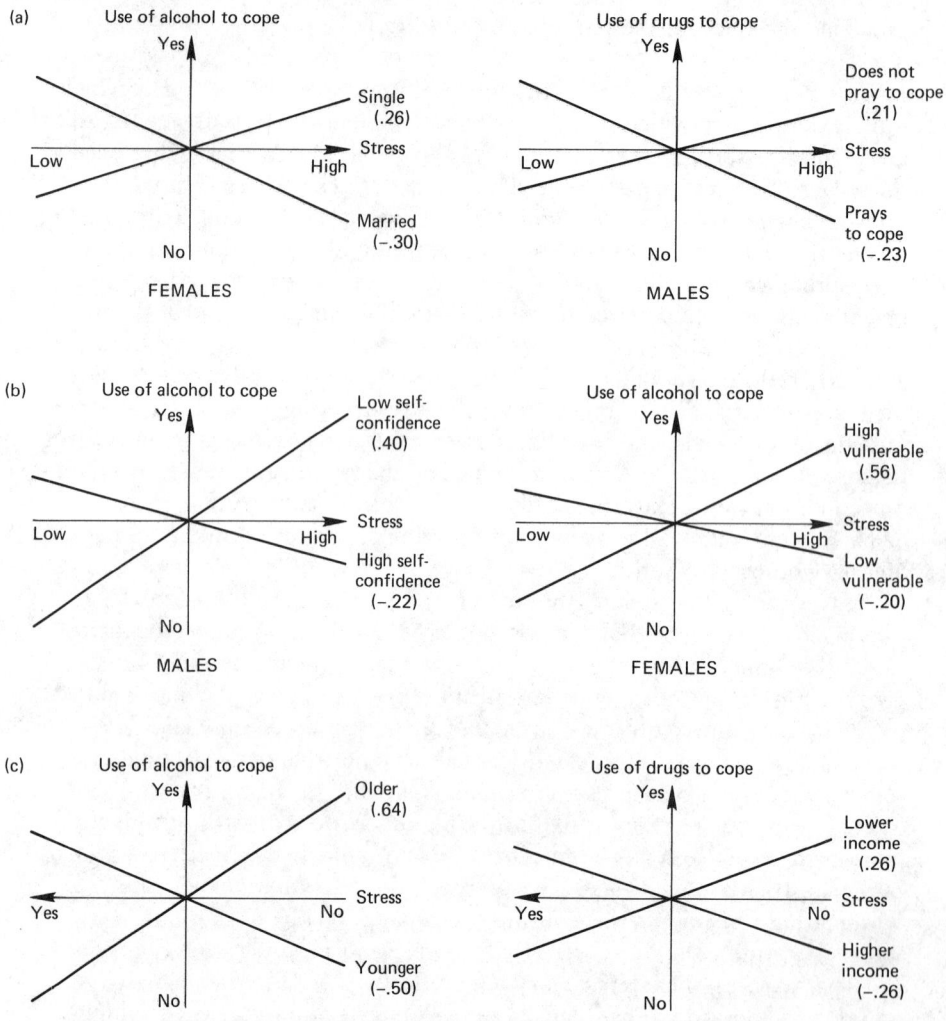

Figure 7.1 Interactions between stressors and substance-use coping. (a), economic worries; (b), marital strain; (c), job stress. Effects are shown in parentheses. Note that job stress variable is inversely scored.

The relationship between drinking to cope with stress and economic worry also varies by women's age. Younger women are more likely to drink to cope when they also mention being worried about finances. Older women are more likely to say they drink to cope with stress when they are not under financial stress. The pattern of relationships here is very similar to those described above. Younger women, with less experience in handling economic crises, might feel somewhat paralyzed when actually faced with these kinds of problems. Under these conditions, drinking may temporarily help to relieve anxiety but perhaps not in the long run. Older women under the same conditions may have developed ways for coping with financial stress so that it does not frighten or discourage them. Older women who do not mention economic worries, possibly like the married women, may view drinking alcohol as a legitimate response to everyday stresses but not to more serious financial stress. Younger and unmarried women have, on the one hand, less experience, and on the other, less financial support (i.e., fewer resources) and may see drinking as a good way to handle severe anxiety.

Economic Worries and the Use of Drugs to Cope

Talking to cope and having access to a social network both represent aspects of social integration. Yet one represents a coping style that may be independent of one's style of social interaction (these results appear in Table 7.1). Men with sufficient access to a social network are more likely to use drugs when faced with economic worries than are men with little access to a social network. Access to a social network may provide men with information about the utility of drugs for coping, legitimation of their use, and the actual access to drugs either through doctors or private sources. The effect of economic worries on the relationship between using drugs to cope and talking as a coping strategy shows that men who do not tend to talk with others as a coping strategy are more likely to say they use drugs to cope with stress when they are also confronted with economic worries (irrespective of their level of social access). Similarly, men who use prayer as a coping strategy are less likely to use drugs to cope when faced with financial pressure. It appears that substance use for men faced with financial pressure is used in lieu of talking or praying.

It is interesting, and somewhat surprising, to note the relationship between using prayer to cope with unhappiness and the use of drugs to cope. Among men, the more likely they are to pray in the face of unhappiness, the more likely they use drugs to cope with stress when they are not under financial pressure (Figure 1a). It seems that for religious men, drugs are legitimate ways to reduce stress (if they can afford them?). Drug use (likely to be prescribed treatment) must not call into question the strength of their faith as alcohol (likely not to be prescribed) seems to do. There are no interactions between economic worries, personal resources, and the use of drugs to cope in women.

Marital Stress and the Use of Alcohol to Cope

The listing of the regression results in Table 7.2 shows that men having problems in their marriage and who are not very confident about themselves drink to relieve tension. One might suppose that a man already unsure of himself might feel particularly vulnerable when under marital tensions. Drinking as a protest to feeling disadvantaged in a marriage can easily result. By contrast, more confident men are less likely to drink to relieve tension if they experience stress in their marriage than if they do not experience such stress (Figure 1b). It is as if these men feel that they need a clear head to handle difficult marital troubles but can appreciate the relaxation of drinking when only minor tensions arise. This represents a recurring pattern in these data. Certain people, while they may use alcohol as a coping device under minimal stress, evidently avoid it when highly stressful conditions prevail. This pattern may be common in many marriages.

The regression analyses in Table 7.2 indicate that women who experience more marital stress and who feel particularly vulnerable, are older or in good physical health report more drinking in response to stress. That women who feel particularly vulnerable respond to stress by drinking is similar to the result about men who lack confidence in themselves (Figure 1b). Drinking can dull a woman's sense of vulnerability that might arise in conjunction with marital discord, just as drinking can give a man a sense of control if he lacks confidence in his marital strife.

Why is drinking in conjunction with marital stress characteristic of older but not younger women? One might speculate that younger women feel particularly responsible for the care of young children. Drinking may be seen as incompatible with that responsibility. As close supervision of children is reduced when women get older, the psychological constraints against drinking may be lifted.

Why are healthy women facing marital problems more likely to drink to relieve tension, whereas those in bad health are less likely to drink as stress increases? Perhaps unhealthy women might attribute any marital distress they encounter as reactive to their poor health and take more drugs instead of drinking. Marital distress that occurs without such an easy objective attribution of difficulty could be more threatening. Given that assumption, we suggest that healthy women feel much more psychologically vulnerable to marital difficulty—and hence respond with drinking—than women in ill health. Unhealthy women, on the other hand, may feel more physically vulnerable in the face of stress—and take more medicine.

Marital Stress and the Use of Drugs to Cope

Regression analyses in Table 7.2 focusing on drug use and marital stress point to two factors that are generally predictive of using drugs to relieve tension among married men and women: poor health and feelings of vulnerability. These two factors reflect issues of general stress—one more physical, the other more psychological. It is interesting to note, however, that the relationship of health to using drugs occurs only among women experiencing marital distress. Thus, ill health in and of itself does not affect drug taking to relieve stress in married women but only if they feel upset about their marital situation. One might speculate that in good marriages, husbands can mitigate some of the feelings of vulnerability that women encounter in their experiences of ill health, enough to dampen interests in turning to drugs.

Although subjective feelings of vulnerability seem clearly tied to drug taking in both men and women, some more objective situations also make married men vulnerable to drug taking. There are two instances in the regression analyses for men in which interactions with marital stress are predictive of drug taking. Better educated men who are experiencing stress in their marriages are more likely to use drugs to relieve tensions than less educated men; and men with more access to a social network are more likely to take drugs when faced with marital stress than are those with little access to a social network. It is probable that men who are less educated or without much outside social support are especially attached to their wives. If they are in a well-functioning marriage, they would be particularly unwilling to disrupt the relationship by doing or saying anything that would hurt their wives. These men probably would resist drinking, since it is often the basis of disruption in marriage. They might accept taking drugs as a way to cope with the tensions experienced outside of the marriage, since legal drug taking is more consonant with the way women cope with tensions than with the way men do.

Work Stress and the Use of Alcohol to Cope

Table 7.3 reports the regression models used to predict alcohol and drug use in employed people. It is clear from Table 7.3 that among men various resources or the lack of them do not affect the relationship of work stress to drinking. In fact, work stress itself is not significantly related to drinking among men.

Although looking for another job is unrelated to the use of alcohol to cope in men, Table 7.3 shows that women looking for another job appear more likely to say they drink to cope with stress if they are young (Figure 1c) and if they generally talk to someone to help them cope with unhappiness. Whether the stress of job dissatisfaction evokes or simply relates to the use of alcohol to cope among younger women and not older women, we might speculate about the meaning and function of the work role to younger and older women. The older women are more likely to be married with grown children and to have been raised with the belief that work is an option for women—not their primary role—and not worth the investment of their self-identity. They may also have had more experience with unsatisfactory jobs. The younger women, in contrast, are better educated and may have higher expectations for advancement from their jobs; they are less likely to have families and more likely to be working. In these ways, work for young women may be a more important source of self-esteem and identity than for older women. If success at work is a source of high self-esteem for young women, then stress or failure in that role must be a source of anxiety and depression. Then younger women, more than older women, feel internal stress and anxiety as a result of failure in a job and are more likely to drink in response to job-related stress.

Table 7.3 also shows that women who say they generally talk to someone when they are unhappy are also more likely to say they drink to cope when faced with job stress. Women who do not talk to others when they are unhappy are less likely to drink to cope as job stress increases. This finding seems to illustrate two different dynamics. The use of alcohol may be a social facilitator for the women experiencing job stress and who generally use social networks to help them cope. For example, they may use a "happy hour" as a time during which they can relax with co-workers and discuss bitter job experiences. Sharing the misery or just having your feelings affirmed in the context of using alcohol may greatly help in the coping process. The person in this example is not likely to be overwhelmed by the job search and is also using other modes for handling the stress. Alcohol is used in a limited and perhaps effective way.

Women who say that they do not talk to others when they are unhappy may not have very well-developed coping strategies for dealing with minor life stress. They may not be very good at taking action; they let things happen to them. Drinking alcohol to cope with stress is a way to feel better and yet not to have to work at figuring how to improve a situation. But the women actually looking for another job have initiated action or have begun actively coping with their job dissatisfaction, and they may not need to use alcohol to cope. The initiation of an active coping strategy may thus decrease the likelihood that they would also drink to cope with the stress.

Work Stress and the Use of Drugs to Cope

Regression analyses in Table 7.3 indicate that there is a positive relationship of work stress to drug taking but only among those employed men who have high incomes (see Figure 7.1c). This finding suggests that it takes money to support that kind of style of adaptation to work stress. The more financially resourceful man who is distressed with his work is the one who turns to drugs. He is, in effect, using a coping style more typical of women than of men. We saw in the section, "Marital Stress and the Use of Alcohol to Cope," that greater income in women permits them to cope with marital stress by drinking. It may be that assuming the coping styles of the opposite sex requires whatever assurance that financial security brings. For employed women, the stress of job dissatisfaction does not relate directly to the use of drugs to cope with stress.

SUMMARY AND CONCLUSIONS

Results of analyses of the moderating effects of personal resources on the relationship between life stress and the use of alcohol and drugs to cope formed some consistent patterns. In general, people under stress or with fewer psychological resources (e.g., lack of self-confidence, feelings of vulnerability) show a greater overall tendency to use alcohol or drugs to help handle tension. However, we also find that among persons who are not under any major life stress, those who appear well adjusted, tend to use alcohol or drugs more often than less well-adjusted people. Putting these patterns together we can say that as stress increases, people who feel vulnerable to stress and lack confidence in themselves are more likely to rely on drinking and drug use to cope, but people who feel efficacious and confident about themselves are less likely to rely on drinking and drug use. This pattern underscores the dual aspect of substance use. It is certainly related to stress but, under everyday circumstances, it may be related to effecting pleasurable activities. In general, however, these findings parallel previously documented connections between low self-esteem and heavy drinking (Pearlin & Radabaugh, 1977). Our results strongly support Marlatt's (1979) formulation about substance use, in particular alcohol use, as a means of coping among people who feel inadequate about their capacities to deal with stress.

These patterns suggest that alcohol and drugs serve very different coping functions for different people. For those who cannot cope with stress very well, alcohol and drugs may be the only way to quiet the internal accusations of incompetence or their anxieties about abandonment. Alcohol and drugs weave a fairy-soft web of illusion about the self and the burdens of life. For people who can generally cope well with severe life stresses, alcohol and drugs may be an effective way to handle minor tensions and anxiety. When the major facet of a problem is merely the physiological tension, then alcohol or drugs may be effective tools to aid in relaxing. We suspect that the amount of alcohol or drugs needed to "escape" when stressed is much greater than the amount of alcohol needed to "relax" when not greatly stressed. Expectations of alcohol or drugs involving moderate use are more healthy than expectations involving heavy use, since after all, alcohol is in many ways a poison.

Beyond these general patterns we were also impressed with how gender conditions many of the findings. For example, results partially support McClelland et al.'s (1972) framework about the importance of power motivation in evaluating drinking in men; no parallel results exist for women. These results are consistent with Brown et al.'s (1978) finding that the expectation that alcohol will enhance physical prowess is related to heavier drinking in general. Men were much more likely to believe that alcohol enhanced sexuality and aggressiveness than were women. Being older is related to drinking in women under marital stress; no parallel results exist for men. In these instances and in others that were discovered, we construed ways in which differential gender proscriptions in the family, in work, or in the proper use of substances for coping can produce very different results for men and women. Similar trends have been documented in relation to family role responsibilities and psychotropic drug use (Cafferata, Kasper, & Bernstein, 1983), suggesting consistent differences between the sexes in the types of stressful contexts that relate to substance use for coping.

We are equally impressed with the ways in which some of the factors affecting the use of alcohol or drugs to cope with stress were specific to the kind of stress considered. Power motivation was relevant for men only when economic stress was an issue. Income was relevant for men only when job stress was being considered. These and other results reinforce Abrams' (1983) contention that the dynamics of substance use, while clearly dependent on people's generalized perceived vulnerability, are highly contextual. Specific factors increase or decrease the likelihood of substance use for each of the types of stress we examined.

Finally, we were impressed that measures of perceived efficaciousness and confidence are strongly related to the use of both kinds of substances. However, we are equally impressed that different factors also come into play, depending on whether we are explaining drug use or alcohol use.

The implication of all these additional impressions is that one cannot generalize too broadly about factors relevant to drug and alcohol use under stress. Researchers and clinicians must be aware of whether they are observing or helping men or women, what kind of stress these people are under, and whether they are using alcohol or drugs as their instruments of coping. Nevertheless, analyses show that, whether male or female, people with few personal resources are more likely to use both alcohol and drugs in general, and that the presence of severe life stress—whatever it may be—increases that propensity even further. People with sufficient personal resources use alcohol and drugs to cope under very different circumstances. We believe that the differences in alcohol and drug use in these two populations stem from their expectations about the effectiveness of alcohol, their coping alternatives, and the degree to which a stressor is perceived as stressful.

REFERENCES

Abrams, D. B. (1983). Psycho-social assessment of alcohol and stress interactions: Bridging the gap between laboratory and treatment outcome research. In L. Pohorecky & J. Brick (Eds.), *Stress and alcohol use*. New York: Elsevier.

Antonucci, T. C., & Depner, C. E. (1982). School support and informal helping relationships. In T. A. Wills (Ed.), *Basic processes in helping relationships*. New York: Academic Press.

Brown, S., Goldman, M., Inn, A., & Anderson, L. (1980). Expectations of reinforcement from alcohol: their domain and relation to drinking patterns. *Journal of Consulting and Clinical Psychology, 48,* 419–426.

Bryant, F., & Veroff, J. (1984). Dimensions of subjective mental health. *Journal of Health and Social Behavior, 25,* 116–135.

Cafferata, G., Kasper, J., & Bernstein, A. (1983). Family roles, structure, and stressors in relation to sex differences in obtaining psychotropic drugs. *Journal of Health and Social Behavior, 24,* 132–143.

Cleary, P. D., & Kessler, R. C. (1982). The estimation and interpretation of modifier effects. *Journal of Health and Social Behavior, 23,* 159–169.

Coyne, J. C., and Lazarus, R. S. (1980). Cognitive style, stress perception, and coping. In I. L. Kutash & L. B. Schlesinger (Eds.), *Handbook of stress and anxiety*. San Francisco: Jossey-Bass.

Deardorff, C. M., Melges, F. T., Hout, C. N., & Savage, D. J. (1975). Situations related to drinking alcohol: A factor analysis of questionnaire responses. *Journal of Studies on Alcohol, 36,* 1184–1195.

Dohrenwend, B. P., Shrout, P. E., Egri, G., & Mendelsohn, F. S. (1980). Nonspecific psychological distress and other dimensions of psychopathology. *Archives of General Psychiatry, 37,* 1229–1236.

Garber, J., & Seligman, M. E. P. (Eds.). (1980). *Human helplessness: Theory and applications*. New York: Academic Press.

Gourash, N. (1978). Help-seeking: A review of the literature. *American Journal of Community Psychology, 6,* 413–423.

Jessor, R., & Jessor, S. L. (1977). *Problem behavior and psychosocial development: A longitudinal study of youth*. New York: Academic Press.

Johnson, P. B. (1982). Sex differences, women's roles and alcohol use: Preliminary national data. *Journal of Social Issues, 38,* 93–116.

Kahn, R. L., & Antonucci, T. C. (1980). Convoys over the life course: Attachment, roles, and social support. In P. B. Baltes & O. Brim (Eds.), *Life span development and behavior* (Vol. 3). New York: Academic Press.

Marlatt, G. A. (1979). Alcohol use and problem drinking: A cognitive-behavioral analysis. In P. C. Kendall & S. D. Hollon (Eds.), *Cognitive behavioral intervention: Theory, research, and procedures.* New York: Academic Press.

McClelland, D. C. (1975). *Power: The inner experience.* New York: Irvington Publishers.

McClelland, D. C., Davis, W. N., Kalin, R., & Wanner, E. (1972). *The drinking man.* New York: Free Press.

Neff, J. A., & Husaini, B. A. (1982). Life events, drinking patterns and depressive symptomatology: The stress-buffering role of alcohol consumption. *Journal of Studies on Alcohol, 43,* 301–318.

Parry, H. J., Cisin, I., Balter, M., Mellinger, G., & Manheimer, D. (1974). Increasing alcohol intake as a coping mechanism for psychic distress. In R. Cooperstock (Ed.), *Social aspects of the medical use of psychotropic drugs.* Toronto: Alcoholism and Drug Research Foundation of Ontario.

Pearlin, L., & Radabaugh, C. (1977). Economic strains and the coping functions of alcohol. *American Journal of Sociology, 82,* 652–663.

Timmer, S. G., Bryant, F., & Veroff, J. (in preparation). Factor analyses of reactions to family roles in *The Inner American.*

Veroff, J., Depner, C., Kulka, R., & Douvan, E. (1980). Comparison of American motives: 1957 vs. 1976. *Journal of Personality and Social Psychology, 39,* 1258–1271.

Veroff, J., Douvan, E., & Kulka, R. (1981). *The inner American.* New York: Basic Books.

Veroff, J., Kulka, R., & Douvan, E. (1981). *Mental health in America.* New York: Basic Books.

Warren, D. T. (1981). *Helping networks: How people cope with problems in the urban community.* Notre Dame, IN: University of Notre Dame Press.

Wills, T. A., & Warshawsky, A. (1983, August). Stressful events, coping behavior patterns, and substance use in middle adolescence. In S. Shiffman (Chair), *Stress and smoking.* Symposium conducted at the meeting of the American Psychological Association, Anaheim, CA.

Wilson, G. T., & Abrams, D. (1977). Effects of alcohol on social anxiety and physiological arousal: Cognitive versus pharmacological processes. *Cognitive Therapy and Research, 1,* 195–210.

Winter, D. *The power motive.* (1973). New York: Free Press.

Chapter 8

Daily Coping and Alcohol Use in a Sample of Community Adults*

ARTHUR A. STONE
SHELLEY LENNOX
JOHN M. NEALE

INTRODUCTION

There are two ideas that are central to this volume: that substance use relates to stress and that the level of substance use may be affected by how people cope with stress. In this chapter we examine data relevant to these issues, using alcohol as an example.

The tension reduction hypothesis (TRH) of alcohol use is clearly an example of substance use as a method of coping. According to the TRH, stressful situations raise the level of a person's tension or anxiety and alcohol is then ingested as an immediate means of reducing these unpleasant affective states. Used this way, alcohol has reinforcing properties that increase the likelihood of repeated use in stressful and/or nonstressful situations. For some persons, alcohol use then develops into a pattern of habitual, problematic drinking. Many laboratory studies have been conducted to explore this model of alcohol abuse and the processes that may account for the effect; for example, investigations of what individuals believe will happen to them if they drink alcohol (see Abrams, 1983).

A second way of viewing alcohol ingestion is as the end point in the stress–appraisal–coping–outcome model that is seen very often in the stress and coping literature. Here alcohol use is viewed as one of many possible consequences of stress, which include physical illness, psychiatric illness, reduced productivity, and low morale. In this approach to the prediction of

---

*The authors thank Lina Jandorf for her contribution to this paper. This material is based on work supported by the National Science Foundation under Grant no. BNS-7923715.

heavy drinking, an individual appraises a situation as stressful and tries to cope with it. When efforts to cope are unsuccessful, increased drinking may occur. Alcohol use at this point may be used to relax or even distract the individual. Thus, increased alcohol use is posited to result from ineffective coping, just as ineffective coping could lead to illness, dysphoric mood, or reduced productivity. If ineffective coping results in increased tension, as most stress investigators would probably agree, then the use of alcohol may be thought of as coping with the tensions that result from poor coping.

Our approach in this chapter is to consider alcohol use as both a direct (primarily coping) and indirect (primarily outcome) method of coping. Thus, some of our analyses treat alcohol as a method of coping with the problematic situation, while others view it as the result of particular coping strategies. We present a model for conceptualizing events, appraisals of events, and coping and describe the measures we have developed for daily assessments of these variables. We then describe how patterns of alcohol use are related to life events appraisals, mood, and coping.

TRANSACTIONAL MODEL OF STRESS AND COPING

A general model of stress and coping, described by R. Lazarus and his associates (Coyne & Lazarus, 1980; Lazarus, 1966), has guided much of our research. In brief, an environmental occurrence is first perceived, and then it may be appraised as threatening, outside control, or undesirable. Because these appraisals of the situation define stress, what is stressful for one individual may not be stressful for another. Just what is appraised as stress for someone may depend on a number of factors, including the person's background, past experience with the occurrence, and the context of the occurrence. Once the situation is appraised as stressful, the person determines how he or she will cope with it. Lazarus discusses many types of coping, including the general classes of problem-focused coping (behaviors or thoughts that directly address the situation) and emotion-focused coping (thoughts that are meant to reduce the distress associated with the situation). Once coping has been initiated, it is then evaluated as to its effectiveness and, if necessary, other ways of coping are used. This dynamic feedback aspect of the model has been termed *transactional*.

Although the transactional model of stress and coping is appealing, and there is some laboratory-based evidence to support its validity, it has not been employed to any great extent in the study of stress and coping in relationship to alcohol use. Most studes of alcohol in the natural environment have used cross-sectional designs wherein stress, coping, and alcohol use have been measured at one point in time. A better design is prospective, in the sense that measurements of the independent and dependent measures are made at two or three points, but these designs have often used retrospective assessments of stress and coping. One common measure, the Holmes and Rahe (1967) Social Readjustment Rating Scale, measures life events over the past 6 or 8 months (see, e.g., Neff & Husaini, 1982). Likewise, the coping inventories that have been used often measure trait-like coping; that is, the questions on the inventory either ask how the individual generally copes with problematic situations or present the subject with a small number of situations and ask how they would cope with them. Neither of these approaches allows coping to vary widely across different kinds of problematic situations. Yet, available research indicates that coping does vary considerably according to the content of the problem (Billings & Moos, 1981; Folkman & Lazarus, 1980; Pearlin & Schooler, 1978). Clearly, these sorts of data cannot address the transactional view of stress and coping. In most published research the assessment of stress has not been specific: A total score on a life event inventory tells us little about what the individual actually experienced—for example, were there many small events or a few major ones? Also, the coping assessments give us no information about how a particular situation was coped with or how the coping changes over time. These problems with the measurement of stress and coping are not limited to studies where alcohol is the outcome measure; similar conceptual and measurement problems are quite evident in general studies of stress and coping (Cohen & Lazarus, 1979; Coyne & Lazarus, 1980).

Our own research has focused on achieving a better understanding of the relationships among environmental occurrences and their appraisal, coping, mood, and symptomatology. To do this, we broke away from the typical design used in life events research, which we considered too coarse to yield interesting data relevant to the transactional model. Instead, we changed the time frame of our designs to use days as the unit of measurement. Questionnaires were not available for doing this; thus, we developed the Daily Life Experiences survey (DLE) and a Daily Coping Inventory (DCI). A brief description of the development of these instruments follows to provide a clear understanding of our approach to stress and coping.

Daily Life Events

Following the general life events checklist strategy, we aimed to create a daily event checklist. To insure that the list of events was representative of people's daily activities, we first had a representative group of 32 couples record in diary format either "meaningful" or "emotionally laden" events for 14 consecutive days. To organize the daily experiences into categories, the 1848 experiences were content analyzed by two research assistants whose task was to organize the experiences into categories arranged in outline form. After much discussion, the outlines generated by each research assistant were combined to yield a 66-item outline with two levels of headings. To provide subjects with a means of rating their appraisals of the events we devised four rating dimensions for each event. Three of the dimensions were derived from a factor-analytic study where it was found that desirability–undesirability, changing–stabilizing (with regard to their lifestyle), and meaningfulness were important concepts for describing events (Redfield & Stone, 1979). Because events out of an individual's control may be related to negative health outcomes, the dimension of control over the event's occurrence was also included.

We next did a pilot study to determine if the questionnaire could be completed properly and to test several hypotheses. One result that is of particular interest from the pilot study is the development of the target–observer procedure. As a check on report validity, husbands monitored their own experiences, and simultaneously, wives rated their husband's experiences. We found that targets occasionally did not record experiences that had happened. As a result, the target–observer procedure was adopted as a routine aspect of data collection. Targets and observers first independently check what they believe happened to the observer; next they review each other's forms and discuss and resolve any disagreements, finally providing a consensus list of the day's events. This procedure increases the accuracy of the daily event reports. A full description of the DLE's development is found in Stone and Neale (1982).

Daily Coping Inventory

In some ways the development of a new coping inventory was a more difficult task than the events checklist because the coping literature is so diverse in both the definition of coping and approaches toward its measurement. For example, measuring the concept of complete denial of a problem would require detailed observations of people and their environment and, thus, was out of the domain of what was feasible to measure on a daily basis.

Our first step was to survey the existing coping questionnaires. A large list of potential items for what we imagined would be a fairly short coping checklist were assembled with the intention of locating the best items repre-sentive of various coping concepts. The individual items were rationally sorted into 10 scales that represented most of the kinds of coping found in the literature. A pilot study was conducted with a sample of convenience in which subjects were asked to describe a recent problem and check items that were used to handle it. However, we found relatively poor internal consistency coefficients (alpha): Several scales were below .60. As this was unsatisfactory, two additional pilot studies were conducted to improve our understanding of how the items fit into coping classes. In these studies, participants sorted individual coping items into conceptually similar categories, thus we could examine individual differences in categorizing the coping items.

To summarize, the results of having individuals sort coping items into conceptual bins showed that various items could be viewed as falling into more than one coping type. For example, the item "asked someone else to handle the problem" was classified as "seeking social supports" one-third of the time and two-thirds of the time as falling into the other coping categories. In other words, for many of the items the intention of what the person thought the action or thought could accomplish could vary depending on both the person and/or the situation.

This information led us to take an unusual route in developing the questionnaire finally used; instead of specifying particular actions or thoughts and letting them be checked in response to a problem, we listed various intentions on the questionniare. For instance, the questionniare asked "Did you do anything to distract yourself from the problem?" to which the subject answered yes or no. If the response was yes, they then described the particular thought or action in a few blank lines immediately following the original question. The final coping categories included in the DCI are found in Table 8.1 (see p. 207). For a more detailed description of this work see Stone and Neale (1984b).

Events, Coping, and Alcohol Use

Our research has been concerned mainly with conceptualizing stressful events and coping and exploring the relationships among stress, appraisal, coping, mood, and symptoms. This chapter examines how people with different levels of drinking perform with our new questionnaires in a prospective study. The results are relevant to general methodological and theoretical issues in studying the relationship between coping and substance use, and with the available data we attempt to test some issues relevant to the tension-reduction model of alcohol use.

METHOD

Overview

Participants in the study were first visited in their homes and trained in the use of the measures that would be collected on a daily basis for the next

16 weeks. This prospective assessment included our measure of daily experiences, mood, symptoms and medication use, and coping. During the home visit subjects also completed a number of other questionnaires concerning demographic characteristics, personality, psychological distress, marital satisfaction, and a retrospective assessment of both life events and symptoms experienced during the previous year. Drinking patterns for the past year were also assessed during the home visit.

Subjects

Subjects were solicited by mail from two communities in eastern Long Island. Postcards with a brief description of the study were initially sent to all residences in the selected areas ($n = 3107$). Subjects who expressed interest in participation ($n = 516$) were subsequently sent more detailed information about what the study entailed. As married couples were the population of interest, volunteers who fulfilled this criterion were selected to be interviewed in their homes and trained in the use of the daily booklet ($n = 149$ couples). Data on the 79 couples who participated for at least 12 weeks total (84 days) were included in most of the analyses to be reported. Three subjects had missing data on the alcohol questions and were not included in the analyses; also, some individuals did not complete the coping section of the booklet for a minimum of 12 weeks, and they were not included in the coping analyses. Moreover, as women were not required to report on daily events and mood, information on these variables was available for men only. The sample is clearly self-selected and should not be regarded in any sense as a random population sample. It is likely, for example, that our participants are better adjusted than a random sample of the population and drink less than an average amount of alcohol.

The mean ages for the men and women were 43.2 years ($SD = 10.1$) and 40.4 years ($SD = 9.5$), respectively. The mean educational level for the men was 14.0 years ($SD = 2.3$), and 13.4 years ($SD = 2.0$) for the women. Mean family income was $30,965 ($SD = $10,532$).

Retrospective and Demographic Data

Drinking patterns over the past year were assessed during our preliminary interview with subjects prior to the start of daily recording. Drinking was measured with a brief questionnaire that asked subjects whether or not they consumed any alcohol during this period and, if they had, the frequency with which they had done so. Subjects also indicated the drink most frequently imbibed (i.e., beer, wine, or liquor) and the typical quantity consumed over a 24-hour period.

Many other questionnaires were completed during the background interview. Socioeconomic status (SES) was quantified with the Duncan Index of Occupational Status (Reiss, 1961), which codes the occupation of the major household wage earner on a scale of 0 to 100. (Information about both average education and income is derived from this scale.) Life events experienced over the previous year were assessed with a revised version of Myers, Lindenthal, and Pepper's (1974) checklist, which also included seven items from Dohrenwend's (1974) form. Physical symptoms (e.g., constipation, stomachache) present during this same time period were measured with a 93-item checklist developed by Wyler, Masuda, and Holmes (1968). Sick-role tendency was evaluated with Mechanic and Volkart's (1961) scale, and hypochondriasis with Pilowsky's (1967) questionnaire. The General Health Questionnaire (GHQ, Goldberg & Hillier, 1979) was used as a measure of psychological distress, Jackson's Personality Research Form (1974, PRF: Form E) assessed 22 personality variables, and the Short Marital Adjustment Test (MAT, Locke & Wallace, 1959) served as a measure of marital satisfaction.

Prospective Assessment

Prospective data were collected through use of a 20-page booklet, a multicomponent instrument that assesses mood, daily events (DLE), symptoms, medication use, and coping in response to problematic situations (DCI).

Mood. Mood was assessed with a revised 12-item version of the Nowlis Mood Adjective Checklist (Nowlis, 1965), originally a 36-item questionnaire that has been factor analyzed into the two main factors of negative and positive engagement (Stone, 1981). Each of the 12 mood items was measured with a 3-point response key, with 1 indicating its definite presence and 3 representing the absence of mood.[1] The Nowlis appears to be a reasonable method for assessing an entire day's mood (Hedges, Jandorf, & Stone, in press). In addition, several aspects of depression were assessed with five questions taken from the Beck Depression Inventory (BDI; Beck, Ward, Mendelson, Mock, & Erbaugh, 1961), a 21-item questionnaire originally designed to assess severity of depression in those already diagnosed with the disorder. These questions were modified so that the time period referred to a single day, rather than being left unspecified as in the original version of the form.

---

[1]Negative engagement includes original Nowlis mood adjectives of angry, clutch up, concentration, skepticism, and sadness, while positive engagement includes playful, elation, energetic, kindly, self-centered, and leisurely (Stone, 1981).

Events. Event information was obtained through subjects' daily use of an 80-item event checklist, a modification of a 66-item instrument developed by Stone and Neale (1982). As discussed earlier, each event was classified in a two-level outline consisting of five major categories (upper case) with secondary classifications (lower case): WORK—concerning boss, supervisor, upper management; concerning co-workers, employees, and so forth; general happenings at work, LEISURE ACTIVITIES—personal; family oriented; social, FAMILY AND FRIEND ACTIVITIES—concerning relatives, friends, and/or neighbors; concerning target and spouse; concerning children; family duties, FINANCIAL ACTIVITIES, OTHER ACTIVITIES. Space was also provided for description of events that could not be classified elsewhere.

Each event that had occurred in the past 24 hours was rated on the four dimensions of desirability–undesirability, changing–stabilizing, meaningfulness, and control. The first two dimensions were bipolar and measured the perceived desirability or undesirability of the event or the degree to which it had changed or stabilized the respondent's life. Each consisted of a 6-point scale with the following adjectives: extremely, 1; moderately, 2; and slightly, 3; for one pole (desirable or changing) and slightly, 4; moderately, 5; and extremely, 6, for the other pole (undesirable or stabilizing). Meaningfulness and control were both unipolar and were assessed with 3-point response keys that measured the perceived meaningfulness of the event and the perceived amount of control over its occurrence. The dimensions for meaningfulness were extremely, 1; moderately, 2; and slightly, 3, and for control they were complete or quite a lot of control, 1; some control, 2; and no control, 3. Each of the dimensions was explained to subjects during the training interview and was printed in several places on the booklet.

Though event information was obtained on men only, increased accuracy of event recording was achieved through the target–observer procedure described above. Initially the spouses worked independently to reproduce the events of the husband's day, then they conferred regarding their lists. Once discrepancies were resolved and a master set of the day's events was produced, the husband again worked independently to appraise these experiences.

Symptoms and Medication Use. Physical symptoms and both their perceived cause (e.g., injury, illness, other) and perceived seriousness were recorded in this section (Verbrugge, 1979, 1980). Any medications being taken were listed and subjects indicated whether they were used prophylactically, to treat current symptoms or past health problems, or for some other

Table 8.1
DESCRIPTION OF THE COPING CATEGORIES

Category	Description printed on the inventory
Distraction	Diverted attention away from the problem by thinking about other things or engaging in some activity
Situation redefinition	Tried to see the problem in a different light that made it seem more bearable
Direct action	Thought about solutions to the problem, gathered information about it, or actually did something to try to solve it
Catharsis	Expressed emotions in response to the problem to reduce tension, anxiety, or frustration
Acceptance	Accepted that the problem had occurred, but that nothing could be done about it
Seeking social support	Sought or found emotional support from loved ones, friends, or professionals
Relaxation	Did something with the explicit intention of relaxing
Religion	Sought or found spiritual comfort and support

reason. When any medication was taken to alleviate a symptom mentioned previously, this information was provided as well.

Coping. The inventory instructed subjects to describe their "most bothersome problem" of the day (which could have been something that had occurred in the past, on the day of recording, or that was anticipated as happening in the future), and then to indicate which (if any) of the eight coping categories they had used in an attempt to handle the problem. Any number of categories could be checked. When a category was used, subjects were required to specify what they had actually done in several blank lines following each category. For coping responses that could not be classified in the existing scheme, a miscellaneous category (Other) was included. Subjects were also asked to identify the category they considered most important to handling the problem. The eight coping categories and their definitions are provided in Table 8.1.

Each problem to be coped with was appraised on the dimensions of desirability–undesirability, meaningfulness, changing–stabilizing, and control. Subjects also indicated the degree to which it was anticipated (completely unexpected, somewhat unexpected, somewhat anticipated, completely anticipated), whether or not it had occurred previously (no, yes), and its chronicity (single event, long-lasting), and frequency of occurrence. Finally, each problem was assessed on a stressfulness dimension scale of 0 to 100.

Procedure

All demographic and retrospective information was collected at a training interview conducted by advanced graduate students in the homes of the participants. During this 2-hour session, couples were instructed in the use of the daily booklets and were then given the opportunity to complete one for that day. This procedure enabled the interviewers to clarify immediately any misunderstanding about proper execution of the task. Each member of a couple them completed one booklet each day for the following 3 months. The 79 couples completing the project mailed in the booklet an average of 110.5 days per subject.

RESULTS

Classification of Subjects According to Reported Alcohol Use

Subjects were classified on alcohol use according to their position in the sample rather than relative to an absolute standard. To ensure an adequate number of subjects in each group, category boundaries were somewhat arbitrary. An alcohol consumption index was derived from the drinking questionnaire. This index was computed by multiplying the number of glasses of preferred beverage (i.e., beer, wine, or liquor) typically consumed over a 24-hour period by the estimated number of drinking days for the year.[2] Based on this index, the sample was divided into the following four

---

[2]Several subjects specified more than one beverage-type when asked about the quantity of beer, wine, or liquor consumed over a 24-hour period. However, our alcohol index was computed by multiplying drinking frequency by the quantity of one's favorite beverage only. Given the information available, we though this would yield the most accurate estimate of consumption. Our assumption was that subjects who specified various beverage-types for the quantity question actually consumed each on a different occasion. Therefore, it made sense to choose the quantity of the most frequently consumed drink as the basis of our index. However, it was possible that we misinterpreted these subjects' responses in that they actually consumed more than one type of beverage on a single drinking occasion. Consequently, to alleviate the concern that we might have underestimated total consumption, another alcohol index was derived. It was computed as the product of the sum of drinks across beverage type and the estimated number of drinking days in the year. As the two indices were almost perfectly correlated ($r = .95$), we decided to use the one originally computed, reflecting our belief in its greater accuracy.

drinking groups: (1) the abstainer or infrequent drinker, whose consumption averaged less than 1 drink per month; (2) the light drinker, whose average ranged from greater than 1 drink per month to less than 2 per week; (3) the moderate drinker, whose average consumption was between 2½ drinks a week and slightly over 1 per day; and (4) the heavy drinker, whose range of average consumption was from slightly under 2 to 12 drinks per day. However, these are self-reports of "usual" amounts of alcohol consumption and should be treated with some caution.

As a result of this method of classification, our categories are not directly comparable to others reported in the literature. For example, Cahalin, Cisin, and Crossley (1969), whose classificatory scheme is used by others in the field (e.g., Barnes & Russell, 1978; Wechsler, Demone, & Gottlieb, 1978), have different inclusion criteria for their light, moderate, and heavy drinking groups. Although total volume of alcohol consumed is an essential consideration in category assignment, the variability in quantity consumed on individual drinking occasions is important as well. Those who drink larger quantities per occasion are classified as relatively heavier drinkers. For example, the average monthly volume for each of two individuals could be 15 glasses of any alcoholic beverage (a moderate drinker according to our scheme). If, however, in any given month, the drinking patterns of these two individuals differ such that one consumed five glasses on each of three occasions while the other has a drink every other day, the former would be classified as a heavy drinker and the latter as a light drinker.

While the Cahalin et al. (1969) method enables the identification of binge drinkers, it also has the potential for assigning to the moderate group an individual whose total consumption is many times that of a heavy drinker. For instance, the moderate group includes those who consume one or two drinks twice daily, while the heavy group has individuals whose drinking pattern is five or six drinks twice or thrice monthly. Similarly, the total volume consumed by a light drinker could be substantially larger than that of a moderate drinker.

Demographic Characteristics of the Alcohol Use Groups

The abstainer–infrequent, light, moderate, and heavy drinking groups comprised 34, 67, 34, and 20 individuals, respectively (see Table 8.2). Women were overrepresented in the light category (54% of the women vs. 33% of the men), while substantially more men were moderate and heavy drinkers (48 vs. 21% of the women, $\chi^2(3) = 13.01; p < .01$).

Comparisons of the four groups on major demographic characteristics, retrospective symptom reports, mood, personality, marital satisfaction, sick-role tendency, and hypochondriasis were computed with one-way anal-

Table 8.2
MEANS OF DEMOGRAPHIC CHARACTERISTICS AND QUESTIONNAIRE DATA BY DRINKING CATEGORY

	Drinking category (means)			
Variable[a]	Abstain or infrequent	Light	Moderate	Heavy
DEMOGRAPHIC CHARACTERISTICS				
Years of education	13.90	13.74	13.96	13.05
Male+	14.00	14.27	14.22	13.13
Female+	13.82	13.40	13.41	12.80
SES	53.82	55.12	52.21	59.30
Income (in $1000)	31.50	27.95	31.92	36.38
Age***	44.12	39.13	39.88	48.60
Male	45.13	42.04	39.91	48.13
Female	43.32	37.29	39.82	50.00
PRF SCALE SCORES				
Abasement	45.47	47.18	44.03	44.85
Achievement	49.59	45.83	48.32	46.10
Affiliation	48.38	51.08	49.44	49.40
Aggression	49.91	52.77	53.21	50.35
Autonomy	43.71	42.15	43.35	43.60
Change	41.97	41.41	41.35	40.75
Cognitive structure	52.15	52.58	52.74	54.00
Defendence	49.88	52.14	53.47	49.75
Dominance+	48.32	48.41	51.82	43.95
Endurance	49.91	46.97	48.71	48.45
Exhibition	48.12	49.80	51.50	46.65
Harm avoidance	60.12	59.65	58.21	59.65
Impulsivity	50.32	49.82	49.53	49.70
Nurturance+	51.18	50.70	52.56	46.10
Order	53.24	54.77	53.47	49.85
Play*	41.65	46.79	46.24	48.70
Sentience	42.74	42.80	47.09	44.85
Social recognition	51.53	52.52	55.74	53.55
Succorance	51.15	52.15	51.53	51.95
Understand	46.00	44.53	42.24	43.00
Desirability*	48.24	48.77	51.32	45.80
Infrequency	50.62	51.23	51.00	51.55
RETROSPECTIVE EVENTS, SYMPTOMS, AND OTHER DATA FROM TRAINING INTERVIEW				
Retrospective symptoms (no.)*	9.47	9.79	8.74	6.90
Male**	9.13	8.77	8.09	6.33
Female**	9.74	10.44	10.09	8.60
Retrospective desirable events (no.)	0.91	0.76	0.79	0.90
Male*	1.13	0.92	0.91	1.13
Female*	0.74	0.66	0.55	0.20

Table 8.2 (*Continued*)

Variable[a]	Drinking category (means)			
	Abstain or infrequent	Light	Moderate	Heavy
Retrospective undesirable events (no.)	1.06	1.63	1.24	1.20
Male	0.93	1.85	1.00	1.13
Female	1.16	1.49	1.73	1.40
Retrospective ambiguous events (no.)	1.41	1.37	1.18	1.20
Male	1.33	1.54	1.30	1.33
Female	1.47	1.27	0.91	0.80
Total Retrospective events (no.)	3.38	3.76	3.21	3.30
Male	3.40	4.31	3.22	3.60
Female	3.37	3.41	3.18	2.40
Marital Adjustment Test	117.38	112.28	105.35	107.60
Male	122.27	109.85	104.30	108.33
Female	113.53	113.83	107.55	105.40
General Health Questionnaire	2.00	2.41	3.41	1.37
Male	1.00	2.40	3.35	1.07
Female	2.78	2.41	3.55	2.50
Sick role tendency	5.85	6.01	6.03	7.05
Male*	4.67	5.96	5.52	7.07
Female*	6.79	6.05	7.09	7.00
Hypochondriasis*	10.97	10.45	9.88	10.70
Male	11.33	10.42	9.74	10.60
Female	10.68	10.48	10.18	11.00
PROSPECTIVE DATA FROM DAILY LIFE EVENTS BOOKLET				
Daily Beck Depression Inv. score	5.61	5.69	5.66	5.58
Male*	5.31	5.53	5.57	5.57
Female*	5.85	5.79	5.85	5.61
Daily negative mood[b]	2.57	2.50	2.45	2.56
Daily positive mood[b]	2.42	2.25	2.27	2.34
Proportion symptomatic days[c]	0.98	0.96	0.89	0.64
Male (INT)+	0.64	0.98	0.91	0.62
Female	1.24	0.95	0.83	0.70
Daily undesirable events (no.)[b]	1.15	1.18	1.36	0.95
Daily desirable events (no.)[b]	3.96	4.35	3.57	4.46
CROSS-TABULATION BY SEX				
N				
Male	15	26	23	15
Female	19	41	11	5

[a](INT) indicates a sex by group interaction is present.
[b]Collected only for males.
[c]Proportions are arc-sine transformations.
+$p < .10$. *$p < .05$. **$p < .01$. ***$p < .001$.

yses of variance (ANOVAs). Income, retrospective symptoms, and age differentiated the groups ($p < .01$), as did several personality dimensions of the PRF and hypochondriasis ($p < .05$; see Table 8.2). Post-hoc comparisons (Tukey's "honestly significant difference") showed that heavy drinkers earned significantly more than light drinkers ($p < .05$), were older than light and moderate drinkers ($p < .05$), and reported fewer symptoms on retrospective reports than the abstainer–infrequent and light drinker groups ($p < .05$). Although the analyses of variance showed an overall difference on the PRF Play dimension, Tukey's procedure did not indicate significant differences between any pair of group means. Post-hoc analyses showed that moderate drinkers scored higher than heavy drinkers on the PRF Desirability scale ($p < .05$), which assesses the degree to which an individual presents a favorable picture of himself or herself. Two interactions between sex and drinking group were also found on the PRF scales of Abasement and Autonomy. Finally, as assessed by Pilowsky's (1967) scale, abstainers and infrequent drinkers were more hypochondriacal than moderate drinkers ($p < .05$).[3] It must be noted, however, that the drinking categories were formed by questionnaire data referring to the previous year, whereas the event and mood data refer to the subsequent 3 months. This temporal lag may weaken the test of TRH.

Daily Event, Mood, and Symptom Measures

There was information contained in the daily assessment that we thought might also differentiate the four drinking groups and test the TRH. Two of these measures are the mean number of daily desirable and undesirable events reported by men over the 16-week period of data collection. We and others have shown that increased numbers of negative events and decreased number of positive events are associated with high levels of negative mood (Lewinsohn & Libet, 1972; Rehm, 1978; Stone, 1981). There were no differences across the alcohol groups on either of these measures tested by ANOVAs. Three mood variables were also assessed on a daily basis: Beck items; Nowlis positive mood (men only); and Nowlis negative mood (men only). No differences by group were found on the means of these variables averaged over the 16-week reporting period. Finally, the proportion of days

---

[3]To determine if there was a linear relationship between our alcohol consumption index and the same variables assessed with the one-way ANOVAs using group status (1–4) as the independent variable, correlational analyses were performed. The findings essentially replicated those of the analyses of variance for age ($r = .21, p < .01$), income ($r = .20, p < .01$), and retrospective symptom reports ($r = -.25, p < .01$). Further, the correlational analysis revealed that marital satisfaction was found to decrease with increases in alcohol consumption ($r = -.19, p < .01$).

on which individuals reported one or more symptoms was also computed. No main effects for sex or drinking group (2 × 4 ANOVAs were computed) were detected.

Another analysis was run to explore further the potential effects of experiencing undesirable daily events. In this analysis, each subject was first placed into one of three groups depending on his overall level of undesirable event reporting (average daily number of undesirable events in each group: low, 0.53; medium, 1.00; high, 2.04), establishing a between-groups factor. Next, within each group, the frequency of daily undesirable events was examined and divided into low, medium, and high groups. Thus, each subject was classified according to their overall level of undesirable event report and each day was classified according to the number of undesirable events reported relative to other days reported by subjects in the same between-subjects group. With these groupings of subjects and days, we could examine daily drinking according to relative levels of undesirable events. The dependent measure in this analysis was a question from the form which asked "Was the amount of alcohol you consumed today: (1) more, (2) the same, or (3) less than you usually consume on this day of the week?" The wording of the question implies that answers are to be relative to consumption levels; absolute consumption is not derivable from this question. Means on this question were examined across subject groups and within subject groups. No differences or trends were observed.

Coping

How Subjects Conceptualize Their Drinking. As mentioned earlier, drinking alcohol is sometimes thought of as a method of coping in its own right. Although our coping assessment did not explicitly include a category for alcohol and drug use, which clearly would have been the most direct way of addressing this issue, we were nonetheless able to explore the question by examining subject's narrative descriptions of their coping.

We chose to explore the responses of the heavy drinking group as we thought they would be most likely to report alcohol use as a method of handling problematic situations. Surprisingly, we found that only 2 individuals (out of 20) reported drinking as a coping response on a substantial number of days, indicating its use 16 and 22% of the time. Of the heavy drinking subjects, 70% (14) reported this response no more than 2% of the time and three of these subjects never reported it. When drinking was reported, it was most frequently perceived as a means of relaxation (77% of the time). It was used as a method of distraction 10% of the time and as direct action and acceptance each 3% of the time. On 7% of the days that drinking appeared on the inventory, it was classified in the Other category, which consisted of coping responses that could not be classified elsewhere. Subjects either did not know they used it to deal with problems or they reallly did not use it.

Appraisals of Coping Problems. According to the transactional model, once an event occurs a person appraises its characteristics. Appraisal may be affected by previous experience with the event, by personality, or by demographic characteristics, and is important to assess because it is associated with differential use of coping. As meaningfulness of events increases, for instance, subjects report using more coping (Stone & Neale, 1984b). If appraisals are not assessed and controlled for in between-group analyses of coping behaviors, one runs the risk of confounding group status with appraisal differences among groups (Stone, 1983).

Means and standard deviations of the eight appraisal questions for the four drinking groups are presented in Table 8.3. As with previous analyses, the unit of analysis was the average appraisal across an individual's responses over the 16 weeks of data collection; thus, the N was the number of subjects and not the number of reporting days. Eight 2 (sex) × 4 (drinking group) ANOVAs were computed to test between-group differences and the possibility of a sex by group interaction. No main effects for drinking group were observed on any of the appraisal dimensions. A single main effect of sex on desirability and an interaction of group by sex on happened before were observed, but given the number of tests performed, these differences are not striking.

Coping Responses to Problems. Assessment of the appraisal dimensions showed that the problems experienced by subjects did not vary across the four drinking groups. Therefore, coping responses to problems may be determined without having to control for appraisals. Table 8.3 presents the average proportion of days subjects used the various coping categories, broken down by sex of respondent and drinking group.

As expected, many sex differences were detected with univariate F tests. Males used less Distraction and Religion, and tended to use more Direct Action. Only one main effect for drinking category emerged: abstainers used more Religion than did subjects in the other three groups. To view the effects of sex and drinking on the eight coping categories simultaneously, a 2 × 4 MANOVA was computed. No main effect for drinking group was found or the interaction term, but a significant main effect of sex was detected. To control statistically for the observed differences on age and the PRF Desirability scale, which could mask group coping differences, a multivariate analysis of covariance was run. The results were the same as those computed without the covariate: The overall test did not show a significant effect across drinking groups.

Table 8.3

MEANS AND STANDARD DEVIATIONS OF COPING RESPONSES BY DRINKING CATEGORY

	Proportion of days subjects used of coping categories							
	Abstain or infrequent		Light		Moderate		Heavy	
Variable[a]	Mean	SD	Mean	SD	Mean	SD	Mean	SD
Distraction	.26	.20	.28	.18	.27	.20	.24	.18
Male*	.25	.22	.24	.18	.22	.15	.23	.18
Female*	.26	.19	.31	.17	.36	.26	.29	.17
Situation redefinition	.25	.15	.25	.19	.26	.19	.28	.25
Male	.27	.14	.23	.18	.23	.17	.23	.22
Female	.24	.16	.26	.20	.30	.24	.44	.30
Direct action	.44	.18	.43	.21	.44	.22	.37	.18
Male+	.48	.17	.51	.20	.42	.25	.37	.16
Female+	.41	.19	.38	.20	.47	.16	.36	.25
Catharsis	.27	.20	.27	.19	.26	.22	.14	.09
Male	.19	.14	.29	.20	.25	.22	.11	.07
Female	.34	.21	.26	.18	.30	.22	.24	.09
Acceptance	.26	.19	.30	.19	.25	.17	.31	.16
Male	.25	.15	.28	.20	.24	.13	.30	.16
Female	.26	.13	.31	.19	.29	.23	.33	.18
Social support	.19	.24	.15	.17	.10	.09	.10	.10
Male	.17	.27	.16	.18	.08	.07	.06	.06
Female	.21	.21	.15	.16	.15	.11	.20	.14
Relaxation	.17	.18	.18	.20	.14	.12	.15	.17
Male	.13	.19	.20	.19	.12	.11	.09	.06
Female	.19	.17	.17	.21	.16	.13	.32	.29
Religion**	.13	.24	.03	.06	.04	.07	.03	.05
Male (INT)**	.10	.27	.02	.02	.02	.04	.02	.04
Female	.16	.22	.05	.07	.08	.09	.07	.09
Other	.07	.12	.06	.13	.03	.04	.11	.13
Male (INT)**	.04	.09	.04	.05	.03	.03	.07	.08
Female	.09	.14	.08	.16	.05	.06	.21	.21

[a](INT) indicates a sex by group interaction is present.
+$p < .10$. *$p < .05$. **$p < .01$.

To assess the existence of possible linear relationships between the coping measures and the alcohol consumption index, correlations were computed. These analyses are not directly comparable to the MANOVA approach, which treats the drinking variable as nominal; correlational analyses are more sensitive for detecting linear relationships, but may capitalize on chance findings. These analyses indicated that heavier drinkers used less

Catharsis ($r = -.20$, $p < .01$) and sought less Social Supports ($r = -.14$, $p < .05$). These findings are suggestive of differences in coping across the drinking groups.

DISCUSSION

We have investigated the relationship among a variety of daily life experience measures and level of alcohol consumption in a sample of community residing, married couples. Although our method of measuring overall alcohol consumption, a series of questions, is not as comprehensive as those used in some studies, the relationships found between the four-category drinking classification and demographic variables were consistent with those found previously. For instance, the heavy drinkers are the oldest group, and males are much more likely to be heavy drinkers than are females. Although we did not replicate other findings on stress and alcohol use, we did find some relationships between coping behaviors and heavy drinking.

On some background variables such as symptoms, events, and personality measures, differences that are worth noting emerged among the drinking groups. Heavy drinkers reported fewer physical illness symptoms over the past year compared to the other three groups. It is not clear why this symptom pattern was found, and it does not follow the often-cited finding that light to moderate drinkers are generally healthier than abstainers or heavy drinkers. All groups had roughly the same number of desirable, ambiguous, undesirable, and total life events, in contrast to findings obtained with random samples (Neff & Husaini, 1982; Pearlin & Radabaugh, 1976). The tension reduction hypothesis suggests that the heavy drinkers should have had a greater number of undesirable events which prompted the drinking, but this idea was not supported. Perhaps a more extreme drinking group, composed of a high proportion of alcoholics, would evince such a pattern of events. Furthermore, drinking patterns have been long established in our sample; the tension reduction hypothesis, focused as it is on the origins of drinking, may not be appropriately tested in a middle-aged sample.

There were several differences in PRF scores found across the drinking groups, and we start with those that were interactions of sex and group status. On the Abasement scale, defined as "showing humility, accepting blame and criticism, and tending to be self-effacing," abstaining males had low scores while males in the remaining groups had higher scores. Female abstainers, on the other hand, had high Abasement scores while female heavy drinkers had lower scores. The interactional pattern was the same for the Autonomy scale, defined as "enjoys being unattached and may be rebellious when confronted with constraints." These results are consistent with other findings on sex differences in the dynamics of coping and substance use, as reported by Tucker (Chapter 6, this volume) and Timmer, Veroff, and Colten (Chapter 7).

Two main effects of drinking groups were observed; on the Play scale, defined as "does many things just for fun, enjoys making jokes or stories, and maintains a light-hearted, easygoing manner," abstainers had the lowest levels while heavy drinkers had higher levels. On the validity scale (Desirability) the heavy drinkers had the lowest score or least tendency to present themselves in a desirable light. The finding for the first personality variable may be viewed as consistent with the function of alcohol use for positive-affect enhancement (Wills & Shiffman, Chapter 1, this volume). We find the difference on the Desirability scale surprising given the general belief that alcoholics tend to present themselves in a socially desirable manner insofar as they underestimate their degree of drinking. This result may indicate that the heavier drinkers in the present sample are not comparable to clinic patients, but this finding needs further replication.

Analysis of data summarizing the environment of the male subjects and the mood and symptoms of both males and females showed remarkably few differences among the four drinking groups. Also, there were no differences on daily relative drinking levels when subjects and days were classified according to the number of undesirable daily events. However, we did find a significant linear relationship between marital dissatisfaction and alcohol consumption. In contrast to the indices of relatively discrete event occurrences, marital discord is a more pervasive stressor that has been characterized as an "enduring strain" (Pearlin & Schooler, 1978). In relatively stable and well-adjusted samples, this type of more enduring role strain may be a better predictor of substance use than other types of measures derived from the life-events paradigm.

To understand how drinking relates to coping behavior, two analytic schemes were used. The first involved tabulating how written-in instances of drinking as a way of handling a problem were used. Consuming alcohol was reported very infrequently in the coping section, indicating that, except for two individuals who reported drinking about 20% of the time, persons in the most heavy drinking group did not explicitly conceive of drinking as a coping mechanism. When it was used, the vast majority of responses were found in the Relaxation coping category. The second most frequent category was Distraction. Consistent with the formulation of substance use as a coping mechanism (Wills & Schiffman, Chapter 1), both of these results support the idea that alcohol is viewed by subjects as a means of reducing tension, presumably created by environmental events although, as was previously noted, subjects in the heavy drinking group reported no more stressful experiences overall compared with the other gorups. The finding is consistent with theories claiming a central role for expectancy as a mediator of alcohol's effects: People expect alcohol to reduce tension. Whether persons with characteristics represented by the present sample (middle-aged, middle-class) explicitly conceive of their alcohol use as a coping mechanism is a question that needs further investigation.

We also explored coping and alcohol use by classifying individuals by their previous years' self-reported drinking data into four groups and then comparing their coping responses to everyday problems. Thus, in this analysis alcohol is an independent, background variable and how problems are viewed and what was done to handle them are the dependent measures. Generally, problems that subjects reported throughout the 16-week reporting period did not vary by drinking group in the way they were appraised. No simple main effects were observed for any of the eight appraisal dimensions; however, there was one significant group by sex interaction indicating that males who drank less reported that the problems happened before more often than men who drank more heavily, whereas the pattern was reversed for women. The lack of group differences here was unexpected: We had believed that heavy consumers of alcohol would report that problems were more undesirable, more out of their control, and more changing than those who consumed less alcohol. On the other hand, these results are entirely consistent with the retrospective life event data and the daily experiences data which also showed no differences in frequency or quality of events experienced by the groups.

The lack of appraisal differences simplified our examination of coping responses to problems in that the difficult process of controlling for appraisal differences was not required. (The one difference did not appear to warrant great concern.) Following the pattern of previous analyses, there was a significant main effect of group on only one coping category, Religion. The positive result was highly significant and, hence, we are fairly confident that it is real. Abstainers used Religion much more than any of the three remaining groups. Several main effects for sex were also observed but are of little interest here.

These results generally provide some evidence that heavy drinkers use different coping than those who drink at more moderate levels or who drink very little or not at all, although the magnitude and extent of differences were not great. It may be that the range of our subjects' drinking was not great enough to reveal extensive coping differences, especially since the sample lacked adequate representation by consumers of extremely large quantities of alcohol. Nonetheless, the fact that any differences at all were detected between the drinking groups suggests that alcohol consumption may be related to how people cope with day-to-day problems.

REFERENCES

Abrams, D. B. (1983). Psycho-social assessment of alcohol and stress interactions: Bridging the gap between laboratory and treatment outcome research. In L. Pohorecky & J. Brick (Eds.), *Stress and alcohol use.* New York: Elsevier.

Barnes, G. M., & Russel, M. (1978). Drinking patterns of western New York State: Comparison with national data. *Journal of Studies on Alcohol, 39*(7), 1148–1157.

Beck, A. T., Ward, C. H., Mendelson, M., Mock, J., & Erbaugh, J. (1961). An inventory for measuring depression. *Archives of General Psychiatry, 4,* 561–571.

Billings, A. G., & Moos, R. H. (1981). The role of coping responses and social resources in attenuating the stress of life events. *Journal of Behavioral Medicine, 4,* 139–157.

Cahalan, D., Cisin, I. H., & Crossley, H. M. (1969). American drinking practices: A national study of drinking behavior and attitudes. *Rutgers Center of Alcohol Studies, Monograph No. 6.* New Brunswick, NJ.

Cohen, F., & Lazarus, R. S. (1979). Coping with the stresses of illness. In G. C. Stone & N. Adler (Eds.), *Health psychology.* San Francisco: Jossey-Bass.

Coyne, J. C., & Lazarus, R. S. (1980). Cognitive style, stress perception, and coping. In I. L. Kutush & L. B. Schlesinger (Eds.), *Handbook on stress and anxiety: Contemporary knowledge, energy, and treatment.* San Francisco: Jossey-Bass.

Dohrenwend, B. P. (1974). Problems in defining and sampling the relevant population of stressful life events. In B. S. Dohrenwend & B. P. Dohrenwend (Eds.), *Stressful life events: Their nature and effects.* New York: Wiley.

Folkman, S., & Lazarus, R. S. (1980). An analysis of coping in a middle-aged community sample. *Journal of Health and Social Behavior, 21,* 219–239.

Goldberg, D. P., & Hillier, V. F. (1979). A scale version of the General Health Questionnaire. *Psychological Medicine, 9,* 139–145.

Hedges, S. M., Jandorf, L., & Stone, A. A. (in press). The meaning of daily mood assessments. *Journal of Personality and Social Psychology.*

Holmes, T. H., & Rahe, R. H. (1967). The social readjustment rating scale. *Journal of Psychosomatic Research, 11,* 213–218.

Jackson, D. N. (1974). *Personality Research Form manual.* Goshen, NY: Research Psychologists Press.

Lazarus, R. S. (1966). *Psychological stress and the coping process.* New York: McGraw-Hill.

Lewinsohn, P. M., & Libet, J. (1972). Pleasant events, activity schedules, and depressions. *Journal of Abnormal Psychology, 79,* 291–295.

Locke, H. J., & Wallace, K. M. (1969, August). Short marital adjustment and prediction tests: Their reliability and validity. *Marriage and Family Living,* pp. 251–255.

Mechanic, D., & Volkart, E. H. (1961). Stress, illness behavior and the sick role. *American Sociological Review, 26,* 51–58.

Myers, J. K., Lindenthal, J. J., & Pepper, M. P. (1974). Social class, life events, and psychiatric symptoms: A longitudinal study. In B. S. Dohrenwend & B. P. Dohrenwend (Eds.), *Stressful life events: Their nature and effects.* New York: Wiley.

Neff, J. A., & Husaini, B. A. (1982). Life events, drinking patterns and depressive symptomatology: The stress-buffering role of alcohol consumption. *Journal of Studies on Alcohol, 43,* 301–318.

Nowlis, V. (1965). Research with the mood adjective checklist. In S. S. Tompkins & C. E. Izard (Eds.), *Affect, cognition and personality*. New York: Springer.
Pearlin, L. I., & Schooler, C. (1978). The structure of coping. *Journal of Health and Social Behavior, 19,* 2–21.
Pilowsky, I. (1967). Dimensions of hypochondriasis. *British Journal of Psychiatry, 113,* 89–93.
Redfield, J., & Stone, A. A. (1979). Individual viewpoints of stressful life events. *Journal of Consulting and Clinical Psychology, 47,* 147–154.
Rehm, L. P. (1978). Mood, pleasant events, and unpleasant events: Two pilot studies. *Journal of Consulting and Clinical Psychology, 46,* 854–859.
Reiss, A. J., Jr. (1961). *Occupation and social status*. New York: Free Press.
Stone, A. A. (1981). The association between perceptions of daily experiences and self- and spouse-rated mood. *Journal of Research in Personality, 15,* 510–522.
Stone, A. A. (1983). Comment on Brown and Parker. *Archives of General Psychiatry, 40,* 1031–1032.
Stone, A. A., & Neale, J. M. (1982). Development of a methodology for assessing daily experiences. In A. Baum & J. Singer (Eds.), *Environment and Health* (Vol. 4). Hillsdale, NJ: Erlbaum.
Stone, A. A., & Neale, J. M. (1984-a). The effects of "severe" daily events on mood. *Journal of Personality and Social Psychology, 46,* 137–144.
Stone, A. A., & Neale, J. M. (1984-b). A new measure of daily coping: Development and preliminary results. *Journal of Personality and Social Psychology, 46,* 892–906.
Verbrugge, L. M. (1979). Female illness rates and illness behavior: Testing hypotheses about sex differences in health. *Women and Health,* 4(1), 61–79.
Verbrugge, L. M. (1980). Health diaries. *Medical Care, 18,* 73–95.
Weschler, H., Demone, H. W., & Gottlieb, N. (1978). Drinking patterns of greater Boston adults: Subgroup differences in the OFV index. *Journal of Studies on Alcohol,* 39(7), 1158–1165.
Wyler, A. R., Masuda, M., & Holmes, T. H. (1968). Seriousness of illness rating scale. *Journal of Psychosomatic Research, 11,* 363–374.

Part IV

COPING AND CESSATION OF SUBSTANCE USE

This part deals with the role of coping in efforts to reduce or stop substance use. Substance use behavior frequently resists permanent change; while achieving initial changes in such behaviors is not easy, maintaining the behavior change is usually the greater problem. The recidivism rates for cigarette smoking, alcoholism, and opiate addiction approach 80% in the first 6 months (Hunt & Matarazzo, 1973). This recidivism cannot be explained in purely biochemical terms; accounting for it is one of the greatest challenges in the study of substance use.

The chapters in this part embody a shift in research focus away from recidivists' enduring traits toward investigation of more immediate events or actions that influence the course of a particular behavior-change effort. Several chapters concern the stimuli which trigger relapse, identifying stress as a prominent antecedent. This suggests that the use of drugs to cope with stress and, perhaps, deficits in more appropriate stress-coping responses, play key roles in relapse.

The chapters' common focus is on substance users' attempts to cope with the temptation to relapse. The coping responses studied encompass a variety of behavioral and cognitive strategies. Some are global strategies for preventing temptation, such as stimulus control strategies (e.g., not keeping alcohol in the house) and strategies to maintain motivation (e.g., self-reinforcement). Others are immediate responses to temptation and include strategies such as escape (e.g., leaving when drugs are offered) and distraction (e.g., doodling instead of smoking).

Consistent with their focus on subjects' efforts to control their behavior, most of the chapters study substance users who are attempting behavior change without formal treatment. The premise is that we have much to learn from people's "natural" behavior-change strategies. This reverses the usual presumed flow of information, in which propositions regarding behavior change arise out of clinical theory. The shift is fueled by the observation that most substance use behavior change occurs outside of treatment (Schachter, 1982).

Despite their methodological differences, the chapters share a common approach to the problem. All are naturalistic correlational studies of change in problematic substance use, and each relates subjects' temptation-coping activities to the outcome of their behavior-change efforts. Shiffman opens with a summary of data on smoking relapse crises obtained from interviews with callers to a relapse-prevention hotline. The data emphasize the role of immediate coping in averting relapse in the face of temptation. Curry and Marlatt report on a study of smokers quitting on their own. Their data replicate Shiffman's finding that cognitive and behavioral coping are both effective, and they also reveal situational differences in coping.

Chaney and Roszell report a series of studies with opiate addicts in methadone maintenance. They find that relapse-promoting situations can be typed on the basis of their affective tone and that most opiate users perceive their drug use as an attempt to cope with stress. Perri reports a prospective study of coping among adults who were trying to curtail their drinking. Successful subjects used a greater variety of coping techniques, especially stimulus control. Perri also reviews his studies of college students' attempts to change smoking and eating patterns. While the impact of many coping strategies was specific to a given problem or population, the use of a broad repertoire of techniques emerged as a consistent correlate of success.

DiClemente and Prochaska introduce a comprehensive "transtheoretical" model of behavior change. One of their contributions is a systematic account of coping processes and developmental stages in behavior change. The model was applied in a study of smokers quitting on their own. A key finding is that coping activities change as the stages are traversed. A second chapter by these authors (Prochaska & DiClemente) draws on the same sample but examines commonalities in coping processes across problems. The data reveal striking similarities in how people cope in smoking cessation, weight control, and control of psychological distress. This supports a general theory of coping encompassing both stress coping and temptation coping. Further investigations of these coping processes may lead to advances in both theory and practice.

REFERENCES

Hunt, W. A., & Matarazzo, J. E. (1973). Three years later: Recent developments in the experimental modification of smoking behavior. *Journal of Abnormal Psychology, 81,* 107–114.

Schachter, S. (1982). Recidivism and self-cure of smoking and obesity. *American Psychologist, 37,* 436–444.

Chapter 9

Coping with Temptations to Smoke

SAUL SHIFFMAN

INTRODUCTION

Most attempts to stop smoking end in relapse. Although initial cessation rates of 66–100% are common in smoking cessation clinics, relapse takes a huge toll on these successes. Despite some recent improvements in smoking cessation techniques, 60–80% of those who quit smoking relapse within a year (Hunt & Matarazzo, 1973; Lichtenstein, 1982; Ockene, Hymowitz, Sexton, & Broste, 1982). Permanently stopping smoking is thus by all accounts a difficult self-control task.

This chapter concerns the role of coping in maintaining abstinence in the face of temptation to smoke. Data from a study of exsmokers' encounters with temptation and relapse are used to illustrate the dynamics of coping with temptation. Although the data focus on smoking, they probably have implications for control of other substance use as well.

A MODEL OF SMOKING CESSATION MAINTENANCE

Awareness of the difficulty of maintaining abstinence following smoking cessation spawned many attempts to identify differences between recidivists and successful exsmokers. A variety of demographic and personality factors were examined. Although some predictive factors were identified, the results of this line of research have been inconsistent and inconclusive, especially in relation to personality differences between recidivists and successes. Excepting extraversion, personality factors do not account for much variance in smoking or in cessation (Smith, 1970).

Implicitly, research on predictors of success viewed relapse as a function of stable individual differences. The focus was on the person who relapsed rather than on the process of relapse itself. An alternative is to view relapse as a specific event or process deserving direct study. During the maintenance phase of cessation, the drug user is faced with repeated temptations to reinitiate drug use.[1] This chapter examines relapse episodes as functions of the temptations the exsmoker encounters following cessation.

I refer to these episodes of temptation as *relapse crises:* situations in which abstinence is threatened by temptation. Some of these episodes lead to relapse, whereas others do not. Successful maintenance thus consists of regularly resisting temptation to smoke in each successive relapse crisis. The data show that coping plays a key role in determining the outcome of relapse crises. Maintaining abstinence from drug use is thus a process of continual coping with temptation.

The study of relapse episodes was initiated by Alan Marlatt and his colleagues (Marlatt, 1978; Marlatt & Gordon, 1980; see Curry & Marlatt, Chapter 10, this volume) and by Lennart Sjöberg (Sjöberg & Johnson, 1978; Sjöberg & Samsonowitz, 1978) and colleagues. Focusing on the stimuli that precipitate relapse, Marlatt (1978; Cummings, Gordon, & Marlatt, 1980) demonstrated that negative mood states and social influences account for most relapse episodes. Sjöberg and colleagues published a series of case histories emphasizing the importance of what they call "cognitive distortions" in relapse episodes. Both investigators emphasize the role of affective states in precipitating relapse and the role of coping in preventing it. Both used retrospective reports to study episodes in which relapses actually took place.

This chapter reports a study of smoking relapse crises which attempted to improve the fidelity of reports of relapse crises by obtaining them soon after their occurrence. A relapse prevention hotline was set up as a means of communicating with exsmokers undergoing relapse crises. Exsmokers who called the Stay-Quit Line were interviewed at length regarding the details of the crisis, including their attempts to cope with the temptation to smoke.[2] Some of those who were interviewed had already smoked and thus provided reports of actual relapses. Others had not smoked but had been faced with a situation in which they experienced very strong temptation. One focus of the present study is on distinguishing these successes and failures.

The chapter briefly examines the situational antecedents of relapse crises, but the major focus is on the dynamics of coping in these situations. Classifying coping responses, for example, may enable one to identify the most effective coping responses or patterns. Other questions concern the factors

[1]Temptation arises when one is faced with a choice between immediate reinforcement and reinforcement which is uncertain or much delayed. Temptation reflects a conflict between what one wants to do and what one ought to do.

[2]Much of the data presented in the current chapter have been or will be included in other publications. The intent here is to integrate findings presented separately elsewhere. Also, it is not possible in every case to cite the published source of each finding; the reader is referred to the references for a list of publications by the author.

that affect coping. Does formal treatment affect coping? How much is coping determined by trait-like individual differences?

METHOD

Subjects

Subjects were 264 exsmokers who called the Stay-Quit Line, a smoking relapse prevention hotline operating in Los Angeles. The hotline was promoted through smoking cessation programs and through broadcast media. The sample was restricted a priori to those who had smoked at least 10 cigarettes per day for 1 year and who reported having been abstinent for at least 48 hours at the time of the call.

Subjects had smoked an average of 33.2 cigarettes per day ($SD = 14.7$) for 20.3 years ($SD = 11.7$) and had been abstinent an average of 88 days. Half had been abstinent less than 10 days. Almost two-thirds of the subjects (65%) had undergone formal treatment for smoking, most under the auspices of the American Cancer Society. A majority of the subjects were female (70%), and female subjects were especially likely to have undergone formal treatment for smoking. Both statistics are consistent with the finding that women are more likely to be help seekers (Wills, 1983).

Procedure

Subjects were interviewed regarding the details of the relapse crisis. Subjects who reported having smoked (41%) were interviewed about the relapse episode, while subjects who had not smoked were interviewed about the current relapse crisis. Interviews typically lasted 30 minutes or more and were conducted by experienced and trained interviewers.

Subjects who called the hotline were encouraged to call again if they experienced further difficulties, and 57 individuals were interviewed more than once, resulting in a total of 365 interviews. (Of these cases, 44 had complete coping data available for both occasions.) Except where otherwise indicated, only one observation per subject is used in each analysis.

Measures

Each caller was thoroughly debriefed regarding the crisis by a trained interviewer. Among the variables recorded were (1) a subjective rating of the stressfulness of the period preceding the crisis; (2) the site of the crisis (home, another's home, work, a restaurant or bar, or other sites); (3) the subject's affect (frustration or anger, anxiety, depression, or positive affect); (4) what, if anything, the subject had recently consumed (food, alcohol, coffee, or drugs); (5) what withdrawal symptoms, if any, the subject was experiencing (physical, psychological, stimulation, appetite, other, or none); (6) what, if anything, the subject was thinking about in the crisis (thoughts relating to demoralization, deprivation, the benefits of smoking, rationalizations for smoking, a conscious decision to smoke, or no thoughts); (7) the stimulus that precipitated the crisis (emotional upset, stress, associations with relaxation, associations with food or drink consumption, smoking stimuli, or other precipitants); (8) whether the antecedent situation was one in which the subject had habitually smoked; and (9) what effect the subject sought or expected from smoking (reduced tension, reduced craving, enhanced positive affect, stimulation, or other effects).

Besides measures describing the situation associated with the relapse crisis, subjects were asked to describe their attempts, if any, to cope with the temptation to smoke. Their responses were categorized by trained judges at two different levels. They were first categorized globally as either *behavioral* coping, which involves an overt activity or action, or *cognitive* coping, which involves only mental activity. Each type of coping was further classified into the following categories, which were formulated from an examination of the data: (Interrater agreement on all measures was assessed as adequate; see Shiffman, 1982a, 1984a.)Behavioral coping included:

1. Consumption of food or drink (e.g., eating a carrot instead of smoking),
2. Physical activity (going for a walk),
3. Relaxation (deep breathing),
4. Distracting activity (doing the dishes),
5. Escaping the situation,
6. Delaying action, or
7. Other behavioral coping.

Cognitive coping included:

1. Thinking about the positive health consequences of not smoking,
2. Thinking about the negative health consequences of smoking,
3. Thinking about the negative consequences of smoking unrelated to health ("My kids will be disappointed."),
4. Using Willpower (coded only when the report could not be reduced to more specific coping activity),
5. Self-punitive thoughts ("I'm such a weakling."),
6. Thoughts related to Delay ("I'll just wait this out."),
7. Distraction ("I thought about my trip to Hawaii."), or
8. Other cognitive coping.

Data

Most variables allowed for multiple responses; that is, a respondent could report more than one affect or coping response. The data were coded by transforming the information on each variable into a series of binary-coded variables indicating the presence or absence of an attribute. Thus, someone who was depressed and anxious but not angry would have values of 1, 1, and 0 for each of these respective variables.[3]

RESULTS

Situational Antecedents of Relapse Crises

WITHDRAWAL

An important theory of addiction and relapse posits that conditioned withdrawal symptoms are the major factor in relapse. It has been proposed that relapses are motivated by attempts to get relief from withdrawal symptoms that emerge as a conditioned response to stimuli previously associated with them (Wikler, 1965). Research has supported the possibility of conditioning withdrawal symptoms (O'Brien, 1975).

One implication of this theory is that most relapses should occur in the presence of withdrawal symptoms. In these data, however, only 45% of the subjects reported withdrawal symptoms in association with the crisis. Among those experiencing withdrawal, physical symptoms were most common (21%), followed by psychological symptoms (19%), appetite disturbances (10%), and disturbances of arousal (8%). The reports of exsmokers undergoing relapse crises are thus not consistent with a purely biological view of drug use.

AFFECTIVE ANTECEDENTS

In contrast to the biological view discussed above, an "adaptive" orientation to drug use and relapse (see Alexander & Hadaway, 1982) suggests that drugs are used in an attempt to cope with stress. Exsmokers' reports of smoking relapses are more consistent with this view. Some form of negative

---

[3]An implication of this method of recording is that although the variables are conceptually at a nominal level of measurement, the binary-coded variables may be treated by analyses such as discriminant function, which do not typically handle nominal data. The data were also analyzed using chi-square statistics more typically applied to nominal data. Log-linear analysis is a multivariate extension of chi square which tests the fit of hypothetical models to the data in multiway contingency tables. In some applications, it can be used to estimate a pattern of interrelationships in a manner similar to path analysis.

affect at the time they were tempted to smoke was reported by 75% of the subjects. While anxiety was the negative emotion most frequently reported (41%), anger was also reported by about 25% of the subjects. A like number reported depressed or low mood. Moreover, these affects or stresses were identified as the precipitants of the crisis in more than half of the cases.

In addition to immediate emotional upsets, the overall level of stress experienced in the period preceding the crisis was related to relapse. While only half the subjects reported substantial levels of stress, these stressed subjects were more likely to relapse (53 vs. 30%). On average, relapsing subjects reported greater antecedent stress than surviving subjects, 2.0 versus 2.6, $t(242) = 3.4$, $p < .001$.

These data imply that subjects may have been attempting to use smoking to cope with stress, and subjects' reports confirm this. More than half of the subjects who relapsed reported seeking to reduce tension (56%). (This was significantly less common among subjects who were tempted, but did not relapse, $\chi^2[1, N = 143] = 6.92$, $p < .01$.) Also, subjects who were feeling depressed were likely to report seeking stimulation from smoking ($r = .23$, $p < .01$). Thus, exsmokers are drawn to cigarette smoking in an attempt to cope with negative affect. These data support an adaptive view of drug use and relapse.

Not all relapse crises occur under stressful or negative circumstances, however. Positive affects, particularly in social situations, may also precipitate temptations to smoke. Indeed, the relationship between stress and relapse is significantly curvilinear: Relapse is more likely under conditions of either very high or very low stress.[4] Of subjects reporting "no stress at all", 34% relapsed as compared to 27% of those who reported a little stress; $r = .12$, $p < .10$.) The data on the role of smoking in happy circumstances are unclear (but see Wills & Shiffman, Chapter 1, this volume). Although most smoking typologies (e.g., Ikard, Green & Horn, 1969) include enhancement of pleasure as a smoking motive, less than 1 in 10 subjects reported wanting to smoke to enhance positive experience, and subjects who were feeling good were more likely to cite other, unclassified motives.

Coping with Temptation to Smoke

What distinguishes those crises that result in smoking from those in which relapse is averted? Analysis shows that situational antecedents do not account for the difference. Coping does. The performance of a coping re-

---

[4]Cluster analyses of the relapse data confirm the importance of affect in relapse-promoting situations. In two differing solutions based on different statistical methods, the affective tone of the situation emerged as the single most critical dimension for classifying relapse crises.

9. COPING WITH TEMPTATION

sponse in the face of temptation is the single best predictor of outcome in a relapse crisis. Of those who produce a coping response, 70% survive (i.e., do not relapse) compared with only 18% of those who do not cope. The situation seems important in promoting temptation to smoke; coping with the temptation seems to be the key to averting relapse.

Cognitive and behavioral coping responses were equally effective in averting relapse when either was performed alone (60% survival; $\chi^2[1, N = 46] = 1.3$, ns). The number of coping responses performed had no effect on relapse. Subjects who limited themselves to one response were as likely to succeed as those who performed many responses; $\chi^2(1, N = 221) < 1$, ns. The specific combination of cognitive and behavioral coping responses *was* more effective (82% survival), exceeding the success rate seen for either strategy alone; $\chi^2(1, N = 56) = 7.2, p < .01$. Each class of coping may have specific effects that work synergistically when they are performed together. Alternatively, this finding may reflect unknown differences between persons who favor a single kind of coping and persons who tend to combine them.

SPECIFIC COPING RESPONSES

The preceding data establish that coping is generally effective, but they do not identify the kind of coping that is most effective. To address this question, coping responses were classified into the 15 categories shown in Table 9.1. Engaging in substitute consumption is by far the most frequent behavioral response, with distracting activity close behind. Among cognitive responses, willpower and thoughts about the nonhealth negative consequences of smoking were most popular.

The effectiveness of each specific coping response was evaluated relative to two standards. A comparison with subjects who did no coping tested whether the response was effective at all. Comparison with other responses in the same global class (cognitive or behavioral) tested whether the response was differentially more or less effective than the others. Table 9.1 summarizes both comparisons.

The results for all behavioral responses and for most cognitive responses were surprising: All coping responses were equally effective. That is, the survival rates associated with each response were significantly higher than those among subjects who did no coping, showing each response to be effective. But the responses did not differ from each other, suggesting that the coping responses were not *differentially* effective. With the exceptions discussed below, this implies that one cannot distinguish better coping styles from worse coping styles.

The two exceptions to this surprising uniformity were willpower and self-punitive thoughts. Willpower was somewhat effective in that subjects who

Table 9.1
FREQUENCY AND EFFECTIVENESS OF SPECIFIC COPING RESPONSES

Coping response	Frequency (%)	Not smoking (%)	Outcome compared to[a]	
			No response	Other responses
BEHAVIORAL RESPONSES ($N = 228$)				
Eating or drinking	24.3	84.8	.52	.07
Distracting activity	12.1	89.3	.48	.10
Escape	3.4	100.0	.37	.12
Delay	4.3	70.0	.23	.09
Physical activity	8.6	80.0	.37	.02
Relaxation	5.2	83.3	.33	.01
Other behavior	10.8	75.0	.33	.08
Any behavioral response	55.6	81.7	.51	—
COGNITIVE RESPONSES ($N = 221$)				
Positive consequences (health)	4.0	88.9	.37	.11
Negative consequences (health)	8.9	84.2	.44	.12
Negative consequences (other)	11.2	84.0	.46	.14
Distraction	3.1	85.7	.32	.15
Intent to delay	3.1	100.0	.32	.08
Willpower	17.0	55.3	.24	−.20**
Self-punitive	3.6	37.5	.05*	−.18**
Other cognitions	38.1	70.0	.40	.00
Any cognition	63.8	80.5	.39	—
Any coping response	71.5	70.3	.47	—

[a]Columns 3 and 4 are phi coefficients, measures of effect size for 2 × 2 contingency tables. Column 3 compares subjects who performed each response to those who performed no response, while column 4 compares the same subjects against subjects who performed any of the other coping responses. All phi coefficients in column 3 are significant and those in column 4 nonsignificant unless otherwise noted. From Shiffman (1984a).
*Not significantly superior to no response.
**Significantly inferior to other responses.

reported using willpower to resist smoking were less likely to smoke than those who reported no cognitive coping. These subjects were more likely to smoke, however, than those who used other cognitive coping responses. Willpower is less effective than more specific coping cognitions. Self-punitive coping thoughts were not only less effective than other cognitive responses, they were totally ineffective: Subjects who used self-punitive cognitions were as likely to relapse as those who used no cognitive coping at all.

But for these two exceptions, the coping responses studied were comparable in effectiveness. It appears to be the act of trying to cope, rather than the character of the response, that determines outcome. This suggests that the importance of coping *skill* may be minimal and implies that the choice of a specific coping response or strategy may be relatively unimportant, especially compared to the simple performance of a coping response. This focuses attention on the factors that relate to the performance of coping.

Influences on Coping

THE EFFECTS OF TREATMENT

The coping of smokers who had participated in formal smoking cessation treatment was different from that of smokers quitting on their own but not dramatically so. Treated subjects more frequently reported using behavioral coping (71 vs. 52%; $\chi^2[1, N = 197] = 5.25, p < .03$) and also more frequently reported using more than one behavioral response (40 vs. 12%; $\chi^2[1, N = 73] = 8.00, p < .005$). These results do not represent a simple preference for behavioral coping but rather a tendency to use it in combination with cognitive coping. Untreated subjects were likely to rely on cognitive coping alone, while treated subjects typically combined it with behavioral coping. (There were no differences between the groups in the percentage who did not cope or in the percentage who relied only on behavioral responses.)

Among the treated smokers, cognitive and behavioral coping are asymmetrically related: Behavioral coping seldom occurs without cognitive coping, but cognitive coping may occur without any behavioral accompaniment; $\chi^2(1, N = 64) = 9.0, p < .005$. Among subjects quitting on their own, the two kinds of coping are unrelated; $\chi^2(1, N = 59) = 1.1$, ns. This suggests that treatment facilitates a transition from cognitive coping to behavioral coping.

Subjects who had received formal treatment also preferred two particular behavioral responses. They were more likely to use relaxation techniques, which are often taught in smoking cessation clinics (Fisher's exact test, $p < .002$) and indeed, were the sole users of these techniques. Nevertheless, only 12% of these subjects reported using relaxation techniques, which are heavily emphasized in many treatments. These data suggest that compliance with coping suggestions made in treatment may be quite poor. Treated subjects also were more likely to engage in physical activity as a way of forestalling relapse (18 vs. 2%, Fisher's exact test, $p < .001$.)

One might have expected trained subjects to be more effective copers, but this was not so. Both groups had comparable survival rates overall and among those using either cognitive or behavioral coping. In sum, smoking cessation treatment appears to facilitate the use of behavioral coping, especially in combination with cognitive coping, but does not systematically improve coping.

SITUATIONAL INFLUENCES ON COPING

It may be that the performance of coping is influenced by transient situational factors rather than by stable individual differences. Our contacts with callers to the Stay-Quit Line suggested, for example, that coping might diminish over time following the initial period of maximum involvement and motivation. Analysis showed that coping is indeed time-dependent. Performance of behavioral coping is correlated ($r = -.27$) with the amount of time elapsed since smoking cessation; for cognitive coping, the correlation is $-.16$.[5] This finding highlights the importance of maintaining coping vigilance and preparedness.

Another contextual variable suggested by our clinical experience on the hotline also concerned the person's preparedness to cope with a relapse crisis. It was hypothesized that exsmokers would be more likely to cope when faced with temptation in a situation where previously they would have smoked habitually. Since temptation is expected in such a situation, the person might be better prepared to cope with it. In contrast, an exsmoker confronted with temptation in a novel situation might be taken by surprise. This hypothesis was tested using subjects' simple self-reports about whether the situation in question was one in which they would have smoked habitually. Both behavioral and cognitive coping were less likely in situations that were not habitual. (Behavioral coping was reported in 60% of the habitual smoking situations and in 38% of the nonhabitual ones; $\chi^2[1, N = 153] = 7.3$, $p < .01$. For cognitive coping, the figures were 69 and 53%; $\chi^2[1, N = 148] = 3.9$, $p < .05$.) Thus, coping performance may depend in part on the person's preparedness to cope with a particular situation.

Another variable which affected coping was alcohol consumption, one of the few situational variables that was related to smoking in a relapse crisis. This could be a direct effect of drinking but might also be mediated by coping: If alcohol inhibits coping, it could have an indirect effect on relapse. The data showed that alcohol does indeed affect behavioral coping. Of the subjects who were drinking, 43% performed behavioral coping, whereas 62% of those not drinking coped behaviorally. Cognitive coping was not affected by alcohol. Thus, alcohol might affect outcome directly or indirectly by reducing the likelihood of coping. Log-linear analyses were used to test these two models. The analysis showed that a model positing that

---

[5]In both cases, the time variable was the log number of days elapsed since cessation. The log transformation was used because of the skewness of the time variable.

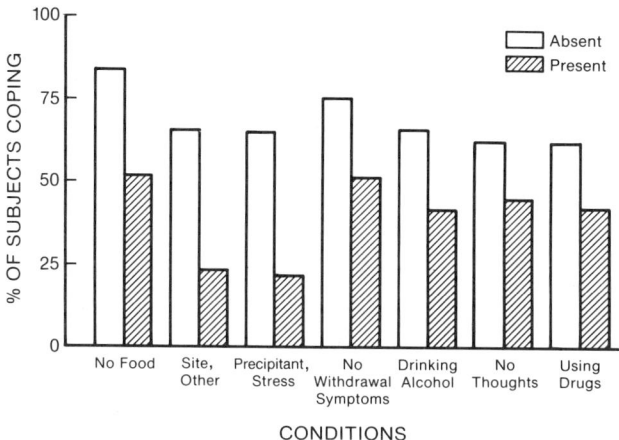

Figure 9.1 Effect of situational conditions on behavioral coping.

alcohol influences outcome only through its effects on behavioral coping (and *not* directly) fits the data. Situational influences on coping thus explain the effects of some situational factors on relapse.

To investigate other situational determinants of coping, a stepwise discriminant function analysis was performed. The analysis compared the situations in which coping had been performed and those in which it had not. No situational predictors of cognitive coping were identified. In contrast, the function identified six situational variables that jointly accounted for 36% of the variance in the performance of behavioral coping. Behavioral coping was least likely when (1) the person had been drinking alcohol; (2) the person had been using drugs; (3) the person was neither at home, at work, at a bar or restaurant, nor at a friend's home;[6] (4) the person was not experiencing withdrawal symptoms; (5) the person identified stress as the precipitant of the crisis; (6) the person had not eaten recently; and/or (7) the person reported that no thoughts were associated with the relapse crisis. The effects of these situational conditions on behavioral coping are illustrated in Figure 9.1.[7]

---

[6]Typically, these crises occurred either in an automobile or in an unusual location such as a hospital.

[7]Close analysis of the data showed that the effect of these conditions was additive rather than interactive or synergistic. A simple count of how many of these conditions were present yielded a correlation of $-.525$ with behavioral coping. Subsequent analysis showed that this index correlates substantially with time elapsed since cessation. When the variance due to the index is removed through partial correlation, time since cessation is no longer related to coping. The index thus accounts for the effects of time on coping.

Table 9.2

CONSISTENCY IN BEHAVIORAL AND COGNITIVE COPING IN TWO SITUATIONS

	Comparison case		
Index case	Coped	Did not cope	Total
BEHAVIORAL COPING			
Coped	15	12	27
Did not cope	3	14	17
	18	26	44
	$\kappa = .34$		
COGNITIVE COPING			
Coped	22	11	33
Did not cope	6	8	14
	28	19	47
	$\kappa = .22$		

TRANSSITUATIONAL CONSISTENCY IN COPING

The above data show that coping is influenced by situational factors. This in turn implies a limit on the influence of stable individual differences on coping and suggests that individuals' behavior lacks consistency across situations. A test of this issue requires that the same individuals be observed on at least two separate occasions.

Data from 47 exsmokers who had called the Stay-Quit Line more than once were used to test the transsituational consistency of coping behavior.[8] Since the hypothesis concerns the correspondence between the two observations, Cohen's kappa (Cohen, 1960) was used to analyze the data. Kappa is a measure of agreement that corrects for the degree of agreement that would be expected by chance alone. Table 9.2 shows the relationship between the cognitive and behavioral coping reported for the two occasions. For cognitive coping, the two observations agreed 64% of the time, but chance alone would be expected to produce 54% agreement. The value of kappa was .22, which is not significant (ns, 95% confidence interval was −0.08–0.51). Behavioral coping shows 66% agreement, with chance agreement of 48% and a kappa value of .34, which is significant ($p < .01$, 95% confi-

---

[8]Where more than two observations were available for a given subject, temporal proximity to the index case and completeness of the data were used as criteria for selecting the comparison case. The index and comparison cases were not necessarily collected in a particular order.

dence interval was 0.08–0.61) but not very high. Thus, there appears to be only modest consistency in coping performance across situations.[9]

DISCUSSION

These data on the details of the relapse process confirm the importance of coping processes in control of smoking and support the stress reduction model of smoking. The data show that attempts to cope with temptation were the single best predictor of outcome in a relapse crisis. At the same time, the data contradict several widely held ideas about coping, suggesting that most coping responses are of comparable effectiveness and that the performance of coping responses may be controlled more by situational factors than by individual differences.

Limitations of the Data

These data are limited in several respects. Most of the limits result from the reliance on exsmokers' self-reports. Although the use of the hotline method minimized the interval over which events were recalled, self-reports nevertheless may be subject to conscious or unconscious distortion. For example, subjects may have reported coping when they were successful to claim credit for their success, and subjects who smoked may have preferred to present themselves as not having made any effort. The use of a hotline to collect the data could also have introduced other biases. Clearly, it results in a sample of help seekers. Finally, the correlational nature of these observations limits the causal inferences that may be drawn.

The data on coping are also limited in scope. Although coping was categorized, there was no attempt to measure how well coping was enacted. The study's focus on single episodes also limits its scope. The study provides a snapshot view of relapse crises, capturing a critical moment in time but divorcing it from its context. Little information was collected regarding subjects' past histories or subsequent fate. Nevertheless, the study does provide an intensive view of relapse episodes.

[9]To the extent that the hotline interviews influenced callers to use coping, their changed behavior would exaggerate transsituational inconsistency. To test for this effect, the observation collected first was compared to that collected later. In this analysis, cognitive and behavioral coping were combined. Only 19% of the subjects who coped on the first occasion failed to cope on the second, whereas 52% of those who did not cope the first time reported a coping response on the second occasion. McNemar's chi-square test for change over time (Siegel, 1956) shows that this change was only marginally significant; $\chi^2(1, N = 44) = 3.06$, $p < .10$. Thus, the counseling interview may have had some very small effect on coping and thereby increased inconsistency.

Biological versus Coping Models of Drug Use and Relapse

The data are generally consistent with a coping model of cigarette smoking and relapse and inconsistent with a purely biological–addictive view of smoking relapse. Simple biological models of smoking relapse propose that the drug use itself sets up physiological processes that motivate further drug use. Although this model attributes relapse to withdrawal symptoms, the data show that such symptoms were often absent in smoking relapse situations. Similar findings have been reported for relapse to other substances, including heroin. Cummings et al. (1980), for example, report that only 9% of heroin addicts attributed their relapses to negative physical states associated with previous drug use (see also Chaney & Roszell, Chapter 11, this volume).

The reports of exsmokers suggested that the management of affect was the driving force behind temptation to relapse. Exsmokers were most tempted to smoke when they were anxious, angry, or depressed, and most indicated that they hoped smoking would reduce these negative feelings. It is possible, of course, that these feelings themselves were emotional symptoms of nicotine withdrawal, since anxiety and irritability have been associated with this syndrome (Shiffman, 1979; Hughes & Hatsukami, 1984).

The smokers themselves, however, attributed their emotional stress to interpersonal or other psychological sources but felt that smoking would relieve them. Whether cigarette smoking actually reduces negative affect is a matter of some controversy (see Gilbert, 1979). In any case, a series of experiments conducted by Marlatt and his colleagues (see Marlatt & Rohsenow, 1980) on alcohol suggest that the user's expectations of drug effects may actually be more important than the drug's pharmacology in determining a drug's functional value. In the present study, only 25% of the recidivists who expected to be tranquilized by smoking reported actually experiencing the hoped-for sedation. In sum, the use of tobacco to cope with stress and unpleasant emotion seems to frequently motivate smoking relapse. Other data suggest that management of affect plays a key role in relapses among alcoholics (see Litman, Eiser, Rawson, & Oppenheim, 1977) and opiate addicts (see Chaney & Roszell, Chapter 11, this volume).

One implication of these findings is that interventions that reduce stress or provide the drug user with alternative techniques for reducing stress may be effective in curbing drug use. Indeed, Marlatt and Marques (1977) successfully demonstrated this effect in alcoholics trained in meditation. Most smoking cessation programs now include a stress management component but its contribution to treatment has yet to be demonstrated. Relaxation training has produced some disappointing results (Pechacek, 1976); more research is needed on this question. Perhaps anger management techniques would help, since frustration and anger are prominent precursors of relapse, both in this study and in Marlatt's (1978) study of alcoholics.

Coping with Temptation to Smoke

Attempts to use smoking to cope with stress promote the temptation to smoke in stressful situations. The data show, however, that such factors do not by themselves determine outcome. The data suggest a two-stage process of relapse. Temptation is a product of situational factors, including specific smoking stimuli and stress. (Temptation is probably also affected by individual differences such as the degree of drug dependence.) But temptation itself does not necessarily result in smoking; relapse can be averted by coping. Thus, given temptation, coping determines whether drug use occurs.

Though nearly all coping techniques were effective, there were notable exceptions. Coping with self-punitive thoughts was ineffective, probably because it increased negative affect (see Velten, 1968) and decreased self-efficacy, which has been shown to affect smoking cessation outcome (e.g., Condiotte & Lichtenstein, 1981). Another prominent finding was the relative ineffectiveness of willpower. Consistent with the findings of Burling, Stitzer, Bigelow, and Russ (1983) subjects who said they relied on willpower fared better than those who did no cognitive coping but worse than subjects using other coping responses. The ineffectiveness of this response is important in light of its popularity: It was cited by 17% of the subjects in this study and was the single most frequently cited coping response in Baer, Foreyt, and Wright's (1977) study of smokers quitting on their own.

Given its popularity and its impaired effectiveness, willpower deserves greater study. The use of willpower may reflect an orientation toward self-control that is antithetical to a coping-oriented approach. Heavy reliance on willpower may indicate a belief that no activity is necessary to achieve one's goal—one simply has to be sufficiently motivated. A planful coping orientation to self-control, in contrast, holds that having "a will" still requires "a way," a specific method of coping (see Shiffman, Read, Maltese, Rapkin, & Jarvik, in press; Curry & Marlatt, Chapter 10, this volume). Identifying people who consistently hold a willpower orientation might pave the way for interventions directed to this attitude.

The differential (in)effectiveness of willpower and self-punitive thoughts were exceptions to a surprising uniformity in the effectiveness of coping responses. These results suggest that the choice of a particular coping response may be less important than the act of coping itself. Although traditional problem-solving approaches (D'Zurilla & Goldfried, 1971) emphasize the importance of generating alternative responses to a situation and then choosing among them, these data imply that such choices may not be critical.[10] Clinically, these findings imply that treatment ought to focus on increasing the *likelihood* of coping, rather than its appropriateness. They imply that mastering a few responses thoroughly may be superior to having a broad repertoire of responses.

Determinants of Coping

Although exsmokers who performed nearly any coping response were likely to survive the relapse crisis, many exsmokers relapsed because they performed no coping response at all. What determines whether coping is performed or not? The data indicate that coping performance is determined by contextual or situational variables. Behavioral coping proved to be highly related to such contextual factors. One unifying theme may be the importance of vigilance, which may be the common link among several diverse determinants of coping. Exsmokers may become less vigilant or less practiced in coping as time passes following cessation. The disappearance of withdrawal symptoms may lull them into a false sense of security from relapse. Vigilance may also be impaired when temptation arises in situations which are unusual or which were not habitually associated with smoking. Finally, drinking alcohol may impair readiness to cope and thereby hasten relapse.

Other predictors of coping may relate to the deliberateness inherent in performing a coping response. Sjöberg and Johnson (1978; Sjöberg & Samsonowitz, 1978) observed that disruption and distortion of thinking is a hallmark of relapse crises. Subjects who reported they were not thinking anything at the time of the relapse crisis were unlikely to cope, as were subjects who reported that stress precipitated the crisis. Both of these factors may relate to thoughtless or impulsive action. (A phrase commonly heard on the relapse hotline was "I was smoking before I realized what I was doing.") More research on these predictors, including replication of the present findings, is needed before firm conclusions can be drawn.

Given the many correlates of behavioral coping responses, it is remarkable that cognitive coping could not be predicted at all. One explanation might be that cognitive coping, because of its ephemeral nature, is more subject to distortions in recall and is thus less predictable from other variables. However, it may be that cognitive coping is actually under less situa-

---

[10]One way to conceptualize this is to consider that when one is faced with temptation, indulgent impulses (to drink, smoke, etc.) are activated. Coping responses, especially those which are behaviorally incompatible with indulgence, block out the indulgent behavior. If, however, coping is delayed, there is no force to block the indulgent impulses from being expressed in behavior and relapse results. This model thus posits a race between coping and indulgence in which delay may be fatal.

tional control. Behavioral coping requires effort and, often, planning. Moreover, because it is observable, it often carries social costs (e.g., the embarrassment of leaving a social situation). In contrast, cognitive coping is relatively automatic. Thoughts come to us unbidden, and even coping thoughts may not require conscious effort or planning. As a result, cognitive coping may be less vulnerable to disruption by situational influences.

Much remains to be determined about styles of coping. If people could be characterized according to their preference for cognitive or behavioral coping, how might these coping styles relate to other individual differences? It seems plausible, for example, that those who rely on cognitive techniques to cope with temptations might also prefer similar stragegies in coping with stress. Several theorists (Moos & Billings, 1981; Pearlin & Schooler, 1978) have divided coping responses (though not necessarily individuals) into problem-focused coping (aiming to affect the source of stress) and emotion-focused coping (aiming to affect one's internal reactions). Perhaps a propensity to use cognitive coping is associated with reliance on emotion-focused strategies. This area deserves further study.

Transsituational Consistency in Coping

The finding that coping performance is context-dependent suggests that coping performance will vary from one situation to another. The data confirm that coping performance is not highly stable across situations. Although the analysis indicated statistically significant stability, the actual degree of stability was relatively low. This finding bears much resemblance to the typical finding in studies of transsituational consistency, where significant but disappointing correlations hovering about $r = .30$ are found (Epstein, 1979).

If coping performance is indeed unstable, this would be a severe blow to all theories of coping that deal with individual coping styles because it suggests that coping is more a matter of context than of individual style (see Folkman & Lazarus, 1980). Research on transsituational consistency in other behaviors has suggested that consistency emerges only with many observations (Epstein, 1979). Further research might focus on assessing coping behavior over a greater number of relapse crises. Consistent coping styles may emerge under those conditions. Even so, simple concepts of individual consistency in coping seem unlikely to be supported.

CONCLUSIONS

Data from exsmokers undergoing relapse crises emphasize the importance of stress and coping in smoking relapse. The data are more consistent with an adaptational view of smoking—that it is used to deal with stress—

than with a simple biological model of drug dependence. Moreover, the data highlight the importance of coping in resisting temptations to smoke: Coping was the strongest determinant of survival in a relapse crisis. Coping processes deserve much attention from both researchers and clinicians concerned with drug use.

REFERENCES

Alexander, B. K., & Hadaway, P. F. (1982). Opiate addiction: The case for an adaptive orientation. *Psychological Bulletin, 92,* 367–381.

Baer, P. E., Foreyt, J. P., & Wright, S. (1977). Self-directed termination of excessive cigarette use among untreated smokers. *Journal of Behavior Therapy and Experimental Psychiatry, 8,* 71–74.

Burling, T. A., Stitzer, M. L., Bigelow, G. E., & Russ, N. W. (1983). Techniques used by smokers during contingency-motivated smoking reduction. *Addictive Behaviors, 8,* 397–402.

Cohen, J. (1960). A coefficient of agreement for nominal scales. *Educational and Psychological Measurement, 20,* 37–46.

Condiotte, M., & Lichtenstein, E. (1981). Self-efficacy and relapse in smoking cessation programs. *Journal of Consulting and Clinical Psychology, 49,* 648–658.

Cummings, C., Gordon, J. R., & Marlatt, G. A. (1980). Relapse: Prevention and prediction. In W. R. Miller (Ed.), *The addictive behaviors.* New York: Pergamon Press.

D'Zurilla, T. J., & Goldfried, M. R. (1971). Problem solving and behavior modification. *Journal of Abnormal Psychology, 78,* 107–126.

Epstein, S. (1979). The stability of behavior: On predicting most of the people much of the time. *Journal of Personality and Social Psychology, 37,* 1097–1126.

Folkman, S., & Lazarus, R. S. (1980). An analysis of coping in a middle-aged community sample. *Journal of Health and Social Behavior, 21,* 219–239.

Gilbert, D. G. (1979). Paradoxical tranquilizing and emotion-reducing effects of nicotine. *Psychological Bulletin, 86,* 643–661.

Hughes, J. R., & Hatsukami, D. (1984). *Signs and symptoms of tobacco withdrawal.* Manuscript submitted for publication.

Hunt, W. A., & Matarazzo, J. E. (1973). Three years later: Recent developments in the experimental modification of smoking behavior. *Journal of Abnormal Psychology, 81,* 107–114.

Ikard, F. F., Green, D., & Horn, D. (1969). A scale to differentiate between types of smoking as related to the management of affect. *International Journal of the Addictions, 4,* 649–659.

Lichtenstein, E. (1982). The smoking problem: A behavioral perspective. *Journal of Consulting and Clinical Psychology, 50,* 804–819.

Litman, G. K., Eiser, J. R., Rawson, N. S. B., & Oppenheim, A. A. (1977). Towards a typology of relapse: A preliminary report. *Drug and Alcohol Dependence, 2,* 157–162.

Marlatt, G. A. (1978). Craving for alcohol, loss of control, and relapse: A cognitive-behavioral analysis. In P. E. Nathan, G. A. Marlatt, & T. Lobert (Eds.), *Alcoholism: New directions in behavioral research and treatment.* New York: Plenum Press.

Marlatt, G. A., & Gordon, J. R. (1980). Determinants of relapse: Implications for the maintenance of behavior change. In P. O. Davidson & S. M. Davidson (Eds.), *Behavioral medicine: Changing health lifestyles.* New York: Brunner/Mazel.

Marlatt, G. A., & Marques, J. K. (1977). Meditation, self-control, and alcohol use. In R. B.

Stuart (Ed.), *Behavioral self-management: Strategies, techniques, and outcomes.* New York: Brunner/Mazel.

Marlatt, G. A., & Rohsenhow, D. J. (1980). Cognitive processes in alcohol use: Expectancy and the balanced placebo design. In N. K. Mello (Ed.), *Advances in substance abuse: Behavioral and biological research.* Greenwich, CT: JAI Press.

Moos, R. H., & Billings, A. G. (1981). Conceptualizing and measuring coping processes. In L. Goldberg & S. Breznitz (Eds.), *Handbook of stress: Theoretical and clinical aspects.* New York: Macmillan.

O'Brien, C. P. (1975). Experimental analysis of conditioning factors in human narcotic addiction. *Pharmacology Reviews, 27,* 533–543.

Ockene, J. K. Hymowitz, N., Sexton, M., & Broste, S. K. (1982). Comparison of patterns of smoking behavior change among smokers in the Multiple Risk Factor Intervention Trial (MRFIT). *Preventive Medicine, 11,* 621–638.

Pearlin, L. I., & Schooler, C. (1978). The structure of coping. *Journal of Health and Social Behavior, 19,* 2–21.

Pechacek, T. F. (1976, August). *Anxiety and smoking cessation: The search for specialized treatment packages.* Paper presented at the meeting of the Western Psychological Association, Los Angeles.

Shiffman, S. (1979). The tobacco withdrawal syndrome. In N. M. Krasnegor (Ed.), *Cigarette smoking as a dependence process* (Monograph 23, National Institute on Drug Abuse). Rockville, MD: U.S. Department of Health, Education, and Welfare.

Shiffman, S. (1982a). Relapse following smoking cessation: A situational analysis. *Journal of Consulting and Clinical Psychology, 50,* 71–86.

Shiffman, S. (1982b). A relapse prevention hotline. *Bulletin of the Society of Psychologists in Substance Abuse, 1,* 50–54.

Shiffman, S. (1984a). Cognitive antecedents and sequelae of smoking relapse crises. *Journal of Applied Social Psychology, 14,* 296–309.

Shiffman, S. (1984b). Coping with temptations to smoke. *Journal of Consulting and Clinical Psychology, 52,* 261–267.

Shiffman, S. (in press). A cluster-analytic classification for smoking relapse episodes. *Addictive Behaviors.*

Shiffman, S., & Jarvik, M. E. (in press). Situational determinants of coping in smoking relapse crises. *Journal of Applied Social Psychology.*

Shiffman, S., Read, L., & Jarvik, M. E. (1983, August). Stressful life events, everyday stress, and relapse in smokers. In S. Shiffman (Chair), *Stress and smoking: Effects on initiation, maintenance, and relapse.* Symposium presented at the annual meeting of the American Psychological Association, Anaheim, CA.

Shiffman, S., Read, L., & Jarvik, M. E. (1985). Smoking relapse situations: A preliminary typology. *International Journal of the Addictions, 20,* 311–318.

Shiffman, S., Read, L., Maltese, J., Rapkin, D., & Jarvik, M. E. (in press). Preventing relapse in ex-smokers. In G. A. Marlatt & J. R. Gordon (Eds.), *Relapse prevention: Maintenance strategies in addictive behavior change.* New York: Guilford Press.

Siegel, S. (1956). *Nonparametric statistics for the social sciences.* New York: McGraw-Hill.

Sjöberg, L., & Johnson, T. (1978). Trying to give up smoking: A study of volitional breakdowns. *Addictive Behaviors, 3,* 149–164.

Sjöberg, L., & Samsonowitz, V. (1978). Volitional problems in trying to quit smoking. *Scandinavian Journal of Psychology, 19,* 205–212.

Smith, G. M. (1970). Personality and smoking: A review of the empirical literature. In W. A. Hunt (Ed.), *Learning mechanisms in smoking.* Chicago: Aldine.

Velten, E. (1968). A laboratory task for induction of mood states. *Behavior Research and Therapy, 6,* 473–482.

Wikler, A. (1965). Conditioning factors in opiate addiction and relapse. In D. M. Wilner & G. G. Kassebaum (Eds.), *Narcotics*. New York: McGraw-Hill.
Wills, T. A. (1983). Social comparison and help-seeking. In B. M. DePaulo, A. Nadler, & J. D. Fisher (Eds.), *New directions in helping: (Vol. 2). Help-seeking*. New York: Academic Press.

Chapter 10

Unaided Quitters' Strategies for Coping with Temptations to Smoke*

SUSAN GOLDSTEIN CURRY
G. ALAN MARLATT

INTRODUCTION

Despite the fact that over 90% of the people who quit smoking do so on their own (i.e., without participating in a treatment program), there is little research on the experiences of this population. In light of Schachter's (1982) recent report that over time people seem to be relatively successful at modifying their smoking behavior, this group may provide a rich source of information about successful smoking cessation. In this chapter we discuss findings from a recent investigation of the experiences of unaided quitters: people attempting to quit smoking on their own, without participating in a treatment program. The particular findings discussed relate to the strategies these individuals reported using to cope with situations in which the risk of smoking is high.

Psychologists working in the area of smoking cessation have acknowledged that better understanding of the factors associated with the high relapse rates following smoking cessation is needed (Gritz, 1980; Lichtenstein, 1978). Our investigation of unaided quitters was guided conceptually by the model of relapse developed by Marlatt and Gordon (1980). The Relapse Prevention Model is a cognitive-behavioral approach to addictive behaviors derived from both contemporary social learning theory and self-control theory.

From a social learning perspective, cigarette smoking is one of a general class of addictive behaviors including problem drinking, substance abuse, overeating, compulsive gambling, and the like. The social learning model

*This research was supported by National Institute on Drug Abuse Grant #R01-DA02572, G. Alan Marlatt, Principal Investigator.

emphasizes the importance of both the determinants and consequences of addictive behavior. Determinants of substance use are posited to include situational and environmental antecedents, beliefs and expectations, and the individual's past learning history or prior experiences with the substance. Understanding the consequences of a given behavior can provide insights into the reinforcing effects that may contribute to an increase in the behavior and to negative consequences that may inhibit the behavior.

One of the central assumptions of the self-control model is that addictive behaviors consist of overlearned, maladaptive habit patterns. With repetition of behavior patterns over time, behaviors become associated with a range of situational and affective cues. We call situations and feelings that can trigger the desire to engage in an addictive behavior high-risk situations. The essence of the self-control approach is learning and practicing new behavioral skills and cognitive strategies that enable one to cope effectively with high-risk situations without engaging in substance use.

Drawing from the above conceptual framework, there are two key assumptions of the relapse prevention model. The first is that relapse is situation-specific. In contrast to other approaches which may relate relapse to physical withdrawal or to stable personality characteristics, the relapse prevention model focuses on the types of situations and feelings that act as cues for smoking. We assume that the urge to resume smoking is greatest in situations that have been most often associated with the behavior. Research on the precipitants of relapse (Marlatt & Gordon, 1980) has shown that it occurs most often in the following three situations or mood states: (1) intrapersonal negative emotional states such as frustration, anger, depression, and boredom; (2) interpersonal conflict situations such as an argument with one's spouse; and (3) social pressure situations. The second key assumption is that whether an individual engages in a coping response when in a high-risk situation is a critical determinant of the situation's outcome (abstinence or relapse). There is evidence that while many people trying to maintain abstinence from cigarettes encounter these high-risk situations, only some smoke in them (Goldstein, 1981; Shiffman, 1982). Shiffman (1982) found that the primary distinguishing factor between high-risk situations that resulted in smoking and those that did not was whether an individual performed a coping response.

Shiffman (1982) established that both cognitive and behavioral strategies are effective for preventing smoking in high-risk situations. He also found that engaging in both cognitive and behavioral coping responses is most effective for preventing smoking. Although cognitive coping could not be predicted from situational variables, Shiffman and Jarvik (1983) found six situational variables that discriminated subjects who performed behavioral coping. The consumption of alcohol, absence of the consumption of food prior to the situation, identification of stress as the situation's precipitant, report of no identifiable thoughts associated with the situation, presence in a place coded as "other," and the absence of withdrawal symptoms were found to be associated with inhibition of behavioral coping. An additional finding in their study was that the likelihood of coping in a high-risk situation was lower with increased time elapsed since cessation.

Marlatt's and Shiffman's work provided a foundation for research on coping in high-risk situations. The issues explored in the present study have both theoretical and practical importance. Pertinent questions include: (1) What types of coping strategies do individuals use in high-risk situations? (2) How effective are these strategies in comparison to each other and in comparison to no coping? (3) Is coping more likely in some types of situations than in others? (4) Is coping related to time elapsed since cessation? The coping data reported in this chapter were explored with respect to these questions. Additionally, we looked for relationships between the type of high-risk situation and the type of coping strategy used. Shiffman (1982) found that with few exceptions the coping responses he investigated were equally effective. One possible explanation for this finding is that individuals were choosing the best strategy for the particular situation they faced. If this were the case, we might expect some degree of correspondence between type of situation and type of coping strategy.

The general analytic approach used in this study warrants some explanation. Subjects were asked to report episodes in which they were tempted to smoke but did not actually smoke (temptations) or episodes in which they were tempted and smoked one or more cigarettes (relapses). Note that both temptations and relapses involve the experience of an urge to smoke, but they differ with regard to outcome. Together, temptations and relapses are referred to as high-risk situations. These episodes, rather than the individual subjects, are the major unit of analysis in this study.

METHODS

Subject Recruitment

Smokers who planned to quit smoking on or before January 1, 1981, were recruited from the general public via public service newspaper and radio ads. Interested individuals were asked to call the University of Washington. A total of 227 individuals responded to the recruitment ads. Staffing and time constraints prevented our contacting all of these individuals prior to the January 1 quit date. Sixty-nine individuals were enrolled in the study and interviewed prior to their quit date. An additional 84 individuals were interviewed approximately 1 month after their quit date. The remaining 74 individuals were lost either through refusal to enroll in the study or through inability to reach them. The total number of subjects was 153; however, 35 subjects failed to quit smoking, so that the effective number of subjects was 118.

Assessment

Background Information. Demographic and smoking history information was obtained from all participants. Demographic variables assessed included age, sex, employment status, and income. Smoking history variables included baseline smoking rate, number of years of continuous smoking, number of prior quit attempts, whether subjects had participated in prior treatment for cessation, longest period of prior abstinence, and presence of smoking-related physical symptoms. In addition, participants were asked whether they lived with any smokers and what percentage of their friends and acquaintances were smokers.

Beliefs and Expectancies. Beliefs and expectancy variables were assessed with the subsample of participants who were interviewed prior to their quit date. Ten-point scale ratings were obtained for the following variables: desire to quit, expected difficulty of quitting, expected difficulty of maintaining nonsmoking, and confidence for being able to smoke a single cigarette post-quit without relapsing. Three-item scales regarding participants' beliefs in smoking as an addiction, a habit or both, and beliefs about quitting smoking as a matter or willpower, learning, or both, were also included.

High-Risk Situations. At two times after the quit date (1 month and 4 months), participants were interviewed by phone and asked about high-risk situations and coping strategies. It was first established whether the subject had resumed smoking or had maintained nonsmoking. At each assessment, relapsers were asked to describe the situation in which they smoked their first cigarette (relapse situation). Abstinent subjects were asked whether they had any "close calls" and, if so, to describe the most tempting situation they could recall (temptation situation). Subjects who had relapsed and described the relapse situation at Month 1, and who had remained smokers, were not asked for a description at Month 4. Subjects who described a relapse at Month 1 and reestablished abstinence by Month 4 were reinterviewed at Month 4. Figure 10.1 summarizes the number of subjects describing high-risk situations at Months 1 and 4.

The following characteristics of the high-risk situation were assessed: (1)

10. UNAIDED QUITTERS' COPING STRATEGIES

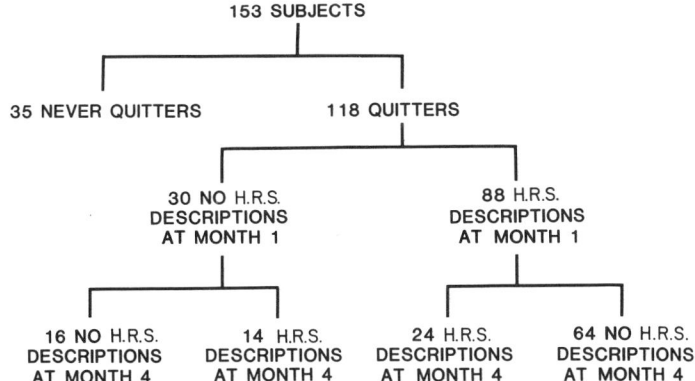

Figure 10.1 Number of subjects providing descriptions of high-risk situations (H.R.S.) at Months 1 and 4.

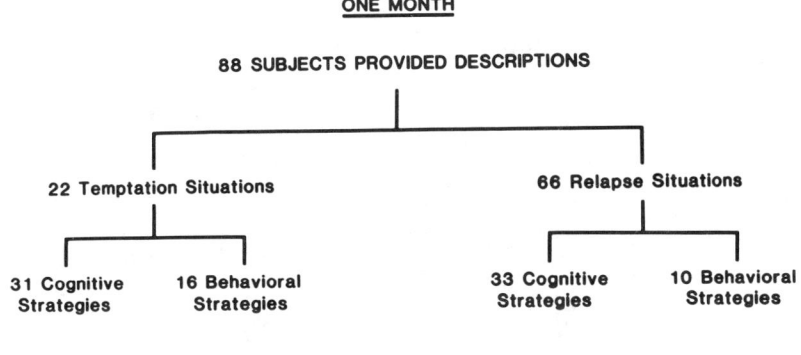

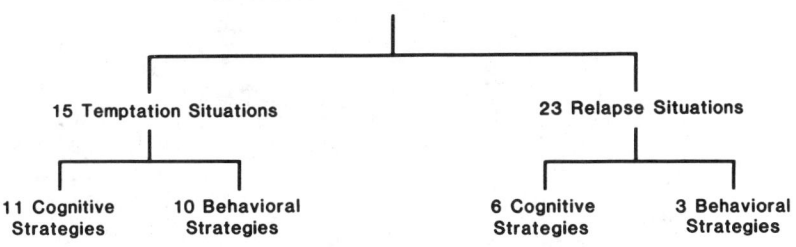

Figure 10.2 Number of cognitive and behavioral coping strategies reported as part of high-risk situation descriptions at Months 1 and 4.

the time of day; (2) whether any other individuals were present and the number who were smoking; (3) whether the individual had been exposed to the situation before; (4) whether food and/or alcohol were present; (5) the number of days since quitting (Month 1 only); (6) ratings on a 10-point scale of how much wanting to smoke in the situation was due to lack of willpower, social influence, and situational factors, respectively, how much self-control the individual was feeling after the situation was over, and how stressful the situation was; (7) separate yes or no questions on whether the main reason for smoking was social influence or negative affect; and (8) whether anger–frustration, stress–tension, boredom, craving, or social influence, respectively, were reported as precipitating thoughts or feelings.

Coping Strategies. The descriptions of coping strategies were obtained from two questions included as part of descriptions of both temptation and relapse situations. These were: "Did you focus on any thoughts or images to try and help you resist smoking?" (cognitive coping) and "Did you take any actions to try and help you resist smoking?" (behavioral coping) A total of 120 coping strategy descriptions were obtained. Figure 10.2 summarizes the number of cognitive and behavioral coping strategies reported for these situations at Months 1 and 4.

RESULTS

Equivalency of Pre- and Post-Quit Samples

Overall, our sample included adult smokers with a long history of heavy smoking. Their average age was 38 years. They had been smoking an average of 27 cigarettes per day for 19 years. Participants reported an average of three prior attempts to quit smoking; their longest period of prior abstinence ranged from less than 1 day to 10 years ($M = 356$ days).

The sample of subjects recruited into the study prior to their quit date was compared to the sample recruited 1 month after their quit date on demographic and smoking history variables to assess the appropriateness of combining their data. The samples differed significantly on two variables: sex and participation in prior treatment for smoking cessation. There was a larger percentage of females than males in the pre-quit sample (65%). Males and females were more evenly represented in the post-quit sample (48% females). A larger percentage of the pre-quit sample had participated in prior treatment (39% pre-quit compared to 17% post-quit).

Additionally, both samples were compared with regard to the initial outcome of their quit attempt as assessed at Month 1. While both groups were equally likely to quit (88% pre-quit, 75% post-quit), more of the pre-quit group relapsed by Month 1 (46% compared to 27% in the postquit sample). Given these similarities and differences, time of the initial interview for enrollment in the study is included as a subject variable in explorations of the relationships between subject variables and coping.

Types of Coping Strategies

The coping strategy descriptions were content analyzed, and category systems for classifying both the cognitive and behavioral strategies were developed on the basis of this examination of the data. All responses were coded into these categories by two coders with 89% interrater agreement. Disagreements were arbitrated by the investigator.

The cognitive coping strategies were classified into the following categories:

1. Fear of relapse thoughts: thinking that all would be lost if just one cigarette were smoked (e.g., "I don't want to begin smoking again as I don't think I could stop again.").
2. Achievement thoughts: thinking about how far one has come with quitting and not wanting to have to begin that process over again (e.g., "I've got it made, why do I need this?").
3. Self-instruction: telling oneself that smoking is unnecessary and unwanted, instructing oneself not to take a cigarette, or other pep talk thoughts like "I must not smoke," "I will not take a cigarette."
4. Health consequences thoughts: thoughts that focus on the negative health consequences of smoking and/or that focus on the positive health consequences of not smoking (e.g., "Health before desires.").
5. Social concern thoughts: thoughts about letting other people down, not wanting others to be upset with you for smoking, not wanting to harm others by smoking (e.g., "I thought of all the people I would be letting down if I were to start smoking again.").

The behavioral coping strategies were classified into the following categories:

1. Alternative behaviors: engaging in behaviors that are incompatible with or can take the place of smoking. Individuals reported primarily consumption behaviors in this category (e.g., eating, drinking) and other oral behaviors (e.g., chewing toothpicks, sucking on a small straw).
2. Avoidance behaviors: engaging in behaviors that range from removing oneself totally from the situation to remaining in the situation but engaging in a distracting or diverting activity (e.g., dancing, knitting).

Table 10.1

PERCENTAGE OF COPING STRATEGIES CODED INTO COGNITIVE AND BEHAVIORAL SUBCATEGORIES FOR MONTH 1 AND MONTH 4 COPING DESCRIPTIONS[a]

Strategy	Month 1 (%)	Month 4 (%)
COGNITIVE STRATEGIES		
Relapse thoughts	12	12
Achievement thoughts	25	17
Self-instruction	42	35
Health thoughts	12	24
Social concern thoughts	9	12
	100	100
N	64	17
BEHAVIORAL STRATEGIES		
Alternative behaviors	46	62
Avoidance behaviors	42	23
Enlisting social support	12	15
	100	100
N	26	13

[a] At Month 1, 50 of the 88 subjects who described high-risk situations provided descriptions of one or more coping strategies. At Month 4, 27 of the 38 subjects who described high-risk situations provided descriptions of one or more coping strategies. Ns and percentages are based on number of responses rather than number of subjects.

3. Enlisting social support: using social support or enlisting the help of other people to resist the temptation to smoke (e.g., "I asked for support from my family").

Table 10.1 shows the percentage of coping strategies coded into each of the cognitive and behavioral subcategories for temptation and relapse situations at Months 1 and 4. The percentages for each strategy are calculated from the total number of strategies reported in their general category (cognitive or behavioral).

At Months 1 and 4, Self-instruction was the most commonly reported cognitive coping strategy. Achievement thoughts were the second most commonly reported strategy at Month 1, whereas Health Consequences thoughts were the most commonly reported cognitive strategy at Month 4. Alternative behaviors and Avoidance behaviors were reported as behavioral coping strategies with equivalent frequency at Month 1. By Month 4, individuals were reporting using Alternative behaviors with more frequency than Avoidance behaviors. Because there is no appropriate statistical model for testing many nominal dependent measures, these statements are based on simple frequencies and have not been tested statistically.

Coping and Outcome of High-Risk Situation

To test for a relationship between reporting coping in a high-risk situation and whether or not that situation resulted in smoking, the percentages of subjects reporting particular coping strategies for temptation (nonsmoking) situations were compared with those for relapse (smoking) situations. Contingency table analyses compared (1) people who reported coping and those who reported no coping; and (2) those who reported no coping, cognitive coping only, behavioral coping only, and both types, respectively. Separate analyses were performed for Month 1 and 4 coping data.

Significantly fewer subjects reported coping strategies in relapse than in temptation situations for both measures of coping at Months 1 and 4; $\chi^2(1, N = 88) = 18.05, p < .001$, and $\chi^2(3, N = 88) = 26.76, p < .001$, respectively, for Month 1 data. For Month 4 data, $\chi^2(1, N = 38) = 4.59, p < .03$, and $\chi^2(3, N = 38) = 11.13, p < .01$, respectively. Figure 10.3 illustrates the percentage of relapse and temptation situations in which no coping, only cognitive coping, only behavioral coping, and cognitive plus

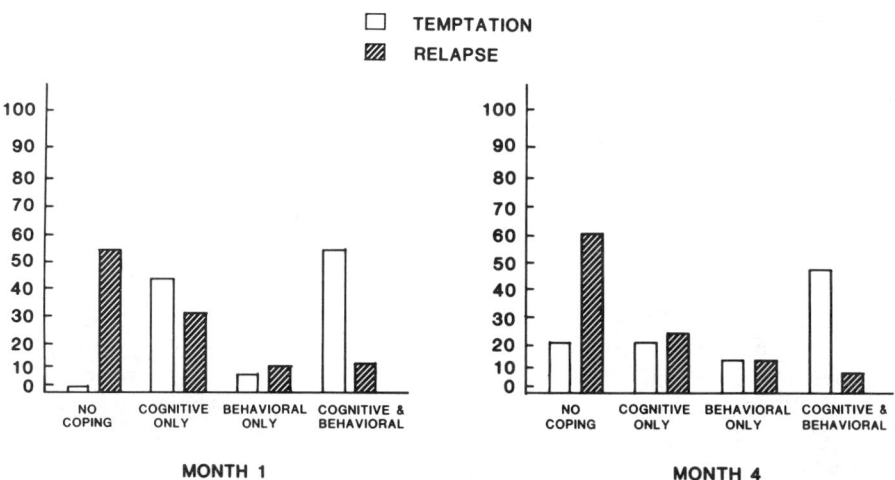

Figure 10.3 Percentage of relapse and temptation situations in which no coping, only cognitive coping, only behavioral coping, and cognitive plus behavioral coping were reported at Months 1 and 4.

behavioral coping were reported at Months 1 and 4. At Month 1, participants who reported using either cognitive or behavioral coping were more likely to have described temptation situations (i.e., situations in which smoking did not occur) than participants who reported using no coping; $\chi^2(1, N = 69) = 7.09, p < .01$). Also, participants who reported using both cognitive and behavioral strategies were more likely to describe temptations than participants who reported using only one type of coping; $\chi^2(1, N = 50) = 4.31, p < .05$. These findings clearly indicate that engaging in no coping response in a high-risk situation increases the probability that the situation will result in smoking, and that a combination of cognitive and behavioral strategies is more effective than either type of strategy used alone.

Relative Effectiveness of Specific Coping Strategies

In addition to assessing the overall effectiveness of the use of coping strategies, we were interested in whether specific types of cognitive and behavioral strategies are more effective than others. Our approach to this question is modeled on recent work by Shiffman (1984). He assessed the relative effectiveness of specific types of coping strategies by analyzing the survival rate for each type of cognitive and behavioral coping strategy. Survival rate is defined as the percentage of individuals who reported using the strategy in situations that did not result in smoking (i.e., temptation situations). Two statistical analyses were conducted: (1) contingency table analysis comparing the percentage of subjects using a specific strategy who survived (i.e., remained abstinent) versus the percentage using any other strategy who survived; and (2) contingency table analysis comparing the percentage of subjects using the specific strategy who survived versus the percentage using no coping strategy who survived. These analyses were done separately for cognitive and behavioral strategies. All analyses were conducted for Month 1 coping data only, since too few descriptions of specific coping strategies were collected at Month 4 for meaningful analysis.

The results for Month 1 coping data are summarized in Table 10.2. The individual coping strategies are equally effective, and, with one exception, the strategies are all significantly more effective than no coping. Although the survival rate for enlisting social support is similar to other coping strategies, it was not significantly more effective than using no behavioral coping strategy; however, only two individuals described this strategy, making any interpretation difficult.

The seemingly low survival rates (ranging from 40 to 64% for the specific strategies are a reflection of the ratio of relapse to temptation situations (3:1). We systematically sampled only one episode per person at Months 1

Table 10.2

EFFECTIVENESS OF COGNITIVE AND BEHAVIORAL COPING STRATEGIES AT MONTH 1[a]

Response	Cases[b] (%)	Survival rate (%)	Compared with no response	Compared with other coping response
COGNITIVE RESPONSES				
Relapse thoughts	7	50	.49*	.05
Achievement thoughts	17	40	.44*	.05
Self-talk	30	46	.49*	.06
Health thoughts	7	50	.49*	.05
Social concern thoughts	7	50	.49*	.05
No cognitive strategies reported	68	5	—	—
Only cognitive strategies reported	31	30	—	—
BEHAVIORAL RESPONSES				
Alternate behaviors	13	55	.36*	.04
Avoidance behaviors	13	64	.43*	.18
Enlisting social support	2	50	.17	.04
No behavioral strategies reported	72	14	—	—
Only behavioral strategies reported	5	25	—	—
Neither cognitive nor behavioral strategies reported	42	3	—	—
Both cognitive and behavioral strategies reported	22	63	—	—

[a]Survival rate is defined as the percentage of individuals who reported using the strategy in situations that did not result in smoking. The percentages reported for individual strategies include any subject reporting a particular response, regardless of other strategies they have reported. Comparisons of individual responses with no responses refer to the relationship between the percentage of subjects using a specific strategy who survived (i.e., remained abstinent) and the percentage using no coping strategy who survived. Comparisons of individual responses with other responses refer to the relationship between the percentage of subjects using a specific strategy who survived and the percentage of subjects using any other strategy who survived. For cognitive responses, "no response" refers to no cognitive response; for behavioral responses, "no response" refers to no behavioral response. The phi coefficient indicates the degree of the relationship between the survival percentages being compared. Significant coefficients reflect comparable survival rates. For cognitive responses, the total number of strategies reported was 64; for behavioral responses, 26.
[b]Percentages figured from 88 subjects reporting either a temptation or relapse.
*$p < .05$.

and 4. If a participant had smoked on any occasion, we specifically obtained a description of this smoking episode. In these instances, we did not ask participants who had smoked for descriptions of situations in which they were tempted but did not smoke. In this way, our sample was biased towards obtaining descriptions of relapses. Thus, it is unlikely that our data reflect the true ratio in the population of temptations to relapses. Nonetheless, the base rate of relapses in this sample necessarily affects the apparent survival rate among those who cope. The most relevant comparison, then, is the relative one between coping and no coping. In this sample only 5% of individuals who did not use cognitive coping survived compared to 40–50% of those who coped cognitively. Similarly, only 14% of those who did not use behavioral strategies survived compared to 50–64% of those who coped behaviorally. To summarize, the effectiveness of different cognitive and behavioral coping strategies were comparable. And, consistent with our discussion of the relationship between coping and the outcome of high-risk situations, survival was much less likely if no coping strategies were used.

Type of High-Risk Situation and Coping

To see if there was any relationship between the type of temptation or relapse situation and the type of coping strategy used, we first categorized the stimulus that precipitated the temptation according to Marlatt and Gordon's (1980) categories for classifying relapse episodes. Following this, Kendall's coefficient of concordance (W) was computed for both cognitive and behavioral strategies using the rank order of the frequency with which each coping response was used in the four most commonly reported precipitants. If the situations are concordant with respect to coping, this implies that coping is applied uniformly, without regard to situational antecedents. In contrast, low concordance implies that coping varies with the situation. In order to increase the number of situations included in our analyses, we combined the Month 1 and 4 situation descriptions.

For both temptations and relapses, the four most commonly reported types of precipitants were:

1. *Intrapersonal negative affect.* These are situations in which the individual experiences a negative emotional state such as anger or frustration that is primarily associated with intraindividual factors or is a reaction to a nonpersonal environmental event. For example, "I was in a service station late in the morning. The main reason for wanting to smoke was because of bad news, the possibility of having an expensive car repair."

2. *General urges or cravings.* These are situations in which the individual experiences an internal urge or craving in the absence of specific emotional states, withdrawal symptoms, or interpersonal factors. For example, "The main reason for being tempted to smoke was seeing a cigarette advertisement in a magazine. I felt a longing for a cigarette—remembered it as soothing, comforting."

3. *Interpersonal conflict.* These are situations in which the individual

experiences a negative emotional state such as anger or frustration that is primarily in response to a conflict with another person or persons. For example, "The main reason for wanting to smoke was stress created by family anger and disagreement over major decisions."

4. Social pressure. These are situations in which the individual experiences a craving or urge to smoke in response either to the presence of others smoking or to direct offers of cigarettes. In the former instance, other smokers act as a cue for smoking, without exerting any specific pressure. For example, "The main reasons for wanting to smoke were companionship, my smoking buddies were visiting, and relaxation. Being with former smoking friends made me want to smoke. I thought of how relaxing it would be."

The coefficients of concordance for both the cognitive and behavioral coping strategies reported in relapse situations were significant (cognitive coping strategies, $W = .72$, $p < .01$; behavioral strategies, $W = .83$, $p < .05$), indicating uniformity across situations with regard to the types of coping strategies reported. This reflects the fact that most subjects reported using no coping strategies in relapse situations.

The coefficients of concordance for both the cognitive and behavioral coping strategies reported in temptation situations were nonsignificant (cognitive strategies, $W = .37$, ns; behavioral strategies, $W = .22$, ns), indicating that coping strategies were used with different frequencies in different

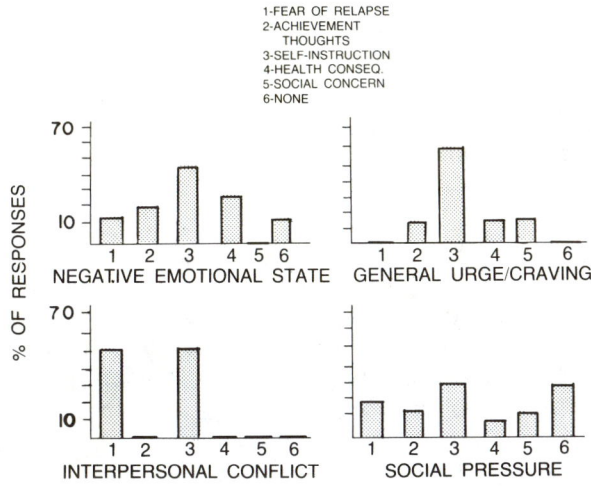

Figure 10.4 Percentage of specific cognitive coping strategies reported in four types of temptation situations.

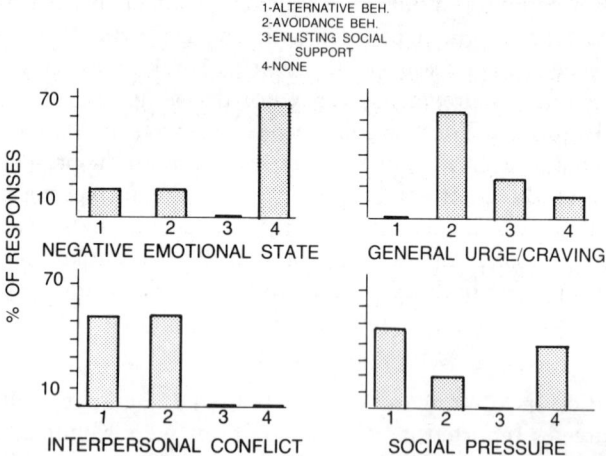

Figure 10.5 Percentage of specific behavioral coping strategies reported in four types of temptation situations.

types of situations. Figure 10.4 shows the percentage of each type of cognitive coping strategy used in each of the four types of temptation situations. This figure reflects the earlier observation that Self-instruction is the most commonly used cognitive strategy. It is used with some frequency in each type of temptation situation. Individuals tended to think about the health consequences of smoking primarily in intrapersonal negative emotional state situations. The widest variety of cognitive coping strategies was reported in social pressure situations; the least variety in interpersonal conflict situations. These findings must be viewed as tentative at best because of the small number of situations involved in some of the categories.

Figure 10.5 shows the percentage of each type of behavioral coping strategy used in each of the four types of temptation situations. This figure indicates that individuals tend not to use behavioral coping strategies in intrapersonal negative affect situations. In these situations, 92% of the subjects reported engaging in cognitive coping, suggesting that successful coping with negative affect is generally cognitive. Avoidance behaviors are used primarily in response to general urges–cravings and in interpersonal conflict situations. Alternative behaviors are used primarily interpersonal conflict and social pressure situations. Enlisting social support was used only in response to general urges–cravings. Again, these findings must be viewed as tentative at best because of the small number of situations involved in some of the categories

Relationship of Coping to Situation Variables

Separate stepwise discriminant analyses were performed with reported cognitive coping and behavioral coping as the outcome variables.[1] A significant function was found for cognitive coping only. The function had a significant Wilk's lambda, $F(3, 61) = 2.74, p < .05$; however, the classification results with this function were relatively poor, with only 59% of the cases classified correctly. Subjects who reported feeling bored in the high-risk situation and who rated the situation as due to external factors were more likely to report cognitive coping (standardized discriminant coefficients were .74 and .30, respectively). Additionally, cognitive coping tended to be reported in situations occurring in the afternoon (standardized discriminant coefficient was .52).

Relationship of Coping to Subject Variables

In addition to exploring relationships between characteristics of situations and whether coping strategies were reported, we also looked for relationships between subject characteristics and both cognitive and behavioral coping.[2] As indicated earlier, data on several belief and expectancy variables were obtained only from subjects who were interviewed prior to their quit date (i.e., the pre-quit subsample). Separate discriminant analyses were performed with pre-quit subjects only for these variables.

Two sets of stepwise discriminant analyses were performed. The first included all subjects and demographic and smoking history variables. The second included only pre-quit subjects and belief and expectancy variables. For the discriminant analyses including all subjects, a significant function was found for the prediction of cognitive coping. The classification results with this function were fair, with 67% of the cases classified correctly. The variables included in the function and their standardized discriminant coefficients are presented in Table 10.3. Individuals who had received prior treatment for smoking cessation were less likely to report cognitive coping strategies. Subjects who were initially interviewed post-quit were more likely to report cognitive coping strategies at Month 1. Individuals who reported cognitive coping had slightly more previous quit attempts on the

---

[1]For all discriminant analyses reported, minimization of Wilk's lambda was the selection criterion; no additional variables were entered into the analysis when F ratios to enter the equation failed to exceed 1.00 for each remaining variable.

[2]As with situation variables, discriminant analyses were performed with Month 1 data only, as the number of subjects providing information on coping strategies at Month 4 was insufficient for meaningful multivariate analyses.

Table 10.3

SUMMARY OF STEPWISE DISCRIMINANT ANALYSES PREDICTING COGNITIVE AND BEHAVIORAL COPING FROM SUBJECT VARIABLES

Variable	Standardized discriminant function coefficient
All subjects: cognitive coping	
Prior treatment	−.688
Smoking acquaintances	.461
Time of enrollment	.449
Longest prior abstinence	.373
Number prior quit attempts	.339
Canonical $R = .373$ Wilks's lambda $= .860, p < .035$ $N = 84$	
Pre-Quit subjects: behavioral coping	
Willpower or learning	.854
Quit difficulty	.609
Canonical $R = .454$ Wilks's lambda $= .794, p < .025$ $N = 35$	

average than individuals who did not report cognitive coping ($M = 2.64$ and 2.35, respectively); cognitive copers had longer periods of prior abstinence ($M = 1.95$ and 1.81, respectively); and cognitive copers reported a larger percentage of smoking friends and acquaintances ($M = 2.34$ and 1.97, respectively. (This is a four-category variable with higher numbers representing larger percentages.)

For the discriminant analyses including subjects interviewed pre-quit only, a significant function was found for predicting behavioral coping which correctly classified 67% of the cases. The variables included in the function and their standardized discriminant coefficients are presented in Table 10.3. The findings suggest that subjects' beliefs about the quitting process and their orientation toward it affects their subsequent coping behavior. Subjects who reported behavioral coping tended to believe that quitting was going to be more difficult than those who did not report behavioral coping strategies ($M = 8.71$ and 6.86, respectively); behavioral copers were more likely than noncopers to believe that quitting smoking involved learning as opposed to willpower ($M = 2.71$ and 2.00, respectively). As indicated above, this was a three-category variable with higher numbers indicating a belief that learning was involved. Scale ratings on expected difficulty maintaining nonsmoking were also higher for subjects who reported behavioral coping than for those who did not ($M = 7.28$ and 5.86, respectively).

Reported Coping and Time Elapsed since Cessation

As stated in the Introduction, Shiffman and Jarvik (1983) found that the likelihood of coping in a high-risk situation decreased with the time elapsed since cessation. We address this issue by comparing the number of coping strategies reported at Months 1 and 4. First, as is evident from Figure 10.2, fewer subjects described high-risk situations at Month 4. This finding is primarily because subjects who had relapsed at Month 1 and who remained smokers were not asked for any subsequent descriptions. Approximately the same percentage of subjects who had maintained complete abstinence at each follow-up described temptation situations (56 and 60%, respectively). Thus, the decrease in the number of reported high-risk situations from Months 1 to 4 does not necessarily indicate that abstinent individuals were experiencing less temptation over this time period. Given this reduction in the number of high-risk situation descriptions, it follows that fewer coping strategies would be reported over time. However, because some of the same subjects were interviewed at Months 1 and 4, it is possible to see whether subjects reporting high-risk situations at both intervals reported less coping at Month 4.

Two separate repeated-measures analyses of variance were run with total number of cognitive coping strategies reported and total number of behavioral strategies reported at Months 1 and 4 as the respective dependent measures. There were 24 subjects who described high-risk situations at both assessments. A significant difference was found between the average number of cognitive coping responses reported at Month 1 ($M = 1.13$) and at Month 4 ($M = 0.58$); $F[1, 23] - 6.8, p < .02$). A marginally significant difference was found between the average number of behavioral responses reported at Month 1 ($M = 0.72$) and Month 4 ($M = 0.36$); $F[1, 23] = 3.0, p < .10$).

Although the findings for cognitive coping are consistent with those reported by Shiffman and Jarvik (1983), they leave open the interpretation that the reason for the difference between Months 1 and 4 is that individuals who reported temptation situations at Month 1 were reporting relapse situations at Month 4. In this case, the difference in the number of responses reported could be due to a difference in the type of situation being described, rather than due to time elapsed since cessation. To address this issue, cases were classified by type of high-risk situation (temptation or relapse) reported at Months 1 and 4 and a second set of repeated measures

ANOVAs were performed on these data. Three groups of subjects were identified: (1) subjects describing temptations at both Months 1 and 4; (2) subjects describing a temptation at Month 1 and a relapse at Month 4; and (3) subjects describing relapses at both Months 1 and 4.[3]

Analysis limited to the subjects who reported temptations on both occasions ($N = 11$) showed a reduction in cognitive coping from Month 1 to Month 4 ($M = 1.54$ and 0.82, respectively). Subjects reporting relapses at both time intervals ($N = 8$) reported equally low rates of cognitive coping on both occasions ($M = 0.38$ and 0.50, respectively). All subjects reported less behavioral coping at Month 4 ($M = 1.00$ and 0.0, respectively).

DISCUSSION

As stated in the Introduction, a key assumption of the model of relapse underlying this investigation was that individuals' coping responses when in a high-risk situation are critical determinants of the situation's outcome (maintenance or lapse). In support of this, we found that unaided quitters who survived high-risk-for-relapse situations reported using coping strategies significantly more often than those who did not survive. Survival rates calculated from these data suggest that the absence of coping leads to almost certain relapse, but the performance of coping does not guarantee survival. The individual effectiveness of the several types of cognitive and behavioral coping strategies identified in this investigation were roughly equal.

These findings are remarkably consistent with those reported by Shiffman (1982). Although Shiffman reported higher survival rates for the individual types of coping strategies, the average phi coefficients for cognitive and behavioral strategies are comparable. Differences between survival rates are probably due to differences in the ratios of relapse (smoking) to temptation (nonsmoking) situations compared in each study. Of the descriptions obtained in this investigation, 75% were of relapse situations compared with 40% of those obtained in Shiffman's investigation. Sample differences between the two investigations could account for this discrepancy. Our sample included individuals who had volunteered to participate in a research project. Participants were explicitly told that we would not provide help for quitting smoking. In contrast, Shiffman's sample consisted of individuals who were seeking help with cessation. In addition, our participants described events that occurred near Months 1 and 4 post-quit. Most of the

---

[3]Eight subjects who described relapse situations at Month 1 reestablished abstinence. These subjects subsequently relapsed again and provided descriptions of their more recent relapse episodes at Month 4.

events described in Shiffman's study occurred during the first 2 weeks postcessation.

The different percentages of relapse situations described in each investigation suggest very different overall survival rates for high-risk situations. Our data suggest that the survival rate during the first 30 days post-quit is low, although it can be improved by engaging in cognitive and/or behavioral coping strategies in high-risk situations. However, the issue could be better addressed if those individuals reporting relapse situations were also asked to describe any close calls they had encountered before the situation in which they smoked. If questions about any strategies they used to resist the temptation to smoke were included, it would be possible to assess whether these relapsers uniformly failed to cope in high-risk situations and managed to survive by other means (e.g., the intervention of a concerned friend, the social norms prescribed by the situation) or whether engaging in coping strategies was the prominent distinction between the situations that resulted in smoking and those that did not.

Building from our assumption that relapse is situation-specific, we found tentative evidence that survivors use different coping strategies in different types of high-risk situations. We also found that the survival rates for the various coping strategies were equivalent, suggesting that the type of coping strategy used in a situation is less important than the fact of using one. These findings highlight the importance of exploring further whether coping is shaped by the demands of the situation.

The variables that predict coping are consistent with a social learning model of the nonsmoking maintenance process. With this model we could expect that (1) prior experience would be related to present behavior; (2) the use and/or acquisition of skills could be mediated by individuals' beliefs and expectations; and (3) newly acquired skills would be refined over time (i.e., more trial and error behavior would occur early in the learning process). This investigation was not designed to test these propositions specifically. Nevertheless, it is useful to consider the pattern of our findings with them in mind.

Consistent with the first proposition, three of the subject characteristics that predicted cognitive coping are related to smoking history. Individuals with a larger number of prior attempts to quit smoking and longer prior periods of abstinence from cigarettes were more likely to use cognitive coping strategies in high-risk situations. Individuals who had participated in prior cessation programs were less likely to cope cognitively. It is interesting to note that the number of previous quit attempts and participation in prior treatment are significantly positively correlated, yet they relate to cognitive coping in opposite directions. These differing relationships suggest two ways that experience can influence coping. First, with experience and some success, people learn the value of cognitive coping and therefore use it more. Second, in contrast to experience gained from unaided quit attempts, individuals who have enrolled in formal treatment programs are most often encouraged to focus on behavioral coping (Shiffman, 1984). This treatment emphasis (or overemphasis) on behavioral coping could reduce the likelihood that unsuccessful participants will use cognitive coping in future quit attempts.

Other subject variables that contributed to the prediction of cognitive coping were time of the initial interview for enrollment in the research project (pre- vs. post-quit) and the reported percentage of smoker friends and acquaintances. Subjects who were enrolled after their quit date were more likely to report cognitive coping strategies than subjects enrolled pre-quit. Two factors probably contribute to this difference. First, the post-quit sample included a higher percentage of abstainers. Abstainers reported temptation situations, and coping was reported more often in these situations. A second consideration is the sample differences in prior treatment. Participants who were enrolled pre-quit reported more participation in prior treatment than the post-quit sample. As we indicated above, participation in cessation programs was negatively related to cognitive coping.

Subjects who reported cognitive coping strategies also reported a larger percentage of smoking friends and acquaintances. Being around other smokers can certainly make the task of quitting smoking more difficult (see Eisinger, 1971; Goldstein & Marlatt, 1983; Ockene, Benfari, Nutall, Hurwitz, & Ockene, 1982). A possible explanation for this is that people may tend to choose between cognitive and behavioral coping. When other people, particularly other smokers are present, they may be inhibited from coping behaviorally. For example, it would be inappropriate to work on a needlepoint project at a party and equally embarrassing to explain that you are leaving the party because you are tempted to smoke. When behavioral coping in inhibited, this could force an increase in cognitive coping. A relevant finding is that cognitive copers tended to attribute high-risk situations more to external factors than subjects who did not cope cognitively. It is possible that the situations perceived as externally precipitated were social situations where behavioral coping had been inhibited.

The variables that predict behavioral coping in subjects enrolled prior to their quit date support the second proposition that beliefs and expectations can mediate performance. Subjects who expected that quitting smoking would be difficult and believed that it involved learning new skills rather than just exercising willpower were more likely to use behavioral coping strategies in high-risk situations. One explanation for why these variables predicted behavioral but not cognitive coping is that most people tend to define *coping* as behavioral coping, since observable behavior is more substantial. Moreover, behavioral coping requires more deliberate effort. Thus, subjects who believed that quitting smoking is difficult and involves learning and not just willpower may be more likely to make deliberate, behavioral efforts to cope.

This finding points to the importance of individuals' initial orientation to the quit process for their subsequent behavior while trying to maintain abstinence. Treatment could capitalize on this and target initial interventions at helping clients to articulate their orientation and, for example, point out the advantages of a skill acquisition approach and the potential pitfalls of viewing quitting primarily as a test of willpower.

The final proposition—that coping skills would be refined over time—is supported by the finding that the number of coping strategies reportedly engaged in during high-risk situations decreased significantly over time. These findings are similar to those of Shiffman and Jarvik (1983). By controlling for the types of situations reported at Months 1 and 4, we were able to rule out the explanation that fewer coping strategies were reported at Month 4 than at Month 1 because subjects were describing relapse situations at Month 4 and temptation situations at Month 1. In fact, the majority of cases involved subjects who were describing temptation situations at both 1 and 4 months. A possible explanation for this difference is that during the first month post-quit individuals were experimenting with several types of strategies for coping with their temptations to smoke. By 4 months post-quit, they may have settled on a smaller number of reliable strategies. In this context, fewer strategies would be reported with increased time elapsed since cessation; however, the decreased number of strategies would not be related to decreased survival rates in high-risk situations where coping is attempted. One might even hypothesize that the survival rates would improve.

By lending support to a social learning model of the nonsmoking maintenance process, our findings also support the continued development and implementation of cognitive–behavioral interventions based on this model. These programs (e.g., Marlatt, 1982; Shiffman, Read, Maltese, Rapkin, & Jarvik, 1985) emphasize the importance of engaging in coping strategies when faced with situations posing high risk for relapse. The typology of coping strategies presented here can serve as useful models of how people cope with urges to smoke. Given that engaging in a combination of cognitive and behavioral coping strategies was reported more frequently in temptation than in relapse situations, treatment participants can be encouraged to "think *and* do something" when in a high-risk situation. Evaluations of cognitive-behavioral interventions could also include assessment of coping abilities pre- and posttreatment. By coping ability we mean the capacity to effectively avoid smoking in high-risk situations by using thoughts, behaviors, or their combination. If the ability to use coping is an important part of successful nonsmoking maintenance, then we predict that skill-training approaches would result in improved coping abilities.

CONCLUSION

In this chapter we have focused on the use and effectiveness of coping strategies relative to the outcome of specific high-risk situations reported at Months 1 and 4 post-quit. A crucial question for further investigation concerns the relationship between the ability to use coping strategies in high-risk situations and long-term outcome. Although we followed participants in this investigation for 2 years, we are unable to address this issue because our coping data were collected retrospectively. That is, when subjects were asked to describe their coping attempts, many had already relapsed. Thus, any attempts to relate Months 1 and 4 coping data with 2-year outcome would confound early outcome and use of coping strategies during high-risk situations. This points to the need for prospective rather than retrospective designs.

Future investigations of coping and nonsmoking maintenance could also include more consideration of the mediating role of individuals' beliefs and expectations about quitting smoking. Self-efficacy expectancies seem particularly relevant. Are individuals who believe that learning new skills is an important part of quitting smoking more successful than those who believe that willpower is the main ingredient for success? Do individuals with high confidence in their ability to cope with high-risk situations have better coping skills than individuals with low self-efficacy? If this relationship was found, then coping skills training could be used to increase self-efficacy.

In this investigation we defined coping in terms of strategies individuals reported using to cope specifically with urges to smoke. We asked participants to describe thoughts and actions they used when they were experiencing the desire to have a cigarette. In a broader context, we could also look at how people cope with the precipitators of smoking urges. Negative feelings, such as boredom, loneliness, and frustration, as well as interpersonal conflict situations are examples of common precipitators of relapse. Future investigations could examine the relationship between a more general measure of the ability to cope with these types of feelings and situations and long-term maintenance (see Wills & Shiffman, Chapter 1, this volume).

Our exploration of data on unaided quitters' strategies for coping with temptations to smoke has been fruitful. We are accumulating evidence that supports the concept of nonsmoking maintenance as a learning process in which the acquisition and use of coping skills is central. We have also begun to identify specific variables that are associated with the use of coping strategies in high-risk situations. By continuing to investigate the learning and skill processes involved in smoking cessation and relapse prevention we hope to improve our ability to develop effective interventions.

REFERENCES

Eisinger, R. A. (1971). Psychosocial predictors of smoking recidivism. *Journal of Health and Social Behavior, 12,* 355–362.

Goldstein, S. (1981) Maintenance of nonsmoking following self-initiated cessation. *Dissertation Abstracts International, 43*(2), 524B. (University Microfilms No. DA-82-12,783)

Goldstein, S., & Marlatt, G. A. (1983). *Smokers in one's environment and unaided smoking cessation.* Paper presented at the annual meeting of the American Psychological Association, Anaheim, CA.

Gritz, E. (1980). Smoking behavior and tobacco abuse. In N. K. Mello (Ed.), *Advances in substance abuse* (Vol. 1). New York: JAI Press.

Lichtenstein, E. (1978). Future needs and directions in smoking cessation. In J. Schwartz (Ed.), *Progress in smoking cessation. Proceedings of the International Conference on Smoking Cessation, New York, June 21–23, 1978.* New York: American Cancer Society.

Marlatt, G. A. (1982). Relapse prevention: A self-control program for the treatment of addictive behaviors. In R. Stuart (Ed.), *Adherence, compliance and generalization in behavioral medicine.* New York: Brunner/Mazel, Inc.

Marlatt, G. A., & Gordon, J. (1980). Determinants of relapse: Implications for the maintenance of behavior change. In P. O. Davidson & S. M. Davidson (Eds.), *Behavioral medicine: Changing health lifestyles.* New York: Brunner/Mazel.

Ockene, J. K., Benfari, R. C., Nuttall, R. L., Hurwitz, I., Ockene, I. S. (1982). Relationship of psychosocial factors to smoking behavior change in an intervention program. *Preventive Medicine, 11*(1), 13–28.

Schachter, S. (1982). Recidivism and self-cure of smoking and obesity. *American Psychologist, 37,* 436–444.

Shiffman, S. (1982). Relapse following smoking cessation: A situational analysis. *Journal of Consulting and Clinical Psychology, 50,* 71–86.

Shiffman, S. (1984). Coping with temptation to smoke. *Journal of Consulting and Clinical Psychology, 52,* 261–267.

Shiffman, S., & Jarvik, M. (1983). *Situational determinants of coping in smoking relapse crises.* Unpublished manuscript.

Shiffman, S., Read, L., Maltese, J., Rapkin, D., & Jarvik, M. (1985). Preventing relapse in ex-smokers: A self-management approach. In G. A. Marlatt & J. R. Gordon (Eds.), *Relapse prevention: Maintenance strategies in addictive behavior change.* New York: Guilford Press.

Chapter 11

Coping in Opiate Addicts Maintained on Methadone*

EDMUND F. CHANEY
DOUGLAS K. ROSZELL

INTRODUCTION

This chapter focuses on coping during the stage of opiate abuse in which an addict has reduced or eliminated use and is attempting to avoid or minimize relapse. The data presented here are from subjects in methadone maintenance treatment. The study of coping and relapse in opiate addicts maintained on methadone is conceptually similar to the study of obesity or controlled drinking in that substance use continues and relapse is a matter of type and quantity. Since there is evidence that methadone maintenance is the best available treatment for many addicts (Cooper, Altman, Brown, & Czechowicz, 1983), the study of the determinants of illicit opiate use during treatment has important implications both for improving treatment outcome and for suggesting interventions that increase the likelihood of a successful outcome following detoxification.

COPING, SUBSTANCE ABUSE, AND AN ADAPTIVE ORIENTATION

Recent years have seen a proliferation of theoretical positions on the important concepts and issues in the high relapse risk stage of substance abuse (Lettieri, Sayers, & Pearson, 1980). Alexander and Hadaway (1982) suggest that recognition of two fundamental orientations about opiate ad-

---

*Preparation of this chapter was supported in part by the General Medical Research Service of the Veterans Administration Medical Center, 1660 South Columbian Way, Seattle, WA 98108.

diction can help to organize the multiplicity of theoretical perspectives. In the exposure orientation, addiction is posited to occur because use of opiate drugs engenders dependence; in the adaptive orientation, addiction is construed as an attempt to adapt to distress. Alexander and Hadaway have argued that the exposure orientation is inconsistent with experimental and clinical evidence.

Adaptation theories predict that an individual attempting to moderate or eliminate opiate use will be at risk to resume drug use as a coping mechanism unless other coping strategies are available or can be developed. Coping is defined here as attempts by the individual to resolve life stressors and emotional pain (Ilfeld, 1980). In this orientation, opiate addiction is coping gone awry as the coping strategy of substance use is substituted for more adaptive coping patterns. As Alexander and Hadaway (1982) point out, there is not much evidence available on opiate addiction from an adaptive orientation. The study of coping and relapse in alcoholism, however, is more developed and can serve as an illustration of the hypothesized relationships between relapse and coping in opiate addiction.

First, stress is clearly related to relapse. Well-controlled research has shown that negative life events, such as the death of a friend or economic or legal problems, are more prevalent among relapsed alcoholics than among recovered patients or demographically matched community controls (Moos, Finney, & Chan, 1981). Also, it appears that the impact of life events on treatment outcome is mediated in part by the individual's coping responses. After equating for background factors, relapsed alcoholics show poorer mood and health-related functioning, less social competence and self-confidence, and use less effective coping responses (such as denial and avoidance) than recovered patients or matched community controls. The use of more positive coping responses (such as active behavioral or cognitive coping) is related to better functioning on outcome criteria (Cronkite & Moos, 1980; Moos et al., 1981).

RELAPSE AND COPING MODELS

Marlatt and Gordon's (1985) conceptualization of relapse is the most comprehensive theory consistent with an adaptive orientation. Their model offers a typology of the "relapse environment" and delineates factors that affect the probability of a lapse associated with stressful or high-risk situations (those in which resuming substance use is likely). Marlatt and Gordon's typology classifies relapse situations as those in which relapse is a response to primarily psychological, physical, or nonpersonal environmental events (intrapersonal) versus those in which the relapse is influenced by the behavior of other individuals (interpersonal). (For more detailed discussion see Curry & Marlatt, Chapter 10, this volume.) Two distinctions particularly relevant for opiate addiction are (1) that frustration and/or anger is distinguished from other negative emotional or interpersonal states, and (2) that coping with physical states associated with prior substance use is distinguished from coping with other physical states.

Besides a theory of relapse, a typology of coping strategies is needed to study the relationship between coping and relapse. That presented by Moos and Billings (1982) examines both the focus of coping and the method of coping. Appraisal-focused coping attempts to define or redefine the meaning of a situation and is divided into three categories: (1) logical analysis, (2) cognitive redefinition, and (3) cognitive avoidance. Problem-focused coping attempts to modify or eliminate the source of stress, to deal with the consequences of a problem, or to develop a more satisfying situation by (4) seeking information or advice, (5) taking problem-solving action, or (6) developing alternative rewards. Emotion-focused coping attempts to maintain affective equilibrium and is divided into (7) affective regulation, (8) resigned acceptance, and (9) emotional discharge.

COPING AND RELAPSE IN ALCOHOLISM

Research in alcoholism illustrates the interaction of coping and relapse. Litman, Eiser, Rawson, and Oppenheim (1979; Litman, Stapleton, Oppenheim, & Peleg, 1983) combined a relapse model similar to Marlatt and Gordon's with a coping typology that overlaps Moos and Billings's to study the relationship between coping and alcoholic relapse.

Studying groups of alcoholic relapsers and survivors using the Coping Behaviours Inventory (CBI), Litman et al. (1979) found that individuals who used multiple coping responses and styles were less likely to relapse. The coping styles that the CBI identifies are (1) positive thinking, (2) thinking of negative aspects of drinking, (3) avoidance–distraction methods, and (4) seeking social supports. The use of positive thinking as a coping strategy was the only significant univariate discriminator between relapsers and survivors.

Sanchez-Craig and Walker (1982) treated alcoholics with a "reappraisal therapy" designed to change their appraisals of stressful high-risk situations and to teach problem solving. In an outcome study, however, halfway house residents treated in this way did no better than a control group. One contributing factor was that 1 month later only 13% of the subjects could recall each of the problem-solving steps taught in treatment.

An intervention study that was a precursor to the work reported in this chapter had a more positive outcome. Focusing on the remediation of coping skills deficits, Chaney, O'Leary, and Marlatt (1978) tested a problem-solving skills training intervention for inpatient alcoholics. Relapse-related coping skills were assessed using a role play measure called the Situational Competency Test (SCT). An audiotape recording of high-risk situations was presented to subjects, who were instructed to respond as if they actually were in each situation. The stimulus situations were based on Marlatt and Gordon's (1980) analysis of relapse determinants. Responses were scored for duration and latency (time to respond) and dichotomously for compliance (drinking or failing to solve the problem), and specification (degree of articulation of the proposed problem solution). The duration and specification scores increased from pretest to posttest for the skill training group but not for the two control groups. Outcome results of the intervention were reflected in decreased amount of alcohol consumed, fewer number of days on which a person was drunk, and shorter average drinking period length over a 1-year follow-up period.[1] Although it did not show a training effect, the SCT latency measure obtained by Chaney et al. (1978) at the end of treatment was as predictive or more predictive of a variety of treatment outcome indicators including employment, duration of rehospitalization, retention in aftercare, and several measures of drinking behavior than the significantly predictive pretreatment baseline measures of the behaviors.

Although not prospective in design, two other studies also have found significant relationships between alcoholic relapse following treatment and role play coping skills measures (Jones & Lanyon, 1981; Rosenberg, 1983). Rosenberg also reported that relapsers experienced more negative life events than nonrelapsers.

COPING IN OPIATE ADDICTS

In comparing and contrasting coping and relapse in opiate addicts with coping and relapse by users of other substances, the following factors should be considered: cognitive and behavioral competencies; evaluation or appraisal of the stressful or high-risk situation; overall goals, intentions, and plans; efficacy and outcome expectancies; and the relevant environmental resources and demands (Mischel, 1981). These factors probably interact to determine whether environmental demands stress the available coping resources and create a potential relapse situation. Although opiate addicts share with other substance users the life-style habit of using a drug to cope, they are different from alcoholics, smokers, and users of other substances on

---

[1] Jones, Kanfer, and Lanyon (1982) failed to replicate these findings, perhaps because of methodological difficulties, including a high rate of subject attrition.

some of the factors mentioned above. Crucial differences are discussed in the following sections.

Cognitive and Behavioral Competencies

Perhaps the most important characteristic that differentiates opiate addicts from members of other substance-abusing populations is the need to engage in illicit activities to obtain their drugs. However, participating in this counterculture is not equivalent to lacking the behavioral repertoire necessary for adequate performance in the dominant culture. Amount or style of narcotic use is to some degree independent of level of social competence or behavioral adequacy. For example, user groups that are on opposite ends of the spectrum of involvement with narcotics, that is, those who seldom use daily versus those who usually use daily, both with low rates of incarceration, had greater job stability and lower crime rates prior to narcotic use than intermediate use groups (Nurco, Cisin, & Balter, 1981a, 1981b). Although poor interpersonal skill is undoubtedly an important factor in particular classes of relapse, it is not warranted to generalize that all drug addicts have globally deficient interpersonal repertoires (Van Hasselt, Hersen, & Milliones, 1978).

Deficiencies in cognitive competencies, on the other hand, may be a specific factor in central nervous system (CNS) depressant substance use. For example, Platt, Scura, and Hannon (1973) compared the interpersonal problem-solving thinking of youthful heroin addicts and nonaddict offenders. They found that addicts demonstrated poorer cognitive problem solving, in spite of the fact that they were significantly older and better educated than the nonaddicts. Appel and Kaestner (1979) compared a sample of older male narcotic abusers in "good" standing in an outpatient treatment program with those in "poor" standing. The former group showed greater quantity and quality of cognitive problem-solving abilities.

Any factors that degrade such cognitive competencies as the ability to remember recent events, to process new information, and to engage in abstract thinking negatively influence a person's use of cognitively based coping strategies. Clearly, learning, abstraction, and problem-solving abilities are impaired by chronic CNS depressants such as alcohol (Chelune & Parker, 1981). Narcotic use per se does not appear to have deleterious effects on cognitive functioning that are detectable by neuropsychological testing (Rounsaville, Jones, Novelly, & Kleber, 1982). Many opiate addicts, however, use multiple drugs, including CNS depressants. The use of nonnarcotic drugs and alcohol may increase dramatically during detoxification and in the initial stages of abstinence from opiates (Waldorf, 1983; Wille, 1983).

Goals, Intentions, and Plans

Illicit drug use as a coping strategy has profound effects on the individual's long-term goals, plans, and intentions. For opiate addicts the difficulty and enormous expense involved in securing drugs sets constraints on all other aspects of an abuser's life and becomes a primary factor in determining family and social relationships as well as vocational and avocational activities (Nurco et al., 1981a, 1981b). When addicts attempt to quit by replacing drugs with other coping responses, several different patterns emerge. Waldorf (1983) studied patterns of recovery in 100 treated and 101 untreated exaddicts who had been off opiates for at least 2 years. Subjects were found through 'chain referral' and were given structured interviews by trained personnel. Waldorf's findings emphasize the importance of change in life goals or intentions. Approximately one-third of his sample described their recovery in terms that suggest maturation or transition from one life stage to another. A second category identifed by Waldorf was "drifting out," which combined passive intentional change with involvement in conventional or mainstream social networks. Other categories represented affiliation with antidrug groups, reappraisal of the risks and benefits of addiction, becoming mentally ill, or situational change (for individuals whose drug use was situation-specific behavior).

Environmental Stressors, Depression, and Social Support

Attempts to study the intervening processes linking stress and drug use have emphasized the relationship of depression to stressors, conceptualizing depression as an indicator of failed coping. Chronic and transient disturbances in affect are related to the resumption of drug use as coping behavior. For example, increased depression may be found in the initial stages of attempting to abstain from narcotics (Kosten, Rounsaville, & Kleber, 1983). Depression may influence not only efficacy expectations (learned helplessness) but also the appraisal process and the individual's goals (relieving the depression might become a primary goal), making resumption of drug use more likely. Aneshensel and Huba's (1983) study illustrates the potential relationships between depression and substance use. They interviewed a normal, adult community sample four times over a 1-year period. Although their sample's self-reported alcohol use and smoking was quite stable over the year and depression moderately stable, they found causal interrelationships. Although smoking did not seem to be directly influenced by either factor across time, high levels of alcohol use of relatively long duration appeared to contribute to increased depression. In turn, depression had a short-term effect on alcohol use, suggesting that alcohol was used as a coping mechanism for presumably transient episodes of depression. Although the immediate effects of alcohol use may be perceived to alleviate depression for some people, their data suggest that the long-term impact is a further deepening of depression. These relationships are likely to be even stronger in populations of substance abusers.

With regard to opiate addicts, Krueger (1981) studied life events and return to heroin use in 48 patients on methadone maintenance. Relapsing patients' Social Readjustment Rating Scale (Holmes & Rahe, 1967) scores were significantly higher than those of the control group and than their own previous scores during a period of heroin-free stabilization. Krueger (1981) found that events such as a recent loss, depression, or exacerbation of intense affect coincided with the reoccurence of heroin use. These results suggest that for many addicts stresses that might otherwise lead to depression are met with coping mechanism such as returning to drug use in an attempt to prevent depressive affect. Similarly, Kosten et al. (1983) used a prospective design over a 6-month period and found that, as in previous studies (Prusoff, Thompson, Scholomskos, & Riordan, 1977; Winstead, Whitworth, & Lawson, 1981), addicts had considerably more recent life events than other depressed patients or normal controls. Kosten et al. (1983) also found significant relationships among negative life events, depression, and illicit drug use. Exit events were related most strongly to illicit drug use; arguments were related more strongly to poorer occupational functioning and increased psychological symptomatology. Kosten et al. suggest that addicts' drug use may drive important people away from them and drug use may act as a form of self-medication (coping) for the depressive affect that loss of a support system may engender. Arguments, in contrast, may reflect the negative consequences of the use of drugs for coping.

Stressors, Coping, and Relapse in Drug Abusers

What do we know about the processes of coping with high-risk relapse situations in drug addicts? Sjöberg and Olsson (1981) studied relapse in a small sample of young drug abusers who primarily used amphetamines and marijuana. They focused on the decision making or volitional aspects of returning to drug use after a period of attempting to abstain. Of the "volitional breakdowns" (relapses) reported, 50% occurred under emotional stress. They classified coping techniques used to combat volitional breakdowns into seven categories. For comparison purposes, we reclassified the techniques into three categories. Of the 28 techniques mentioned by the subject group, 48% appeared to be behavioral in nature, 27% cognitive, and 25% avoidant. Sjöberg and Olsson (1981) previously had studied smokers, obese individuals, and alcoholics using similar procedures and found that, comparatively, the drug abusers were rather unaware of coping techniques but were not as impoverished as a skid row alcoholic group.

The drug abusers showed a unique type of voilitional breakdown in response to situations involving stimuli associated with previous drug use. Mere exposure to the appropriate cues apparently was sufficient to produce an extremely aroused state (craving). This reaction led to a unique coping technique, escape, in which the subject literally ran away from the tempting situation. This observation suggests that physiological drug cues may be more important in relapse for drug addicts than for other substance using groups.

Waldorf's (1983) sample of heroin addicts in a recovery phase reported differential use of coping strategies in different types of high-risk situations. For instance, avoidance was the primary coping mechanism used for parties or social gatherings where opiate users might be present and for encounters with drug-using friends. The second most popular strategy in social situations was "casual treatment," using social skills appropriately to appear friendly but at the same time to avoid protracted conversations. Active problem solving and development of alternative rewards also were mentioned as coping strategies for dealing with excess spare time (57% of the sample reported developing hobbies or recreational interests). Substitution of other drugs was mentioned as a coping mechanism by 41% of the sample for situations or needs that had been associated previously with opiate use.

PROSPECTIVE STUDY OF COPING IN OPIATE ADDICTS

Building upon previous studies of stress, coping, and relapse, our own research has focused on relating a typology of relapse situations based on Marlatt and Gordon's (1980) relapse theory to opiate addicts' coping strategies, categorized using Moos and Billings' (1982) system. The balance of this chapter reports four related studies.

1. Study 1 uses multidimensional scaling to investigate subjects' perceptions of relapse situations with a perceptual set that they are attempting to cope with the situation.
2. Study 2 relates high-risk situation categories to the subjects' role-played coping behavior in those relapse situations.
3. Study 3 investigates coping and efficacy expectations in relation to illicit drug use during methadone maintenance treatment.
4. Study 4 examines failed coping in volitional breakdowns for a group of opiate addicts stabilized on methadone maintenance.

Table II.1
SITUATIONAL COMPETENCY TEST (DRUG REVISION) SITUATIONS

INTRAPERSONAL NEGATIVE EMOTIONAL STATES

You have been working toward a goal (like getting enough money together to buy something), when circumstances beyond your control mess up your plans.

You are bored.

You are feeling depressed or down about how things have been going in your life.

You have an appointment (job interview, court hearing, etc.) tomorrow morning that you are uptight or worried about.

INTRAPERSONAL NEGATIVE PHYSICAL–PHYSIOLOGICAL STATES

It has been quite a while since you used drugs (or alcohol), but your body starts feeling like you are going into withdrawal.

You are in physical pain or discomfort (from a toothache, sore throat, strain, or old injury acting up).

You are having difficulty getting to sleep (or staying asleep).

INTRAPERSONAL TESTING CONTROL OR GIVING IN TO TEMPTATION

You taste, smell, or see something that instantly reminds you of using drugs or drinking.

Some time ago you were using enough drugs or alcohol so that you were physically addicted or dependent on them. You stopped for a while. You think about what you are missing and that you should be able to use some without getting hooked again.

ENHANCEMENT OF INTRA- OR INTERPERSONAL POSITIVE EMOTIONAL STATE

You think about using drugs or drinking to get high or feel good.

You are feeling good and having a good time with another person, and there is some of your preferred drug available.

You are with a group of people who are having a good time.

INTERPERSONAL CONFLICT

You have had several hassles with people lately.

The person you have been living with leaves against your wishes.

You are feeling nervous, tense, or "hyped up" about being around people.

Someone you are close to gets seriously hurt.

SOCIAL PRESSURE

Someone offers you drugs or alcohol of the kind that you prefer.

Someone is trying to persuade you to use drugs or alcohol.

You run into old friends with whom you used to use drugs. They act friendly.

You happen to be around another person who is using some of your preferred drug or alcohol.

Revision of the Situational Competency Test for Opiate Addicts

A coping skills assessment technique for drug abusers was based on earlier research done with the Situational Competency Test (SCT; Chaney et al., 1978). The SCT had been designed as a role play measure of alcoholics' response competencies in situations that appeared to be particularly difficult to cope with by means other than alcohol use. Several steps were taken to adapt the instrument to a drug-using population in treatment, with the goal of validating its use as a screening instrument for assessing weaknesses and strengths in subjects' coping behavior in high-risk relapse situations. We sought to insure that relevant high-risk situations were sampled and that the situations were exemplars of all of the categories in Marlatt and Gordon's (1980) revised relapse situation typology. The sample of situations from which the SCT originally had been generated was reviewed by drug treatment clinicians from several programs. They were asked to suggest changes in wording to reflect the demographic and substance use differences between alcoholic and opiate addict populations.

To further insure that a relevant set of situations was obtained, 38 opiate addicts in a methadone maintenance treatment program who had a relapse episode following at least 1 month of no unauthorized drug use were interviewed about that episode. These reports (Chaney, Roszell, & Cummings, 1982) indicated that of the 38 relapses, 31% were due to coping with negative physiological states not associated with prior substance abuse and 16% involved coping with physiological states that were associated with prior substance use; 16% followed social pressure; 5% were enhancement of positive emotional states; 8% were coping with frustration or anger in interpersonal situations, and 24% were due to coping with negative emotional states other than frustration or anger. There were no relapses in the other categories. Marlatt and Gordon (1980) reported a similar relapse distribution for their sample of opiate addicts.

Based on feedback from drug treatment program staff and the results of the Chaney et al. (1982) study, the SCT was enlarged from 16 situations to 20 situations (the SCTDR). The situation prompts and the categories they are designed to represent are given in Table 11.1. Situations were added representing intrapersonal negative physical–physiological states, enhancement of positive emotional states, interpersonal conflict, and intrapersonal negative emotional states. These situations reflected characteristics of relapses reported by the addict sample but not by previous alcoholic samples.

Study I

Although Marlatt and Gordon's (1980) relapse categories have theoretical appeal, there are few data to suggest either that subjects' appraisals of relapse situations are along the lines suggested by the theoretical categorization or that the content or outcome of subjects' coping attempts is usefully differentiated by these categories. Does this type of category scheme organize relapse determinants in a naturalistic manner in accord with subjects' (as well as experimenters') perceptions? To investigate subjects' perceptions of relapse situations, a study was undertaken using a sample of 20 drug abusers in a Veterans Administration Drug Treatment Program, who were in good standing and judged by the staff to be making satisfactory progress on their treatment goals.

SUBJECTS

The demographic characteristics of the group from which this sample of 20 was drawn are representative of and not significantly different from the sample means and standard deviations of the samples upon which succeeding discussions are based, so will not be repeated. Subjects were all male, reflecting the usual composition of the treatment program. The average age was 34 ($SD = 7$); 40% were single, 20% divorced, and the balance married. The majority were white (70%), 24% black, and 6% Asian or Hispanic. Fifty percent can be described as having a low socioeconomic status, 20% lower middle, 20% middle, and the balance upper-middle status. The average educational attainment was 13 years ($SD = 1.5$), and the current average monthly income (including public assistance and disability compensation) was \$750 ($SD = \$550$). The age of first drug use was 20 ($SD = 5.5$). Duration of drug use averaged 14 years ($SD = 6$). One-third of the subjects reported using only opiates, while the balance used other drugs as well. One-third of the subjects reported one or more arrests. Twenty-four percent of the subjects had no prior drug treatments, 14% had one, 32% had two, and 30% had three or more.

PROCEDURE

Subjects were asked to sort the 20 SCTDR (the drug revision of the SCT) situations presented on cards into as many categories as they liked, putting similar situations together, based on the perceptual set that they did not desire to use drugs or drink alcohol and that they were experiencing the SCTDR situations. Multidimensional scaling and cluster analytic procedures were used to analyze the groupings thus obtained.[2]

---

[2] Multidimensional scaling (Kruskal & Wish, 1978) refers to a class of techniques that use proximities among objects as input. The proximities indicate how similar or different the subjects perceive two objects, or in this case situations, to be. The primary output is a geometric representation of points in which each point represents a situation. This configuration represents the perceptual structure of the data. Cluster analysis refers to a set of techniques that are designed to generate groups of objects under investigation. Different mathematical criteria can be used to generate groups with the goal of retrieving groupings that either reflect the natural structure of the data or have heuristic value for data exploration, hypothesis generation, testing, or prediction. Multidimensional scaling and cluster analysis can complement each other by making possible the display of similarities and dissimilarities among groups of objects.

RESULTS

Subjects used an average of 5.3 categories ($SD = 1.9$) with a range from 2 to 9 to group the situations. The category membership data were transformed into a dissimilarity matrix. The computer program ALSCAL (Young, Takane, & Lewyckyj, 1979), specifying a simple Euclidean model assuming ordinal data, was used to produce two- and three-dimensional scaling solutions. The stress coefficient (Kruskal & Wish, 1978) for the two-dimensional solution was .175 and for the three-dimensional solution was .131. Squared distance correlations were .87 and .90, respectively, suggesting that even though the stress value is somewhat large, the three-dimensional solution was not sufficiently more descriptive than the two-dimensional solution to justify the additional complexity. The two-dimensional solution was judged best and is presented in Figure 11.1.

A cluster analysis (Ward's method using Wishart's CLUSTAN, 1975)

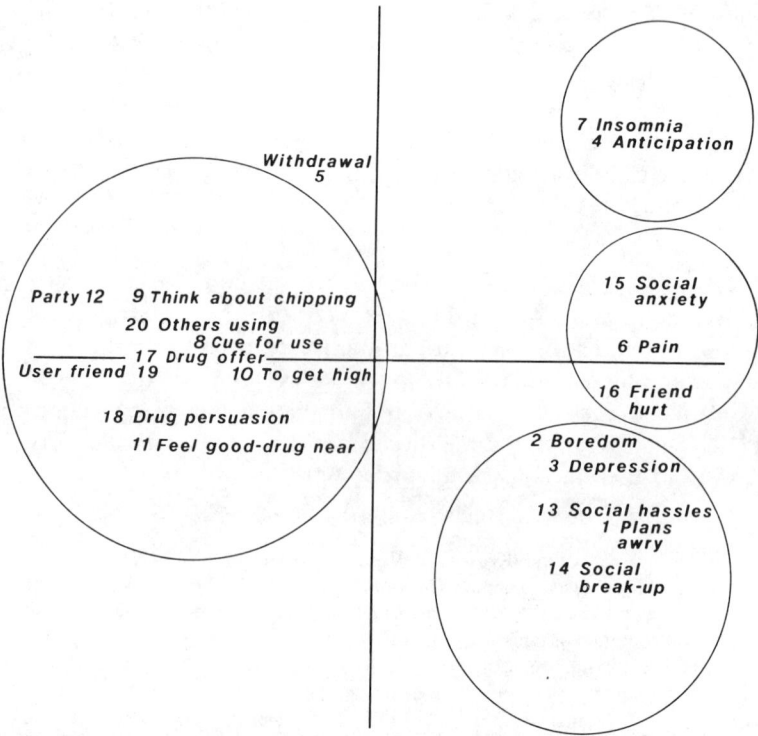

Figure 11.1 Perceptual configuration of relapse situation clusters for 20 opiate addicts stabilized on methadone maintenance.

supported the existence of five different clusters. The circles drawn on Figure 11.1 show the five clusters mapped onto the two-dimensional scaling space. The situation involving feelings of withdrawal appears unique, constituting a cluster of its own. The situations clustered near the horizontal axis to the left of the figure are primarily interpersonal and involve either social pressure, the enhancement of a positive emotional state (interpersonal and intrapersonal), or the ready availability of the preferred drug. On the other end of this horizontal dimension are found clusters involving coping with negative emotional or nonwithdrawal-related physiological states and with interpersonal conflicts. This primary dimension is labeled as positive affect versus negative affect. The vertical dimension appears to differentiate negative affect situations but not positive affect situations. This dimension appears to distinguish intrapersonal negative emotional and physical physiological states from interpersonal conflict types. This typology resembles Shiffman's smoking relapse situations typology (Chapter 9, this volume).

DISCUSSION

The first dimension in subjects' perceptions of relapse situations appears closely related to the distinction between coping with stressful occurrences and coping with the temptation to use drugs. The second dimension, at its extremes, appears to reflect negative affect from either interpersonal or intrapersonal occurrences. At either pole, the use of the drug as a coping response appears to be motivated by its function for regulating affect. The finding that relapse is related to both negative and positive affect is consistent with the theoretical formulation presented by Wills and Shiffman (Chapter 1, this volume) and in some respects with conditioning theories of drug use (Siegel, 1978; Solomon, 1980). Relapses involving negative affect may be motivated by negative reinforcement through the termination of an unpleasant affective state. Relapses involving positive affect may reflect addictive behavior that is maintained by positive reinforcement, that is, the positive effects of the experience of drug taking. Conditioning theories suggest that positive reinforcement is predominant in the early stages of drug use, whereas negative reinforcement becomes increasingly predominant as habituation takes place, particularly if a withdrawal syndrome is experienced. As noted later, the two types of relapse situations tended to occur for different types of clients.

Support for the meaningfulness of the positive affect versus negative affect situational dimension is provided by Chaney et al. (1982). We found that subjects reporting relapses involving a positive emotional state were younger and of lower SES than those reporting relapses involving negative affect. Subjects relapsing in negative affect situations had been abstinent in a treatment program a significantly longer time than those having positive affect relapses. Subjects experiencing positive affect relapses tended to have accepted drugs offered by others, whereas those experiencing negative affect relapses tended to seek drugs or abuse their own or others' prescribed drugs. A negative affect relapse also was more likely to take place at home alone than elsewhere with friends. These findings seem consistent with conditioning theories in that with continued use, situations potentiating relapse shift from coping with temptation to using drugs for coping.

These data lend partial support for the perceptual salience of Marlatt and Gordon's (1980) typological system. The subjects' actual clustering of situations, however, is somewhat different from the theoretical groupings. If the categories "enhancement of intra- or interpersonal positive emotional state," "testing personal control," and "giving in to temptation or urges" are combined to produce five groups, comparing Marlatt's categorization of relapse situations with the subjects' empirical categorization produces a Cohen's (unweighted) kappa of .423. One of the primary differences is that the subjects appear to consider coping with physical withdrawal cues in a category quite distinct from coping with other negative physical states. (This distinction is present in Marlatt and Gordon's system but only as a subclassification.) Also, the intrapersonal–interpersonal dimension does not appear to have much salience when positive emotional states and/or drug cues are involved. The two dimensions suggested by the multidimensional scaling analysis, however, appear to reflect two of the major distinctions or classification rules in Marlatt's system: coping with negative affect and coping with positive affect (also see Wills and Shiffman, Chapter 1). The typology also reflects distinctions in coping with interpersonal conflict and with frustration–anger versus coping with negative emotional states other than frustration–anger and with negative physiological states.

Study 2

The second study related subjects' perceptions of high-risk situations to their predicted coping behavior. The primary hypothesis was that subjects' responses in a role play situation would reflect their perception that different types of relapse situations demand different types of coping responses. Second, we hypothesized that efficacy expectations would be different for different relapse situations. Third, we hypothesized that subjects might have different efficacy expectations related to the coping strategy chosen, both for prevention of relapse and for termination of a relapse episode.

PROCEDURE

The SCTDR was administered as a structured interview. First, subjects were presented all 20 SCTDR situations, physically divided into the six categories shown in Table 11.1. Subjects were asked to rank order the situations within each a priori category from the one most associated with drug and alcohol use for them to the one with least association. The subject was then asked to imagine how the situation ranked highest in each category might happen; to assume that he did not want to use drugs or drink at that time; and to role play what he would do in that situation as if it were actually happening. Thus, six responses were elicited and recorded from each subject. Each reply was analyzed to place it into one of the nine focus-of-coping categories presented by Moos and Billings (1982). Efficacy expectations were operationalized by having the subjects indicate on a 5-point scale how likely they would be to use drugs or drink in that situation (relapse prevention efficacy), how much they would be likely to use, and for how long. Predicted amount of use and duration of use were combined additively into a relapse termination efficacy scale.

A group of 50 military veterans entering an outpatient methadone maintenance treatment program were administered the SCTDR, generating a total of 300 coping responses for analysis. (See Study 1 for demographic characteristics of the subjects.) Content analysis and scoring was done primarily by one trained rater. One of the investigators independently content analyzed and scored a 10% subsample. Interrater agreement was 87% for the coping categorization.

RESULTS

The first hypothesis was evaluated by cross-tabulating the occurrence of each type of coping response in each type of relapse situation; χ^2 (40,N = 300) = 179.5, p = .0001.[3] Table 11.2 gives the frequency of occurrences of coping strategies for each relapse situation category. Cognitive redefinition and affective regulation are coping strategies seldom mentioned by this population. The preponderance of strategies involved problem-focused coping, particularly taking problem-solving action or seeking information or advice. For some relapse situation types, however, responses in other coping categories were predominant. For instance, situations involving coping with negative physical or physiological states produced coping behavior that emphasized resigned acceptance and emotional discharge in addition to seeking information or advice. These situations were perceived by the subjects as beyond their ability, and they either sought help, gave up, or reported they would engage in emotional discharge, which in the majority of instances meant drug use. Situations involving testing personal control or the presence of substance cues were the only categories in which appraisal-

[3] The chi-square test should be interpreted in a descriptive and exploratory manner because (1) the data consist of repeated measures, and (2) several of the cells of the table have an expected frequency less than 5.

Table II.2
RELAPSE SITUATION CATEGORIES AND COPING TYPES FOR HEROIN ADDICTS[a]

Response variable	Relapse situation category						Row total
	Negative emotion	Negative physical	Testing–craving	Positive emotion	Conflict	Social pressure	
FOCUS OF COPING							
Logical analysis	5	1	11	3	2	1	23
Cognitive redefinition	1	0	2	2	1	0	6
Cognitive avoidance	2	2	13	6	5	3	31
Help seeking	12	16	6	4	10	1	49
Problem solving	8	4	10	25	19	41	107
Develop alternatives	15	4	4	4	7	2	36
Affective regulation	0	2	0	0	0	0	2
Resigned acceptance	3	10	0	1	0	1	15
Emotional discharge	4	11	4	5	6	1	31
EFFICACY EXPECTATION							
Relapse prevention							
M	61	77	64	44	67	60	
SD	28	22	23	18	25	24	
Relapse termination							
M	33	48	48	61	42	57	
SD	25	29	29	25	29	24	

[a]Coping cell entries are frequencies. All column marginal frequencies equal 50. Efficacy scores have a range of 0 (low) to 100 (high).

focused coping predominated, although logical analysis and cognitive avoidance were approximately equally prevalent. Help-seeking coping was common in only three of the six categories: negative emotional state, negative physical state, and interpersonal conflict.

The second hypothesis was evaluated by using two repeated-measures analyses of variance, with relapse prevention and termination efficacy expectations as the dependent variables and situation type as the independent variable. Subjects' average self-efficacy expectations were 49% ($SD = 34$) for success in relapse prevention and 50% ($SD = 27$) for success in relapse termination, which in absolute terms reflects a rather pessimistic expectation about one's prospects for maintaining abstinence. Both types of efficacy expectation were related significantly to situation type; $F(5, 100) = 5.82$, $p < .0001$, and $F(5, 100) = 4.80$, $p < .001$, respectively. Table 11.2 gives the means and standard deviations of the efficacy measures for the six situation types.

The third hypothesis concerning the relationship of methods of coping and efficacy expectations was evaluated by grouping the nine coping focus

Table II.3

COPING AND EFFICACY EXPECTATIONS IN HEROIN ADDICTS[a]

Coping method	Efficacy expectations			
	Prevent relapse		Terminate relapse	
	M	SD	M	SD
Active cognitive	69	32.5	49	33.3
Active behavioral	52	31.7	53	27.8
Help seeking	48	31.8	44	25.9
Avoidance	44	37.7	50	25.4

[a]Efficacy scores have a range of 0 (low) to 100 (high).

categories to represent methods of active cognitive coping, active behavioral coping, help seeking, and avoidance or tension-reduction coping. Logical analysis and cognitive redefinition were combined to represent active cognitive coping. Taking problem-solving action and developing alternative rewards constituted active behavioral coping. Affective regulation was added to this category because the two instances reported were behavioral in nature. Seeking information or advice was grouped separately as help-seeking because this may be a particularly important type of coping response for persons in treatment. Finally, cognitive avoidance, resigned acceptance, and emotional discharge categories were combined as reflecting tension reduction or avoidance coping.

Analysis of variance suggested that subjects' efficacy expectations for relapse prevention were significantly different among the four coping method categories, with instances of active cognitive coping related to a significantly higher self-efficacy prediction than the other three categories; $F(3, 46) = 4.27, p < .01$. Efficacy predictions for termination of a relapse once begun were not significantly different among the coping categories. Efficacy expectations means and standard deviations for the four coping method categories are given in Table 11.3.

DISCUSSION

Opiate users beginning treatment appear to select coping strategies depending on the type of situation they are facing. Although their efficacy expectations for the success of alternate coping strategies are quite low, the expectations are actuarially realistic: Although opiate use is significantly reduced in methadone maintenance treatment, use of other drugs and alcohol remains problematic for many clients (Cooper et al., 1983). This perception of inefficacy suggests why avoidance (behavioral, not cognitive) may be an appropriate coping strategy for opiate addicts in many potential relapse situations. Although skillfully applied cognitive techniques may well be among the more effective types of coping (e.g., Litman et al., 1979), the fact that our sample associates cognitive coping with higher efficacy expectations for relapse prevention also may be inaccurate. The process of cognitive coping is less subject to performance scrutiny and feedback than behavioral coping and may be more difficult to learn to do well because it is easy to attribute failed cognitive coping attempts to external causes rather than to faulty execution.

The relationships among situations, efficacy expectation, and coping styles are complex. This exploratory work suggests that situation parameters can account for a part of the variance in coping focus and efficacy expectations. Future research might try to separate the effects of coping methods and efficacy expectations by presenting subjects with a situation and a coping method and asking about their efficacy expectation in that situation with that coping method. This is more artificial than the approach taken here but would allow independent assessment of situation and coping effects.

Study 3

The third study investigates coping and efficacy expectations in relation to illicit drug use over the course of treatment.

PROCEDURE

Random weekly urinalysis data were collected from the 50 subjects whose SCTDR data were reported in Study 2. The subjects were divided into three groups: those with a relatively high level of illicit drug use during their stay in the program (an average of more than one detected use per month), those with a moderate level (use once a month to once every 5 months) and those with a low level (use less than once every 5 months). Since the primary treatment goal for all subjects on this program was to reduce and eliminate all illicit drug use,[4] the extent of this use served as an index of the success of their alternative coping attempts. Of the 50 subjects for whom SCTDRs were collected at intake, 8 were eliminated from this

---

[4] Methadone maintenance programs differ in the extent to which they monitor and focus on the patient's use of nonnarcotic illicit drugs and alcohol. The philosophy of many programs is that eliminating all illicit drug use and problem drinking is necessary for the life-style change that will help prevent relapse following treatment termination.

Table II.4

PREDICTED COPING AND IN-TREATMENT DRUG USE IN HEROIN ADDICTS[a]

Relapse category	Detected illicit drug use groups					
	Low (n = 15)		Medium (n = 14)		High (n = 13)	
	M	SD	M	SD	M	SD
RELAPSE PREVENTION EFFICACY EXPECTATIONS						
Negative emotion	53	33.9	50	32.5	44	32.5
Negative physical	57	35.9	54	35.2	58	38.7
Testing–craving	32	22.1	25	27.7	25	27.0
Positive emotion	53	37.6	43	28.5	50	30.6
Conflict	43	34.7	55	34.2	56	37.0
Social pressure	52	34.7	36	21.3	50	39.5
RELAPSE TERMINATION EFFICACY EXPECTATIONS						
Negative emotion	50	27.0	39	31.3	33	25.8
Negative physical	56	28.0	52	24.3	34	22.1
Testing–craving	55	21.6	53	30.2	51	31.4
Positive emotion	73	19.4	58	29.8	63	25.9
Conflict	57	30.8	50	22.4	23	16.5
Social pressure	67	18.1	67	18.7	54	30.0

[a] Efficacy scores have a range of 0 (low) to 100 (high).

phase of the study because they either did not finish intake procedures or did not remain on the program long enough to become stabilized on methadone (a minimum of 1 month of treatment). Of the remaining subjects, 13 were classified in the high-use group, 14 in the moderate-use group, and 15 in the low-use group. These subjects were monitored until discharge or reinterview 22 months after intake. Average length of monitoring was 17.2 months ($SD = 7.7$).

RESULTS

There were no significant differences in demographic variables or in the types of coping predicted on the SCTDR across the three subject groups. As shown in Table 11.4, relapse prevention efficacy expectations also were not significantly different. Subjects' expectations for terminating a relapse once begun, however, were in the predicted direction for all situation categories. In other words, the low illicit drug use group had the highest mean expectations for relapse termination, the moderate-use group was in the middle, and the heavy-use group had the lowest mean expectations. Univariate analyses of variance showed that the three subject groups had significantly different relapse termination efficacy expectations in the category of interpersonal conflict; $F(2, 29) = 5.85, p = .01$. In the other situation categories, the three subject groups' relapse termination efficacy expectations did not differ at the selected .01 significance level.

DISCUSSION

Our results show that neither aggregated efficacy expectations nor predicted coping responses to role play situations were good predictors of in-treatment outcome. The absence of a relationship between coping category and outcome suggests that one type of coping is not necessarily superior to another (see Shiffman, Chapter 9; Curry & Marlatt, Chapter 10); how well the coping is executed may be the key factor. Though not predictive here, efficacy expectations have been effective predictors of relapse in other studies (e.g., Condiotte & Lichtenstein, 1981) and should be considered for inclusion in comprehensive models of substance use and relapse.

Study 4

Instances of illicit drug use may occur in several distinct relapse episodes or one continuing episode. In studying opiate addicts who are ostensibly committed to eliminating illicit drug use, those situations that result in a new episode of use are of most interest. The fourth study in this series examined failed coping to obtain more information about the types of coping responses associated with actual relapse situations.

METHOD

Of the 42 subjects whose SCTDR data are reported in the previous section, 24 remained in treatment 22 months after admission. Of these, four refused to be reinterviewed and four had no instances of detected illicit drug use during treatment. Comparison of demographic, substance use, coping, and efficacy measures revealed no differences between the 24 subjects available for reinterview and the subjects who were not (16 discharged, 2 transferred to other programs). The data reported here are based on the responses of the 16 addicts who remained in treatment for the full period and who had one or more relapses during the period. A relapse was defined as an episode of illicit drug use detected by the random weekly urinanalysis done on each patient in the program. A relapse was operationally distinguished from continuing illicit drug use by the requirement that it be preceded by at least 1 month of urinalysis results free from illicit drugs. A maximum of two relapses were analyzed for each subject: the one that occurred after the longest time in treatment within the 22-month period and the one that followed the longest interval of abstinence from illicit drug use, if different from the first. For each of the relapses the subject was asked to describe the circumstances that led to the use, what he considered doing instead of using, which of those strategies were actually tried, what the outcome was for each of the alternative coping behaviors attempted, and what his explanation for use was. Subjects also were asked how much they used and for how long a period.

RESULTS

Subjects reported varied ranges of time during which they had considered using drugs as a response to the situation. In 21 of 23 relapse episodes, the subjects reported that they had contemplated substance use well in advance of the actual relapse situation; in 52% of the instances subjects had considered substance use for a 1- to 4-hour period before drug ingestion. In the remaining nine episodes (39%) the period of premeditation varied from 1 day to more than a month.

In 78% of the relapses, subjects' reports suggested that they perceived the drug use as an attempt to cope with a problematic situation. In the remaining five instances, subjects did not appear to view the return to illicit drug use as a volitional breakdown. Of the 18 coping relapses, 6 were perceived as responses to negative emotional states, 6 to negative physical states (pain), 3 to interpersonal conflict, and 3 to social pressure. The latter two interpersonal categories involved important interpersonal relationships (i.e., conflict at work or with significant others, or social pressure from a spouse or girlfriend who was also a user).

Subjects reported that they thought of using some kind of alternative coping behavior in all 23 cases. *In only 38% of the episodes was coping actually attempted.* These attempts were to use over-the-counter drugs (2), to socialize (2), to relax (2), to engage in alternative activity (1), and to cry (1). Of these eight instances of attempted coping, seven were perceived as unsuccessful, and one (socializing) was reported to have helped terminate the relapse eventually.

The coping strategies that relapsing subjects report having considered, but not used successfully were fairly evenly distributed across the domains of appraisal-focused coping (35%), problem-focused coping (39%), and emotion-focused coping (26%). Classifying those 23 coping opportunities in terms of method of coping, 43% were active behavioral strategies, 9% were active cognitive, and 48% were avoidant.

DISCUSSION

This study of failed coping suggests several hypotheses for future research. Subjects' understanding of their own relapse behavior in specific situations appears quite similar to the analysis of those situations based on the categorical system used here. Although subjects think of alternatives to drug use in relapse situations most of the time, they do not use these alternate coping responses. Marlatt and Gordon's (1985) relapse theory suggests that this is because of low efficacy expectations (which these subjects as a group do have) and/or because the anticipated positive benefits of the drug outweigh the possible benefits of other strategies.

None of the relapses that were perceived as volitional breakdowns occurred in positive affect situations. (The social pressure relapse situations were not in the context of positive emotional states.) This finding suggests that few of the relapses of opiate addicts on methadone maintenance are failures in coping with positive temptation to use drugs for positive affective outcomes but rather are based on responses to negative affect. This result may reflect the efficacy of methadone as well as support an adaptational perspective of opiate abuse.

When we examined the coping strategies that subjects considered but did not use successfully, we found that most instances of appraisal-focused coping were avoidant in nature. In fact, avoidance strategies were the most common overall. A topic for future research would be to compare successful coping in opiate addicts with failed coping. Successful coping with negative affect states is probably harder to monitor than coping with specific temptations to use. In the latter situations the stimuli for use should be easily discriminable. In the former, subjects' decisions to try various methods of coping may be sequential. By the time substance use is considered (thereby defining a potential relapse situation as far as the subject is concerned), a coping failure may be highly probable. It may be necessary to monitor subjects continuously and intensively to satisfactorily compare processes leading to successful and failed coping.

GENERAL DISCUSSION

To summarize, we noted previous literature showing a relationship between stress, coping, and relapse among both alcoholics and opiate addicts. Our study of opiate addict clients in methadone maintenance treatment found that their relapse episodes were triggered both by negative emotional states, often based on interpersonal conflict, and on physiological states associated with prior substance use. We found that subjects perceived high-risk situations in terms of dimensions that are consistent with theoretical models of coping, differentiating situations with respect to negative versus positive affect, and intrapersonal versus social settings. In a baseline assessment of our sample, we found that predicted coping behavior, as indicated by a role play situational assessment procedure, varied considerably across different types of situations, and that perceptions of efficacy for resisting relapse were, in absolute terms, rather low. Results from a follow-up conducted 22 months after the baseline assessment indicated that expectations for relapse were related to actual relapse, as indicated by biochemical measures of substance use. Retrospective interviews indicated that in 62% of relapse situations, the clients did not attempt any alternative coping at all. In the instances where coping was attempted, the coping behaviors used (e.g., other drug use, socialization) were not those recommended by theory or taught in treatment. These coping behaviors may have failed to prevent relapse in part because in many instances the subjects had been contemplating substance use for some time before the actual relapse episode. In fact, interviews suggested that clients were using opiates in an attempt to cope with ongoing psychological problems.

Testing personal control, giving in to intrapersonal temptations and urges, and relapses in positive interpersonal emotional situations appear to be fairly rare events for opiate addicts. There are obvious pharmacological reasons why opiate addicts successfully stabilized on methadone maintenance should not have to cope with craving in the absence of withdrawal. If this were not the case, presumably addicts would not stay on maintenance. With craving lessened, testing personal control should occur less frequently—addicts "know" that they could use without having to continue that use. Positive interpersonal emotional situations may not occur as frequently for opiate addicts as for members of other substance-using groups who pay smaller or nonexistent social penalties for use. Intrapersonal negative emotional states, negative physical–physiological states not related to drug use, and interpersonal conflict are likely to be situations in which drugs are used adaptively. Intra- and interpersonal giving-in to temptation and enhancement of positive emotional states may be situations in which individuals must cope with the consequences of past use, that is, the temptation to use.

The differences between coping with positive affect and negative affect relapse situations provide some support for conditioning theories of relapse. Alexander and Hadaway (1982) appear to view conditioning theories of opiate addiction as counter to an adaptive orientation. They point out that the occurrence of withdrawal symptoms is neither sufficient nor necessary to account for addiction. However, since it is obvious that high levels of drug use are self-destructive and therefore not adaptive, they introduce the concept of a positive feedback loop in which drug use creates a need for increased use in the future. They acknowledge that tolerance and physical dependence can play a role in this positive feedback loop.

Studying the behavior of opiate addicts in relapse situations suggests that a resumption of opiate use in fact is viewed as adaptive by the users in the majority of situations, primarily those that involve negative affect. Relapse in these types of situations is consistent with Alexander and Hadaway's suggested positive feedback loop. Opiates are used to cope with stressful situations. The user appraises opiate use as the preferred coping strategy in those situations. The use of this strategy is dysfunctional in that it results in no change to the original situation or in deterioration. However, not all opiate relapse phenomena fit under this rubric. Approximately one-quarter to one-third of relapse situations of the opiate addicts studied here are perceived as resulting from drug-use-related intrapersonal and interpersonal cues. These situations have a different range of coping responses than negatively reinforced situations. Thus, a comprehensive theory of relapse should include attention to drug-specific cues, at least in the case of opiates.

Although opiate addicts exhibit diverse coping strategies, their efficacy expectations for relapse prevention or termination are (realistically) not very high. The research reported here attempted to distinguish efficacy expectations for relapse prevention and for relapse termination. Alcohol relapse research strongly suggests that there are different processes involved (Donovan & Chaney, 1985). The different relationships found for relapse prevention efficacy versus relapse termination efficacy suggest that this is also a useful distinction for opiate relapse.

We are only beginning to relate situational events to cognitive appraisal, efficacy expectations, and the availability of alternative coping strategies. Current cognitive theories suggest that to become more effective in coping with relapse situations, individuals' efficacy expectations must be altered through training processes that result in the reappraisal of opiate use as a maladaptive coping strategy. Accoing to our findings, a primary treatment goal would be to increase the probability that subjects will perform *any* coping behavior (since the majority failed to try alternative coping at all). Findings that coping responses differ across relapse situation types appear rich in treatment implications. Since addicts' efficacy expectations are low for the coping strategies in their repertoire, it may be productive to teach coping strategies that are underchosen in the various situation types. For example, in situations involving testing personal control or craving, logical analysis, which is a high frequency coping choice, simply may be an inappropriate focus for coping. Cognitive redefinition and affective regulation are underchosen specific coping foci that could be taught in a skills training approach (Roskies & Lazarus, 1980; Shiffman, Chapter 9, this volume; Curry & Marlatt, Chapter 10). For some situation types, however, attempts to improve current coping strategies may be most appropriate. For example, if a social pressure situation involves a significant other, a response from the already prevalent problem-solving coping focus category probably is required.

The data reported in this chapter are exploratory in nature and represent only a beginning in the study of coping in opiate addicts. Measurement of drug abusers' coping strategies in specific high-risk relapse situations requires continuing refinement. Replications of multidimensional scaling procedures with different subject groups is needed to determine the stability and generalizability of the results reported here. Research findings are likely to be sensitive to the response set that subjects are asked to adopt (Magnusson & Ekehammar, 1975) and to their intentions and goals. To confirm and extend our findings, prospective studies of successful coping versus failed coping are needed. Subjects in or after treatment need to be monitored more closely and comprehensively and interviewed as soon as possible after actual relapse episodes. Further development of standardized measurement and assessment techniques across types of substance abuse will help refine our knowledge of the similarities and differences in coping with high-risk relapse situations. We think this type of research will be productive for understanding why opiate users relapse and how they can be taught to cope more effectively with relapse situations.

REFERENCES

Alexander, B. K., & Hadaway, P. F. (1982). Opiate addiction: The case for an adaptive orientation. *Psychological Bulletin, 92,* 367–381.

Aneshensel, C. S., & Huba, G. J. (1983). Depression, alcohol use and smoking over one year: A four-wave longitudinal causal model. *Journal of Abnormal Psychology, 92,* 134–150.

Appel, P. W., & Kaestner, E. (1979). Interpersonal and emotional problem solving among narcotic drug abusers. *Journal of Consulting and Clinical Psychology, 47,* 1125–1127.

Chaney, E. F., O'Leary, M. R., & Marlatt, G. A. (1978). Skill training with alcoholics. *Journal of Consulting and Clinical Psychology, 46,* 1092–1104.

Chaney, E. F., Roszell, D. K., & Cummings, C. (1982). Relapse in opiate addicts: A behavioral analysis. *Addictive Behaviors, 7,* 291–297.

Chelune, G. J., & Parker, J. B. (1981). Neuropsychological deficits associated with chronic alcohol abuse. *Clinical Psychology Review, 1,* 181–195.

Condiotte, M. M., & Lichtenstein, E. (1981). Self-efficacy and relapse in smoking cessation programs. *Journal of Consulting and Clinical Psychology, 49,* 648–658.

Cooper, J. R., Altman, F., Brown, B. S., & Czechowicz, D. (Eds.). (1983). *Research on the treatment of narcotic addiction* (NIDA Research Monograph Series). Washington, DC: U.S. Government Printing Office.

Cronkite, R. C., & Moos, R. H. (1980). Determinants of the posttreatment functioning of alcoholic patients: A conceptual framework. *Journal of Consulting and Clinical Psychology, 48,* 305–316.

Donovan, D. M., & Chaney, E. F. (1985). Alcoholic relapse prevention and intervention: Models and methods. In G. A. Marlatt & J. R. Gordon (Eds.), *Relapse prevention: Maintenance strategies in the treatment of addictive behaviors.* New York: Guilford Press.

Holmes, T. H., & Rahe, R. H. (1967). The social readjustment rating scale. *Journal of Psychosomatic Research, 11,* 213–218.

Ilfeld, F. W. (1980). Coping styles of Chicago adults: Description. *Journal of Human Stress, 6,* 2–10.
Jones, S. L., Kanfer, R., & Lanyon, R. I. (1982). Skill training with alcoholics: A clinical extension. *Addictive Behaviors, 7,* 285–290.
Jones, S. L., & Lanyon, R. I. (1981). Relationship between adaptive skills and outcome of alcoholism treatment. *Journal of Studies on Alcohol, 42,* 521–525.
Kosten, T. R., Rounsaville, B. J., & Kleber, H. D. (1983). Relationship of depression to psychosocial stressors in heroin addicts. *Journal of Nervous and Mental Disease, 171,* 97–104.
Krueger, D. W. (1981). Stressful life events and the return of heroin use. *Journal of Human Stress, 7,* 3–8.
Kruskal, J. B., & Wish, M. (1978). *Multidimensional scaling.* Beverly Hills: Sage.
Lettieri, D. J., Sayers, M., & Pearson, H. W. (Eds.). (1980). *Theories on drug abuse: Selected contemporary perspectives* (NIDA Research Monograph 30). Washington, DC: U.S. Government Printing Office.
Litman, G. K., Eiser, J. R., Rawson, N. S., & Oppenheim, A. N. (1979). Differences in relapse precipitants and coping behaviour between alcohol relapsers and survivors. *Behaviour Research and Therapy, 17,* 89–94.
Litman, G. K., Stapleton, J., Oppenheim, A. N., & Peleg, M. (1983). An instrument for measuring coping behavior in hospitalized alcoholics: Implications for relapse prevention treatment. *British Journal of Addiction, 78,* 269–276.
Magnusson, D., & Ekehammar, B. (1975). Perceptions of and reactions to stressful situations. *Journal of Personality and Social Psychology, 31,* 1147–1154.
Marlatt, G. A., & Gordon, J. R. (1980). Determinants of relapse: Implications for the maintenance of behavior change. In P. O. Davidson & S. M. Davidson (Eds.), *Behavioral medicine: Changing health lifestyles.* New York: Brunner/Mazel.
Marlatt, G. A., & Gordon, J. R. (Eds.). (1985). *Relapse prevention: Maintenance strategies in the treatment of addictive behaviors.* New York: Guilford Press.
Mischel, W. (1981). A cognitive-social learning approach to assessment. In T. V. Merluzzi, C. R. Glass, & M. Genest (Eds.), *Cognitive assessment.* New York: Guilford Press.
Moos, R. H., & Billings, A. G. (1982). Conceptualizing and measuring coping resources and processes. In L. Goldberger & S. Breznitz (Eds.), *Handbook of stress: Theoretical and clinical aspects.* New York: Macmillan.
Moos, R. H., Finney, J. W., & Chan, D. A. (1981). The process of recovery from alcoholism: I. Comparing alcoholic patients and matched community controls. *Journal of Studies on Alcohol, 42,* 383–402.
Nurco, D. N., Cisin, I. H., & Balter, M. B. (1981a). Addict careers. I. A New Typology. *International Journal of the Addictions, 16,* 1305–1325.
Nurco, D. N., Cisin, I. H., & Balter, M. B. (1981b). Addict careers. II. The first 10 years. *International Journal of the Addictions, 16,* 1327–1356.
Platt, J. J., Scura, W. C., & Hannon, J. R. (1973). Problem solving thinking of youthful incarcerated heroin addicts. *Journal of Community Psychology, 1,* 278–281.
Prusoff, B., Thompson, W. D., Scholomskos, D., & Riordan, C. (1977). Psychosocial stressors and depression among former herion dependent patients maintained on methadone. *Journal of Nervous and Mental Disease, 165,* 57–63.
Rosenberg, H. S. (1983). Relapsed versus non-relapsed alcohol abusers: Coping skills, life events, and social support. *Addictive Behaviors, 8,* 183–186.
Roskies, E., & Lazarus, R. S. (1980). Coping theory and the teaching of coping skills. In P. O. Davidson & S. M. Davidson (Eds), *Behavioral medicine: Changing health lifestyles.* New York: Brunner/Mazel.

Rounsaville, B. J., Jones, C., Novelly, R. A., & Kleber, H. (1982). Neuropsychological Functioning in Opiate Addicts. *Journal of Nervous and Mental Disease, 170,* 209–216.

Sanchez-Craig, M., & Walker, K. (1982). Teaching coping skills to chronic alcoholics in a coeducational halfway house: I. Assessment of programme effects. *British Journal of Addictions, 77,* 35–50.

Siegel, S. (1978). A Pavlovian conditioning analysis of morphine. In N. A. Krasnegor (Ed.), *Behavioral tolerance: Research and treatment implications.* NIDA Research Mongraph 18. Washington, DC: U.S. Government Printing Office.

Sjöberg, L., & Olsson, G. (1981). Volitional problems in carrying through a difficult decision: The case of drug addiction. *Drug and Alcohol Dependence, 7,* 177–191.

Solomon, R. L. (1980). The opponent-process theory of acquired motivation: The costs of pleasure and the benefits of pain. *American Psychologist, 35,* 691–712.

Van Hasselt, V. B., Hersen, M., & Milliones, J. (1978). Social skills training for alcoholics and drug addicts: A review. *Addictive Behaviors, 3,* 221–233.

Waldorf, D. (1983). Natural recovery from opiate addiction: Some social psychological processes of untreated recovery. *Journal of Drug Issues, 13,* 237–280.

Wille, R. (1983). Processes of recovery from heroin dependence: Relationship to treatment, social changes and drug use. *Journal of Drug Issues, 13,* 333–342.

Winstead, D. K., Whitworth, H., & Lawson, T. R. (1981). Life changes, personality patterns and drug use. *International Journal of the Addictions, 16,* 25–31.

Wishart, D. (1975). *CLUSTAN IC User Manual.* London: University College Computer Centre.

Young, F. W., Takane, Y., & Lewyckyj, R. (1979). *Alscal-4 User's Guide.* Chapel Hill, NC: University of North Carolina Psychometric Laboratory.

Chapter 12

Self-Change Strategies for the Control of Smoking, Obesity, and Problem Drinking*

MICHAEL G. PERRI

OVERVIEW

It is commonly believed that cigarette smoking, obesity, and heavy drinking are highly resistant to change. Reviews of the effectiveness of treatments for these problems typically reveal modest short-term success but high relapse rates over the long run (see Hall, 1980; Hunt, Barnett, & Branch, 1971; Kirschenbaum & Tomarken, 1982; Leventhal & Cleary, 1980; Polich, Armor, & Braiker, 1981; Stunkard & Penick, 1979). Despite the general perception about the intractability of addictive behaviors, there is evidence that substantial numbers of people are able to manage these problems successfully on their own, without professional advice. We are all aware of particular individuals who have had dramatic successes in quitting smoking, losing weight, or controlling their drinking; and there are ample data indicating that successful self-change is a common experience. For example, it is estimated that between 1965 and 1975 approximately 29 million Americans quit smoking, with 70–80% quitting on their own (Center for Disease Control, 1976). Similarly, long-term studies (e.g., Cahalan & Room, 1974; Vaillant, 1983) have shown substantial improvements in drinking behavior for as many as 50% of untreated heavy drinkers in the general population. Although there is less information available regarding self-regulation of

*Support for the study of problem drinkers was provided in part by the Office of Naval Research under Contract N00014-76-C-001 with the Center for Naval Analyses of the University of Rochester. The author gratefully acknowledges the assistance of Ralph Barocas, Fred Brown, Carl Hatch, Gita Krull, Randy Otto, Marjorie Richards, Steven Richards, Karen Schultheis, Robert Shapiro, and David Sieg.

obesity, two studies (Jeffery & Wing, 1983; Schachter, 1982) suggest that substantial numbers of people are successful in self-management of weight problems.

Surprisingly, relatively little research attention has been paid to individuals in the general population who undertake self-initiated efforts to control problem behaviors. Since some naturally occurring episodes of self-change are dramatically successful, study of successful versus unsuccessful self-regulation may show effective elements of successful self-management. It is important to know how self-change occurs in general and what strategies are employed in successful self-management. Presumably certain strategies used by successful self-regulators not only differentiate them from their unsuccessful counterparts but also contribute to their success in self-change. Thus, the study of naturally occurring episodes of self-change may contribute to our understanding of the coping process and may hold heuristic value for improved conceptualization and theory development (see Bandura, 1977; Karoly & Kanfer, 1982). Furthermore, a better understanding of successful self-regulation may suggest clinical applications to improve the efficiency or long-term effectiveness of therapies for problems such as smoking, obesity, or alcohol abuse (see Kirschenbaum & Tomarken, 1982; Lichtenstein, 1982).

This chapter presents and discusses the findings from a series of studies in which my colleagues and I investigated naturally occurring episodes involving self-management of smoking, obesity, and problem drinking. The key question we addressed was: What are the differences in the self-change strategies employed by people who are successful at self-management compared with those who are not? The basic method of our investigations was the use of a structured interview—a procedure that permits a flexible format necessary for an exploratory investigation, yet retains sufficient structure to gather data in a systematic and reliable manner. In our studies of self-management of smoking and obesity (Perri & Richards, 1977; Perri, Richards, & Schultheis, 1977), we conducted retrospective interviews with college students. In our recent study of problem drinking, we studied individuals from the community in a prospective manner over the course of a 6–8-month period. I first present our findings about self-change in college students.

COLLEGE STUDENTS' COPING WITH SMOKING AND OBESITY

For our studies of self-management of smoking and obesity, we solicited subjects from among college students who had a serious problem with smoking or obesity and who made a concerted effort to change the problem behavior. For smoking, a serious problem was operationally defined as smoking at least 20 cigarettes per day for a period of 6 or more months. For obesity, a serious problem was defined as being 20% over ideal body weight for a period of at least 1 year. A concerted effort was defined operationally as an attempt to cope with the problem through the use of a procedural strategy over the period of 1 or more weeks.

Method

We selected 24 individuals who were successful in coping with a smoking problem and 24 who were unsuccessful. Among subjects who coped with weight problems, we selected 12 successful and 12 unsuccessful individuals. (In our original study, Perri & Richards, 1977, we also included groups of individuals who were successful or unsuccessful in coping with study and dating problems.) No individual was interviewed about more than one problem. In each problem area, half of the subjects were male and half were female. The success classification was determined through a telephone-screening procedure with individuals who reported having made a self-control effort and who had volunteered to participate in the study. Subjects classified as successful in coping with smoking were those who reported that they (1) decreased the number of cigarettes smoked by 50%, (2) maintained this lower rate for 4 or more months prior to the interview, and (3) felt happier with their reduction in smoking. Subjects classified as successful in coping with obesity were those who reported that they (1) decreased the amount that they were overweight by 50% or more, (2) maintained this reduction for 4 or more months prior to the interview, and (3) felt happier with their lower weight and the amount of food consumed.

All interviews were conducted in private by one of two clinical psychology graduate students. The interviewer followed a structured, 16-page protocol in soliciting relevant information from all subjects about the following areas and time periods: (1) nature of the problem before attempts to change, (2) method(s) used to deal with the problem, (3) implementation of the method(s), (4) effects of the method(s) on the problem behavior, and (5) current status of the problem. The interview protocol was based on a hypothesized multistage process of self-regulation including the following phases: (1) problem recognition, (2) commitment or decision making, (3) execution of self-control behaviors (e.g., self-monitoring, stimulus control, self-reinforcement), followed by (4) either habit reorganization or self-regulatory failure (see Kanfer & Karoly, 1972; Karoly, 1977). The interview format included yes–no questions, 5-point Likert-type scales, and open-ended questions. Subjects were asked to describe their self-management strategies in their own words; the interviewer then judged whether the procedure used constituted a particular self-control strategy (e.g., self-monitoring, stimulus control) according to predetermined criteria (Thoresen & Mahoney, 1974).

All interviews were recorded on audiotapes. An independent rater was employed to complete comparison answer codes for a sample of 12 interviews; the mean interrater reliability coefficient was .86 (see Perri & Richards, 1977). Thus the structured interviews yielded information that was categorized in a reliable manner.

Results

An examination of the interview data across both target problems revealed the following findings: (1) successful individuals used more techniques for longer periods of time in their self-control efforts, compared with persons who were unsuccessful; (2) the methods used by successful subjects appeared to vary according to whether they were dealing with a smoking or weight problem; and (3) the reported use of certain behavioral strategies, particularly self-reinforcement procedures, differentiated successful from unsuccessful self-management efforts.

Subjects' descriptions of the severity of their smoking and obesity problems as they existed prior to their self-change efforts showed no differences between successful and unsuccessful individuals. Following the self-management effort, however, only the successful subjects described significant improvements. They reported significant decreases in the number of cigarettes smoked ($M = 26.8$ vs. 3.8 fewer cigarettes per day for successful versus unsuccessful subjects) or significant reductions in weight ($M = 36.8$ vs. 9.5 pounds lost for successful vs. unsuccessful subjects). These data supported our screening classification of subjects as successful or unsuccessful.

A comparison of successful versus unsuccessful subjects across both problem areas showed that successful subjects rated themselves as more motivated and committed to personal change than unsuccessful ones. At the outset of their self-management endeavors, successful individuals set their goals and standards for change higher than their unsuccessful counterparts. They used more coping techniques for longer periods of time and also reported more frequent and consistent use of self-control methods. They rated their techniques as more practical and useful, described themselves as more successful, and noted more positive changes and improvements than unsuccessful subjects.

Other significant differences between successful and unsuccessful subjects were specific to whether the target problem was smoking or obesity. Among subjects who atempted to cope with smoking problems, the unsuccessful individuals reported that their smoking followed specific behaviors in a habitual manner (e.g., after meals) more frequently than did successful ones. Smoking had been a longer standing problem for unsuccessful subjects than for successful ones ($M = 29.9$ vs. 14.8 months). During the prechange period, however, successful subjects indicated that significantly more negative consequences (e.g., smoker's cough) influenced their decision to attempt smoking reduction or cessation. In their actual effort at self-control, significantly more successful than unsuccessful subjects reported the use of some form of self-reinforcement procedure, whether overt (e.g., buying oneself a gift for not smoking for a week) or covert (e.g., saying to oneself "I've done a great job in not smoking today"). In addition, successful individuals reported significantly greater use of a general planning or problem-solving strategy in their efforts to cope with smoking. They also reported receiving more positive feedback (especially from their parents) about their smoking reduction efforts than did their unsuccessful counterparts.

Among the college students attempting to cope with obesity, successful individuals reported experiencing a significantly greater number of negative interpersonal consequences (e.g., ridicule from peers) during the prechange period than did unsuccessful ones. In their attempts to lose weight, successful subjects utilized self-reinforcement procedures more often than unsuccessful ones. Successful individuals also reported the use of stimulus control methods (e.g., reducing eating cues by not having any food around their dormitory room) more often than did unsuccessful subjects. During their self-change efforts, successful subjects reported receiving more social support in the form of compliments and positive feedback from peers and parents than did their unsuccessful counterparts.

Discussion

In each problem area, subjects' descriptions of the severity of their problems (number of cigarettes smoked, pounds overweight) as they existed prior to their self-change endeavors showed no significant differences between successful and unsuccessful self-controllers. Yet, successful individuals rated themselves as more motivated and set higher standards and goals for themselves. If both successful and unsuccessful subjects had problems of equivalent severity during their prechange period, what caused the successful individuals to become more motivated in dealing with their problems? The crucial motivating element may not be the severity of the problem per se but rather the manner in which the individual views the problem situation in general and the degree to which each perceives himself or herself as deviating from certain performance criteria or standards. Overeaters who successfully dealt with weight problems cited negative interpersonal reactions as a motivating factor significantly more often than did unsuccessful subjects. Similarly, those individuals who significantly reduced or quit smoking noted a greater number of potential negative consequences, such as damage to health, than did unsuccessful subjects. The greater the perceived discrepancy between what one is doing and what one ought to be doing, then perhaps the greater one's motivation and commitment to change is likely to be (see Bandura, 1977; Kanfer, 1980).

Among college students, the use of self-reinforcement procedures dramatically differentiated successful from unsuccessful self-controllers dealing with *both* smoking and weight problems. The effectiveness of self-reinforcement procedures may derive in part from the result that when they are used in combination with other techniques self-reinforcers probably tend to strengthen the use and lengthen the maintenance of the entire self-control attempt (Kanfer, 1980). Furthermore, the longer an individual attempts to deal with a problem, the greater the chances of working it through successfully (Schachter, 1982). In addition, the use of self-reinforcement may provide a substitute for the inherently reinforcing properties of the smoking and eating behaviors themselves. Thus, the use of self-reinforcement procedures may be partly responsible for the significantly longer and more effective use of self-control strategies by the successful individuals in this study.

Beyond the use of self-reinforcement procedures, the strategies employed by successful individuals varied according to target problem. Among subjects who successfully coped with smoking problems, the use of some form of planning or problem-solving procedure was reported significantly more often than among unsuccessful subjects. For smokers, the development and maintenance of a planned coping strategy may be more important than a particular technique of quitting (Bernstein, 1974; Condiotte & Lichtenstein, 1981). For example, Shiffman (1984) found that among exsmokers the use of a coping response in the presence of temptation was significantly related to maintaining abstinence, but the specific type of coping response used did not appear to be particularly important.

Those individuals who successfully dealt with weight problems reported significantly greater use of stimulus control procedures than did unsuccessful subjects. The stimulus control procedures consisted of making environmental and situational changes toward reducing the prominence of food cues (see McReynolds, Lutz, Paulsen, & Kohrs, 1976). Many of the successful individuals began their self-control efforts immediately following a major environmental change, namely, moving away from their parents' home to attend college. It is interesting to speculate whether the negative interpersonal consequences of the new social environment or changes in the access and availability of food, or both, contributed to their substantial weight losses.

Across both smoking and weight problems, the self-control attempts of successful subjects were more comprehensive and of longer duration. Successful individuals utilized a wider array of strategies than their unsuccessful counterparts. The use of many methods may increase the probability that one or more of the techniques will be effective. If an individual lapses in his or her use of one method but continues in another, he or she is less likely to discontinue in defeat than if he or she were to fail in maintaining his or her one and only method.

Some limitations of the study of successful and unsuccessful efforts of self-control are worth noting. First, the data are based solely on retrospective self-reports. Since an assessment of the accuracy of subjects' recollection was not attempted, the potential influence of recall bias should be considered; after a successful self-management endeavor, some individuals may have tended in retrospect to evaluate their efforts in an overly favorable manner (i.e., halo effect). Second, the difference observed between successful and unsuccessful self-controllers may be accounted for by other unassessed variables (e.g., individual differences) or may be specific to the particular type of assessment format we employed (see Kirschenbaum & Tomarken, 1982). Third, subjects were mostly middle-class college students who were in good health and who had smoking or weight problems that were of briefer history and lesser severity than those of the typical clinic patient.

ADULTS' COPING WITH PROBLEM DRINKING

In the next study in our series on naturally occurring episodes of self-control, we investigated the self-change efforts of adults coping with problem drinking. The subjects for the study were drawn from an adult sample, and the investigation was carried out in a prospective manner over the course of a 6–8-month period. There were several advantages to these sampling and procedural changes from our studies of college students' self-change. First, the subjects were more representative of the U.S. adult population in general and more typical of clinical populations in particular. Second, studying self-change efforts from the point of their initiation alleviates some of the subject bias inherent in a retrospective analysis. Third, following subjects over the course of a 6–8-month period permits an opportunity to observe the effects of self-control on the target problem over time. This gives a particularly important perspective for problems such as alcohol abuse, which are often characterized by temporal instability and high relapse rates.

Method

SUBJECTS

Subjects were recruited from among people attending a film and discussion session on alcoholism at a local community mental health center. The film presentation, which utilized an educational format, was delivered on a weekly basis as a community service and was open to the general public. Each week at the conclusion of the film and discussion session, we solicited volunteers to participate in a study of efforts to cope with problem drinking. Eligibility for participation included two criteria: (1) volunteers had to rate themselves as having a "serious drinking problem" and (2) they had to be planning to stop or reduce drinking without the aid of a formal treatment program. Over the course of a 1-year period, 60 individuals met the criteria noted above and 43 agreed to participate by undergoing an initial interview and two subsequent interviews 3 and 6 months later. Volunteers were not paid for undergoing the initial interview but did receive $5 at each subsequent interview.

All data were collected via structured interviews. The interviews were conducted in private by a clinical psychologist or a trained research assistant. In a subsample of 15% of the interviews, a second interviewer was present to complete a comparison protocol. This procedure allowed for a determination of interrater reliability (all $rs > .80$).

INTERVIEWS

The initial interview, which solicited background data, was adapted from the protocols used in the NIAAA-sponsored Rand studies (Armor, Polich, & Stambul, 1978; Polich et al., 1981) and from instruments developed in the Stanford Social Ecology Laboratory (e.g., Bromet, Moos, Bliss, & Wuthmann, 1977; Moos, Mehren, & Moos, 1978). The types of data collected follow.

1. Demographic data. This included age, sex, marital status, ethnicity, race, religion, education, employment status, occupation, and income.

2. Drinking history. A set of 14 questions was used to assess: how long drinking has been a problem for the subject; the topography of drinking behavior (e.g., where and with whom drinking occurs); positive and negative effects of drinking; reactions of others to the subject's drinking; prior treatments for drinking; and factors that influenced the current decision to stop or reduce drinking.

3. Alcohol consumption. The quantity of alcohol (in ounces of ethanol) from beer, wine, and hard liquor consumed on a typical day during the month prior to the interview was assessed.

4. Behavioral impairment. A set of seven situational and overall frequency items rated on a 5-point scale (from never to often) was used to assess behavioral impairments. Participants were asked: "'How often in the past month did you drink in the morning, at home, on weekdays, on weekends, alone, miss meals because of drinking, and get drunk?"

5. Physical impairment. This set of 12 items rated on 5-point scales (from never to often) assessed alcohol-related physical symptoms. Participants were asked: "How often in the past month did you experience the following symptoms: shakiness in the hands, memory lapses, blackouts, DT's, cold sweats, dry heaves, difficulty sleeping, severe hangovers, upset stomachs, headaches, nervousness or tension, dizzy spells?"

6. Subjective rating. The participant rated on a 5-point scale (from never to quite often) how often drinking was a problem for him or her.

7. Social functioning. This set of five items dealt with social participation. Participants were asked to respond on 5-point scales to the following questions: "How often in the past month did you engage in the following activities: attend parties, spend time with close friends, participate in sports, attend cultural events, engage in community activities?"

8. Psychological well-being. This set of six items was rated on 5-point scales. Participants described themselves on the following items: pleased about accomplishing something, relaxed and comfortale, in control of your life, know where you want to go in life, getting all you want out of life, and feeling on top of the world.

9. Coping plans. Two open-ended items were used to solicit specific plans for coping with problem drinking. They were: "What do you need to change in order not to return to problem drinking?" and "What specific things are you planning to do so as not to return to problem drinking?"

THREE-MONTH FOLLOW-UP

Ten weeks after the initial interview, all subjects were contacted by telephone and scheduled for a second interview. Of our original 43 volunteers, 41 appeared for their scheduled interviews; the other 2 subjects were interviewed by telephone. At the second interview, we repeated our assessment of the subjects' alcohol consumption, behavioral and physical impairments, subjective rating, and social and psychological well-being (i.e., a repeat of items 3 through 9 in the preceding list). The major portion of the second interview was devoted to an assessment of the behavioral strategies the participant used to cope with problem drinking during the 3 months since the initial interview. For this purpose, we adapted the self-control interview protocol we had used in our studies of college students coping with weight and smoking problems (as described previously).

SUBJECT CLASSIFICATION

At the second interview we classified subjects into one of three groups based on alcohol consumption and alcohol-related behavioral impairments. Our three groupings were as follows: (1) abstainers ($n = 16$), individuals who reported no alcohol consumption in the month prior to the second interview and a mean rating less than 2.5 on the behavioral impairment subscale; (2) nonproblem drinkers ($n = 16$), subjects with a mean alcohol consumption less than 1.5 ounces of ethanol per day for the prior month and a mean rating less than 2.5 on the behavioral impairment subscale; and (3) problem drinkers ($n = 11$), individuals with a mean alcohol consumption greater than or equal to 1.5 ounces of ethanol per day for the prior month or a mean rating greater than or equal to 2.5 on the behavioral impairment subscale.

SIX-MONTH FOLLOW-UP

Six months after the initial interview, we contacted subjects to schedule them for a third and final interview. Eight subjects (18.6%) declined to participate; three others (7%) could not be located. The remaining 32 subjects (74.4%) appeared for a final interview 6 to 8 months following their initial contact with us. The third interview included a repeat of items 3 through 9 and the self-control protocol, plus an assessment of any additional outside help the participant may have had in coping with problem drinking (e.g., attendance at Alcoholics Anonymous meetings, participation in formal treatment). In addition, a subsample of 17 individuals were asked without forewarning to take alcohol breathalyzer tests.

Results

SAMPLE CHARACTERISTICS

At the time of their initial interview, the men and women who volunteered to participate in this study displayed many aspects of impairment that are typical of problem drinkers and alcohol abusers. The median alcohol consumption per day for the month prior to their initial interview was 4.7 ounces of ethanol (approximately nine drinks per day). The majority (84%) displayed behavioral impairments associated with problem drinking (i.e., a mean rating >2.5 on the behavioral impairment subscale described previously). Many of the subjects (35%) also reported physical symptoms indicative of alcohol abuse (i.e., a mean rating >2.5 on the physical impairment subscale). At the time of the initial interview 56% were employed, and the median individual annual income was $7000. The median number of years of education was 12. There were 30 males and 13 females; 51% were single, 26% were married, and 23% were divorced. The median age was 33 years with 74% of the sample under age 40. Eighteen subjects (42%) reported that they had been treated previously for alcohol problems.

An examination of the background data from the initial interview revealed more similarities than differences among the three groups. There were no statistically significant differences among the groups with respect to demographics, drinking history, pattern or quantity of drinking or degree of behavioral, physical, social or psychological impairments. There were significant differences among groups, however, in the reasons given for their current effort to control their drinking. At the initial interview, subjects classified later as problem drinkers were more likely to cite "professional advice" (e.g., medical or legal) as their primary reason for self-change than were either the abstainers or nonproblem drinkers ($p < .05$). In addition, at the time of the initial interview, the problem drinkers tended to list a fewer number of plans for coping with their problem drinking than did either the abstainers or nonproblem drinkers ($p < .10$, two-tailed).

THREE-MONTH FINDINGS

An examination of the behavioral self-change strategies employed by the subjects at the 3-month interview revealed a number of significant findings. Overall the abstainers and nonproblem drinkers used a greater number of methods than the problem drinkers ($p < .05$). The abstainers made significantly greater use of certain stimulus control procedures than did either of the other groups. For example, they were more likely to make changes in the people with whom they associated so as to avoid former drinking partners, and they were more likely to remove all alcoholic beverages from their home ($p < .05$). The abstainers also reported more frequently the development of alternative behaviors (e.g., hobbies) to take the place of drinking than did the other groups. Finally, the abstainers rated themselves as more successful at self-control than did either problem or nonproblem drinkers.

SIX- TO EIGHT-MONTH FINDINGS

Considerable change was observed in the drinking status of subjects from the second to the third interview. Subjects' drinking status at the third interview is summarized in Table 12.1. Based on their pattern of drinking over the 6–8-month period from the first to final interview, we categorized subjects as successful or unsuccessful in coping with problem drinking. We classified as successful any subject who was abstinent over the entire period or who was not engaged in problem drinking at *both* the second and third assessment points. The unsuccessful category consisted of those subjects

Table 12.1

DRINKING STATUS OF SUBJECTS AT THE 6–8-MONTH INTERVIEW

Status at 6–8-month interview	Classification at 3-month interview					
	Abstinent		Nonproblem drinking		Problem drinking	
	n	%	n	%	n	%
Abstinent	7[a]	43.8	4[a]	25	1	9.1
Nonproblem drinking	0	0	8[a]	50	1	9.1
Problem drinking	2[b]	12.5	3[b]	18.8	6[b]	54.5
Refused to participate	5	31.3	1	6.3	2	18.2
Could not be located	2	12.5	0	0	1	9.1

[a]These individuals were categorized as successful in coping with their problem drinking.
[b]These individuals were categorized as unsuccessful in coping with their problem drinking.

who were engaged in problem drinking at both the 3-month and 6–8 month follow-ups or who had relapsed to problem drinking during the time from the second to third interview. Using these classification criteria, 19 subjects were categorized as successful and 11 as unsuccessful (see Table 12.1).

A comparison of successful and unsuccessful subjects showed that few statistically significant differences were present at the initial interview. Successful subjects had a significantly higher mean rating on the scale of items assessing psychological well-being ($p < .05$), and they were more likely to have some plan for dealing with their problem drinking ($p < .10$).

Table 12.2 summarizes the various self-control strategies employed by successful and unsuccessful subjects in their efforts to cope with problem drinking. The majority of successful subjects removed all alcoholic beverages from their homes, and many changed their daily routine to lessen the chance of problem drinking. The majority of successful individuals also reported they developed some form of alternative behavior to take the place of drinking. For example, several people mentioned taking up a new hobby, some reported using physical exercise, and others regularly used consumption behaviors such as eating particular snack foods or drinking non-alcoholic beverages.

Overall, successful subjects employed a wider array of strategies in their coping efforts than did unsuccessful subjects. Table 12.3 summarized the ratings by successful and unsuccessful subjects of a number of factors associated with their self-control efforts. Although the successful individuals did not rate themselves any higher on frequency or consistency of technique use, they did rate their self-change methods as more practical and effective than

Table 12.2

PERCENTAGE OF SUCCESSFUL AND UNSUCCESSFUL SUBJECTS USING VARIOUS SELF-CHANGE STRATEGIES FOR PROBLEM DRINKING[a]

Strategy	Successful $n = 19$	Unsuccessful $n = 11$
Self-monitoring	21	0
Self-reinforcement	21	9
Stimulus control procedures		
Remove alcohol from home	63	18**
Avoid former drinking partners	42	27
Avoid former drinking places	42	18*
Change daily routine	56	18*
Use of alternative behaviors	74	27**
Cognitive self-instruction	63	55

[a]Significance levels are for χ^2 or Fisher exact probability test comparing the successful group with the unsuccessful group.
*$p < .10$. **$p < .05$.

Table 12.3

RATINGS BY SUCCESSFUL AND UNSUCCESSFUL SUBJECTS OF FACTORS ASSOCIATED WITH THEIR SELF-CHANGE EFFORTS TO CONTROL PROBLEM DRINKING

Descriptor	Successful $n = 19$		Unsuccessful $n = 11$	
	M	SD	M	SD
Number of strategies[a]	4.26	2.10	2.18**	1.19
Frequency of use	3.71	1.32	3.73	1.21
Consistency of use	4.00	1.11	3.63	1.43
Organization of method	3.63	1.72	2.91	1.31
Practicality of method	4.61	0.76	3.55*	1.37
Effectiveness of method	4.56	0.60	2.45***	1.37
Supportiveness of family	4.50	0.83	2.91**	1.16
Supportiveness of friends	4.00	0.97	3.10*	0.83
Degree of improvement	4.83	0.37	3.18**	1.34

[a]Except for number of strategies, all descriptors were rated by the subjects on the following 5-point scale: 1, not at all; 2, not very; 3, somewhat; 4, very; 5, extremely.
*$p < .05$ (two-tailed t test). **$p < .01$. ***$p < .001$.

did unsuccessful subjects. The support and approval of family and friends was rated differently by our two groups of participants. Successful subjects reported that both family members and close friends were more supportive of them in their self-change efforts than did the unsuccessful subjects. Finally, successful subjects rated themselves as having accomplished a greater degree of improvement than did individuals in the unsuccessful group.

At the final interview, each participant was questioned about additional help or treatment they might have received during the period since the initial interview. Among the successful subjects, eight individuals (42%) reported that they had attended at least one Alcoholics Anonymous meeting as compared with only two individuals (18%) among the unsuccessful subjects (see Cross, Sheehan, & Kahn, 1980). The number of individuals who reported at least one counseling session with a mental health professional was not significantly different across groups (37 and 55% for the successful and unsuccessful categories, respectively). Finally, the most common outside source of help cited by almost all subjects in both groups was the film and discussion session presented by the community mental health center. Many subjects returned on several occasions to attend the discussion sessions using their contact with the mental health workers as a source of support.

BREATHALIZER FINDINGS

At the final interviews, a subsample of 17 subjects were asked to take breathalizer tests. Of the 10 individuals from the successful group whom we approached, one declined, and the remaining nine had negative results. All seven subjects from the unsuccessful group who were asked to take breathalizer tests agreed to do so. In four of the seven cases a positive reading indicating the presence of alcohol was obtained.

COMPARISONS ACROSS PROBLEM BEHAVIORS

Table 12.4 summarizes the self-control strategies employed by successful subjects across three problem behaviors, smoking, obesity, and problem drinking. The smoking and obesity data are those reported by our college student sample. For individuals dealing with smoking or obesity, the use of self-reinforcement differentiated successful from unsuccessful subjects. Stimulus control procedures were implemented more often by those who successfully dealt with overeating or problem drinking, whereas the use of some form of planning or problem-solving strategy was employed more frequently by those individuals who successfully managed their smoking or problem drinking compared with those who were unsuccessful.

Table 12.4

PERCENTAGE OF SUCCESSFUL AND UNSUCCESSFUL SUBJECTS USING VARIOUS SELF-CHANGE STRATEGIES FOR SMOKING, OBESITY, AND PROBLEM DRINKING[a]

	Problem behavior		
Techniques	Smoking	Obesity	Problem drinking
Written self-monitoring			
Successful	4	42	21
Unsuccessful	4	33	0
Self-reinforcement			
Successful	72*	58**	21
Unsuccessful	36	17	9
Stimulus control			
Successful	42	58*	63**
Unsuccessful	33	25	18
Planning or problem solving			
Successful	64*	42	84*
Unsuccessful	20	50	45

[a]Significance levels are for χ^2 or Fisher exact probability test comparing successful versus unsuccessful groups of subjects.
*$p < .10$. **$p < .05$.

Discussion

Before discussing the results of our study of self-change and problem drinking, it may be worthwhile to note some of the study's limitations. First, the findings of the investigation are sample-dependent. The data are derived from a small nonrepresentative group, and the information garnered may not be typical of how Americans in general cope with problem drinking (see Cahalan & Room, 1974). Second, our data are based on self-reports; however, we gathered information from problem drinkers prospectively rather than retrospectively. Presumably, the sampling of self-observations closer in time to the occurrence of the target behavior makes the data less subject to distortion and selective recall. Third, alcohol abuse is typically characterized by a high degree of instability over time (see Polich et al., 1981). It may be argued that 6 to 8 months is too brief a period to assess the stability of changes in problem drinking. Finally, as noted previously, unassessed variables may account for some of the differences between successful and unsuccessful individuals.

Acknowledging the limitations of our investigation, what can we say about the self-change efforts of problem drinkers? Examining the data from the initial interviews, there were few baseline differences between those who would later achieve success and those who would not. Yet several clues were evident. *Self*-change appears to be an important factor. Those subjects urged by others, particularly physicians and lawyers, to cut down on their drinking did less well than those individuals whose motivation for change appeared to be more intrinsic. The effectiveness of a self-change effort may be enhanced if commitment to change is truly self-initiated rather than prompted by others (Brehm & McAllister, 1980; Deci, 1980; Kopel & Arkowitz, 1975).

Those individuals who successfully attained abstinence or nonproblem drinking status were more likely to have plans for self-change in mind at the outset of their self-management endeavor (Kirschenbaum, Tomarken, & Ordman, 1982). The particular content of their plans did not seem as important as whether they had some plan for coping versus those who anticipated relying on willpower or who had no plan at all (Goldstein & Marlatt, 1982; Shiffman, 1982, 1984).

Examining the self-change strategies employed by individuals who were successful in coping with problem drinking, we found that successful individuals reported using a greater array of strategies than did unsuccessful ones. The content of those techniques relied heavily on two procedures: (1) stimulus control, particularly the removal of alcoholic beverages from the home; and (2) the development of alternative behaviors to take the place of drinking. Early on in coping with problem drinking it may be crucial to avoid the temptations inherent in high-risk situations (Marlatt & Gordon, 1980). Thus, the removal of all alcohol from the house and changes in one's routine to avoid former drinking partners and places may be pivotal coping responses. Over the longer haul, success seems linked to the development of substitute behaviors to take the place of drinking and provide alternative sources of satisfaction (Marlatt & Parks, 1982). In a long-term study of the natural course of alcoholism, Vaillant (1983) found that the development of substitute activities (e.g., hobbies, work, prayer, eating) was the single highest factor associated with long-term abstinence.

Vaillant (1983) also reported that help from others, whether through the support of Alcoholics Anonymous or the development of a new love relationship was frequently associated with long-term abstinence. In our study of problem drinkers, some parallel findings were apparent. Successful individuals reported a higher degree of support and approval for their self-change efforts from both family and friends than did unsuccessful subjects (see Mermelstein, Lichtenstein, & McIntyre, 1983). In addition, 42% of the successful subjects reported attendance at one or more Alcoholics Anonoymous meetings as compared with only 18% of the unsuccessful ones. It seems clear that successful coping with problem drinking is often accomplished with the help of others.

IMPLICATIONS FOR THEORY AND PRACTICE

In the present studies we sought to determine what factors distinguish individuals who are successful in the self-management of smoking, obesity, and problem drinking from those who are unsuccessful. Our results suggest that success is associated with, and perhaps mediated by, the active use of self-change strategies. Successful individuals use a wider array of behavioral procedures for longer periods of time than do their unsuccessful counterparts. Furthermore, some coping patterns (e.g., the use of self-reinforcement) appear effective among a variety of problems, whereas other self-change strategies seem specifically effective for particular problems.

In our initial study of self-change efforts we examined the way college students dealt with four different problems, namely, smoking, obesity, studying, and dating. In considering the similarities and differences of self-change strategies across problem behaviors, it may be useful to review briefly our key findings regarding studying and dating. For both of these problem areas, successful individuals used a greater number of techniques and more frequently incorporated self-reinforcement into their self-change efforts than did their unsuccessful peers. Indeed, these two significant differences were consistent across all four problem areas we examined in our college sample. Among students dealing with study problems, we also found that successful individuals were more likely to use some form of written self-monitoring to keep track of the number of hours they spent studying or the number of pages they read each day. Students who successfully increased their dating made significantly greater use of a planning or problem-solving strategy and more frequently used stimulus control in the form of going to new places where they would have an increased chance of meeting members of the opposite sex.

In searching for common threads in the methods used by people who are successful in self-change, we found that few procedural similarities were readily apparent across all problem areas. Once noticeable consistency was evident, however; across each problem we examined, the self-change efforts of successful individuals were more comprehensive and included a greater number of techniques than those of unsuccessful persons. Those individuals who used few or no self-change strategies were less likely to be successful (see Shiffman, 1984). A key question arises: Why are those individuals who implement a greater number of self-change strategies more successful, regardless of whether the problem is smoking, obesity, or problem drinking? Are the number of strategies employed the effective ingredient? Or are there characteristics of the successful individuals (e.g., their skills or motivation to implement the strategies) or the situation in which they find themselves (e.g., negative consequences; feedback from others) that determine success or failure in coping. Clearly, these questions deserve further study.

The very early stages of a self-change effort, wherein the individual recognizes the problem and decides upon a plan of self-change, may be particularly important to eventual outcome. The decision-making process is a complex one that appears to involve at least three components: (1) the "cost" of the problem behavior outweighing the short-term benefits; (2) acknowledgment (vs. denial) of a disparity between the problem behavior on the one hand and personal standards or peer-group norms on the other; and (3) the planning of specific actions to change the problem behavior (see Kanfer, 1980; Karoly, 1977; Kirschenbaum et al., 1982).

In our study of college students' self-change efforts, the use of one particular self-control strategy, self-reinforcement, differentiated successful from unsuccessful individuals across four problem behaviors. In both the negative feedback model of self-regulation (Kanfer & Karoly, 1972) and Bandura's (1977) self-efficacy conceptualization, self-evaluation and self-reinforcement are viewed as key processes in self-change. High rates of self-reinforcement may be crucial to sustaining the chain of behaviors necessary for successful self-regulation (Carroll, Yates, & Gray, 1980; Rozensky & Bellack, 1974). In addition, the use of self-reinforcement may engender expectations for positive outcome (i.e., hope) and may be incompatible with the negative affect (e.g., depression) associated with poor performance (Doerfler & Richards, 1981; Mathews, 1977; Rehm, 1977).

The use of self-reinforcement strategies by problem drinkers whether successful or unsuccessful was dramatically less frequent compared with the college sample. Several factors may account for this. Unlike the college students, the problem drinkers were more typical of a clinical population in terms of the nature, history, and severity of their problem behavior. Unlike smoking and obesity, alcohol abuse often has a thoroughly disruptive impact on an individual's social and occupational functioning. The consequences of problem drinking often include high levels of subjective distress (e.g., anxiety and depression) which are typically associated with low self-esteem and low rates of self-reinforcement (Fuchs & Rehm, 1977; Rehm, Fuchs, Roth, Kornblith, & Romano, 1979). Given the overall low rate of self-reinforcement among the problem drinkers, our sample may have been too small to detect any differential effectiveness. Moreover, the college and community samples also differed on a host of demographic variables as well (e.g., age, education, SES). Many of the college students had taken psychology courses in high school as well as in college and were familiar with learning theory. Consequently, they may have been more likely to incorporate psychological strategies in their self-change efforts, while the community sample relied more on homespun commonsense approaches.

Examining the self-change methods across problem behaviors suggests that the specific strategies used by successful individuals vary according to the problem with which they are dealing (see Table 12.4). Overeaters who successfully dealt with weight problems utilized self-reinforcement and stimulus control procedures more often than their unsuccessful counterparts. Subjects who successfully reduced or quit smoking made greater use of self-reinforcement and problem-solving procedures; and for individuals attempting to deal with problem drinking, the use of stimulus control, planning, and the development of substitute activities were significantly more frequent among successful than unsuccessful subjects.

One implication of differences across problems is a caveat suggesting we be wary of developing uniformity myths about the commonalities of self-management problems. The behavior patterns involved in smoking, overeating, and problem drinking appear to be closely related. In each case, the short-term positive effects of the behavior appear to account for resistance to modification despite obvious long-term negative consequences. The results of behavioral treatment for each indicate some short-term success but remarkably similar relapse rates in the long run. Nonetheless, it is likely that future treatment advances will occur only when greater attention is paid to conceptualizing the unique characteristics of each. For example, an appropriate understanding of smoking must account for the interrelationship of psychological and physiological mechanisms (Leventhal & Cleary, 1980; Lichtenstein, 1982). If treatment merely attends to the overlearned operant of the smoking act but not its conditioned physiological concomitants, then the would-be exsmoker continues to experience discomfort in those situations and emotional states that have come to be associated with smoking. As a consequence, the probability of relapse remains high (Pomerleau, 1979). Similarly, the physiological mechanisms (e.g., set point) in obesity may make it very difficult for the obese individual to achieve continued weight loss despite the maintenance of appropriate eating behaviors (Brownell, 1982). As the dieter becomes aware of this exceedingly high cost–benefit ratio, he or she may conclude that a significant weight loss is beyond his or her capability. Furthermore, they may return to previous patterns of overeating precisely at a time when their bodies are physiologically predisposed to rapid regaining of weight (Garrow, 1978).

We must be cautious in suggesting that the methods useful to individuals coping on their own will be effective for people seeking professional help. The more difficult and complicated cases are the ones typically seen by therapists. With this caution in mind let us briefly examine the implications of our findings for treatment. First, rather than plunging immediately into the implementation of self-control actions, an initial phase of decision making and careful planning seems an appropriate way to undertake a self-change effort. Attention should be paid to long-term goals, the seriousness of the commitment to change, and to careful planning of specific actions to be taken. Second, the self-management program should be comprehensive and multifaceted, covering various aspects of the problem. Using a variety of specific techniques increases the probability that one or more of the procedures will be effective. Third, tailoring the program to the particular target problem appears to be more beneficial than offering generalized suggestions for self-management. For smokers, the development of problem-solving methods to cope with the difficulties of maintenance seems important (D'Zurilla & Goldfried, 1971; Richards & Perri, 1978). For people coping with overeating or problem drinking, the use of stimulus control in general, and stimulus narrowing techniques in particular, appears critical for the early stages of self-management (McReynolds et al., 1976; Miller, 1978). High-risk situations (those associated with previous overeating or problem drinking) should probably be avoided until effective coping skills are well developed (see Marlatt & Parks, 1982; Perri, Shapiro, Ludwig, Twentyman, & McAdoo, 1984). Early in a self-management effort is not the time to test the limits of self-control. For problem drinkers, it appears critical that they develop appropriate, and preferably meaningful, substitute activities (i.e., long-term coping behaviors) to occupy their time and provide an alternative source of satisfaction. Fourth, across problem behaviors it seems appropriate to recommend the inclusion of self-reinforcement strategies. Such procedures may aid in sustaining the entire self-control effort and may enhance positive affect and expectations for success. Finally, the development of sources of social support might aid in the efforts to maintain self-control over the long-run (Colletti & Brownell, 1983). Careful consideration should be given to the contribution that may be made by the involvement of spouses, family members, or friends (Mermelstein et al., 1983). The use of self-help groups (e.g., Alcoholics Anonymous, Weight Watchers) may also provide a useful adjunct to the self-change endeavor (Perri, McAdoo, Spevak, & Newlin, 1984; Stuart, 1977).

Deciding what factors are relevant to success in coping with seemingly intractable behaviors, such as smoking, overeating, and problem drinking, is at best an imprecise process. Continued research efforts are needed to explore coping behavior in its natural context. Future studies might employ an entire cohort to avoid the distorting effect of selective sampling. A long term longitudinal perspective may allow a better understanding of the effect of coping strategies over time. Multiple assessment methods (i.e., interviews, self-reports, corroborated collateral information) would offer an opportunity for consensual validation. In addition, controlled experiments might be undertaken to test whether the strategies employed by successful copers offer improvements in the efficiency or effectiveness of standard treatment (see Heffernan & Richards, 1981). Clearly what is called for is further study so we may better understand the nature of the coping process and improve the efficacy of our treatments for substance abuse.

REFERENCES

Armor, D. J., Polich, J. M., & Stambul, H. B. (1978). *Alcoholism and treatment.* New York: Wiley.
Bandura, A. (1977). Self-efficacy: Toward a unifying theory of behavioral change. *Psychological Review, 84,* 191–215.
Bernstein, D. A. (1974, November). *The modification of smoking behavior: Some suggestions for programmed symptom substitution.* Paper presented at the annual meeting of the Association for Advancement of Behavior Therapy, Chicago.
Brehm, S. S., & McAllister, D. A. (1980). Social psychological perspective on the maintenance of therapeutic change. In P. Karoly & J. J. Steffen (Eds.), *Improving the long-term effects of psychotherapy.* New York: Gardner Press.
Bromet, E., Moos, R., Bliss, F., & Wuthmann, C. (1977). Posttreatment functioning of alcoholic patients. *Journal of Consulting and Clinical Psychology, 45,* 829–842.
Brownell, K. D. (1982). Obesity: Understanding and treating a serious, prevalent, and refractory disorder. *Journal of Consulting and Clinical Psychology, 50,* 820–840.
Cahalan, D., & Room, R. (1974). *Problem drinkers among American men.* New Brunswick, NJ: Rutgers Center for Alcohol Studies.
Carroll, L. J., Yates, B. T., & Gray, J. J. (1980). Predicting obesity reduction in behavioral and nonbehavioral therapy from client characteristics: The self-evaluation measure. *Behavior Therapy, 11,* 189–197.
Center for Disease Control & National Cancer Institute. (1976). *Adult use of tobacco—1975* (Contract No. CDC 21-74-520). Washington, DC: Author.
Colletti, G., & Brownell, K. D. (1983). The physical and emotional benefits of social support: Application to obesity, smoking, and alcoholism. In M. Hersen, R. Eisler, & P. M. Miller (Eds.), *Progress in behavior modification.* New York: Academic Press.
Condiotte, M. M., & Lichtenstein, E. (1981). Self-efficacy and relapse in smoking cessation program. *Journal of Consulting and Clinical Psychology, 49,* 648–658.
Cross, D. G., Sheehan, P. W., & Kahn, J. A. (1980). Alternative advice and counsel in psychotherapy. *Journal of Consulting and Clinical Psychology, 48,* 615–625.
Deci, E. L. (1980). *The psychology of self-determination.* Lexington, MA: D. C. Heath.
Doerfler, L. A., & Richards, C. S. (1981). Self-initiated attempts to cope with depression. *Cognitive Therapy and Research, 5,* 367–371.
D'Zurilla, T. J., & Goldfried, M. R. (1971). Problem solving and behavior modification. *Journal of Abnormal Psychology, 78,* 107–126.
Fuchs, C. Z., & Rehm, L. P. (1977). A self-control behavior therapy program for depression. *Journal of Consulting and Clinical Psychology, 45,* 206–215.
Garrow, J. S. (1978). *Energy balance and obesity in man* (2nd ed.). Amsterdam: Elsevier.
Goldstein, S. J., & Marlatt, G. A. (1982, August). *Unaided quitters' strategies for coping with*

temptations to smoke. Paper presented at the meeting of the American Psychological Association, Washington, DC.
Hall, S. M. (1980). Self-management and therapeutic maintenance: Theory and research. In P. Karoly & J. J. Steffen (Eds.), *Improving the long-term effects of psychotherapy.* New York: Gardner Press.
Heffernan, T., & Richards, C. S. (1981). Self-control of study behavior: Identification and evaluation of natural methods. *Journal of Counseling Psychology, 28,* 361–364.
Hunt, W. A., Barnett, L. W., & Branch, L. G. (1971). Relapse rates in addiction programs. *Journal of Clinical Psychology, 27,* 455–459.
Jeffery, R. W., & Wing, R. R. (1983). Recidivism and self-cure of smoking and obesity: Data from population studies. *American Psychologist, 38,* 852.
Kanfer, F. H. (1980). Self-management methods. In F. H. Kanfer & A. P. Goldstein (Eds.), *Helping people change* (2nd ed.). New York: Pergamon.
Kanfer, F. H., & Karoly, P. (1972). Self-control: A behavioristic excursion into the lion's den. *Behavior Therapy, 3,* 398–416.
Karoly, P. (1977). Behavioral self-management in children: Concepts, methods, issues, and directions. In M. Hersen, R. M. Eisler, & P. M. Miller (Eds.), *Progress in behavior modification* (Vol. 5). New York: Academic Press.
Karoly, P., & Kanfer, F. H. (Eds.). (1982). *Self-management and behavior change: From theory to practice.* New York: Pergamon.
Kirschenbaum, D. S., & Tomarken, A. J. (1982). On facing the generalization problem: The study of self-regulatory failure. In P. C. Kendall (Ed.), *Advances in cognitive-behavioral research and therapy* (Vol. 1). New York: Academic Press.
Kirschenbaum, D. S., Tomarken, A. J., & Ordman, A. M. (1982). Specificity of planning and choice applied to adult self-change. *Journal of Personality and Social Psychology, 42,* 576–585.
Kopel, S., & Arkowitz, H. (1975). The role of attribution and self-perception in behavior change: Implications for behavior therapy. *Genetic Psychology Monographs, 92,* 175–212.
Leventhal, H., & Cleary, P. D. (1980). The smoking problem: A review of research and theory in behavioral risk modification. *Psychological Bulletin, 88,* 370–405.
Lichtenstein, E. (1982). The smoking problem: A behavioral perspective. *Journal of Consulting and Clinical Psychology, 50,* 804–819.
Marlatt, G. A., & Gordon, J. R. (1980). Determinants of relapse: Implications for the maintenance of behavior change. In P. O. Davidson & S. M. Davidson (Eds.), *Behavioral medicine: Changing health lifestyles.* New York: Brunner/Mazel.
Marlatt, G. A., & Parks, G. A. (1982). Self-management of addictive disorders. In P. Karoly & F. H. Kanfer (Eds.), *Self-management and behavior change: From theory to practice.* New York: Pergamon.
Mathews, C. O. (1977). A review of behavioral theories of depression and a self-regulation model for depression. *Psychotherapy: Theory, Research, and Practice, 14,* 79–86.
McReynolds, W. T., Lutz, R. N., Paulsen, B. K., & Kohrs, M. B. (1976). Weight loss resulting from two behavior modification procedures with nutritionists as therapists. *Behavior Therapy, 7,* 283–291.
Mermelstein, R., Lichtenstein, E., & McIntyre, K. (1983). Partner support and relapse in smoking-cessation program. *Journal of Consulting and Clinical Psychology, 51,* 465–466.
Miller, W. R. (1978). Behavioral treatment of problem drinkers: A comparative outcome study of three controlled drinking therapies. *Journal of Consulting and Clinical Psychology, 46,* 74–86.

Moos, R. H., Mehren, B., & Moos, B. S. (1978). Evaluation of a Salvation Army alcoholism treatment program. *Journal of Studies on Alcoholism, 39,* 1267–1275.

Perri, M. G., McAdoo, W. G., Spevak, P. A., & Newlin, D. B. (1984). Effect of a multicomponent maintenance program on long-term weight loss. *Journal of Consulting and Clinical Psychology, 52,* 480–481.

Perri, M. G., & Richards, C. S. (1977). An investigation of naturally occurring episodes of self-controlled behaviors. *Journal of Counseling Psychology, 24,* 178–183.

Perri, M. G., Richards, C. S., & Schultheis, K. R. (1977). Behavioral self-control and smoking reduction: A study of self-initiated attempts to reduce smoking. *Behavior Therapy, 8,* 360–365.

Perri, M. G., Shapiro, R. M., Ludwig, W. W., Twentyman, C. T., & McAdoo, W. G. (1984). Maintenance strategies for the treatment of obesity: An evaluation of relapse prevention training and posttreatment contact by mail and telephone. *Journal of Consulting and Clinical Psychology, 52,* 404–413.

Polich, J. M., Armor, D. J., & Braiker, H. B. (1981). *The course of alcoholism.* New York: Wiley.

Pomerleau, O. F. (1979). Commonalities in the treatment and understanding of smoking and other self-management disorders. In N. A. Krasnegor (Ed.), *Behavioral analysis and treatment of substance abuse* (NIDA Research Monograph 25). Washington, DC: U.S. Government Printing Office.

Rehm, L. P. (1977). A self-control model of depression. *Behavior Therapy, 8,* 787–804.

Rehm, L. P., Fuchs, C. Z., Roth, D. M., Kornblith, S. J., & Romano, J. M. (1979). A comparison of self-control and assertion skills treatments of depression. *Behavior Therapy, 10,* 429–442.

Richards, C. S., & Perri, M. G. (1978). Do self-control treatments last? An evaluation of behavioral problem solving and faded counselor contact as treatment maintenance strategies. *Journal of Counseling Psychology, 25,* 367–383.

Rozensky, R. H., & Bellack, A. (1974). Behavior change and individual differences in self-control. *Behaviour Research and Therapy, 12,* 267–268.

Schachter, S. (1982). Recidivism and self-cure of smoking and obesity. *American Psychologist, 37,* 436–444.

Shiffman, S. (1982). Relapse following smoking cessation: A situational analysis. *Journal of Consulting and Clinical Psychology, 50,* 71–86.

Shiffman, S. (1984). Coping with temptations to smoke. *Journal of Consulting and Clinical Psychology, 52,* 261–267.

Stuart, R. B. (1977). Self-help group approach to self-management. In R. B. Stuart (Ed.), *Behavioral self-management: Strategies, techniques and outcomes.* New York: Brunner/Mazel.

Stunkard, A. J., & Penick, S. B. (1979). Behavior modification in the treatment of obesity. *Archives of General Psychiatry, 36,* 801–806.

Thoresen, C. E., & Mahoney, M. J. (1974). *Behavioral self-control.* New York: Holt, Rinehart & Winston.

Vaillant, G. E. (1983). *The natural history of alcoholism: Causes, patterns, and paths to recovery.* Cambridge, MA: Harvard University Press.

Chapter 13

Processes and Stages of Self-Change: Coping and Competence in Smoking Behavior Change*

CARLO C. DICLEMENTE
JAMES O. PROCHASKA

INTRODUCTION

Traditionally cigarette smoking has been accepted and even promoted in our society as a mechanism for coping with stress. Late-night movies illustrate such coping, with images of soldiers smoking before battle and men and women lighting up as the drama increases. More recent advertising emphasizes the pleasure and status aspects of the smoking habit. Although self-image and chemical stimulation are important factors, the stress and smoking link must not be underestimated. The psychological dependence created by using cigarettes to cope with stressful negative psychological states remains a critical element in the process that turns an occasional smoker into a habitual one and creates a habit resistant to modification (Benfari, Eaker, Ockene, & McIntyre, 1982; Leventhal & Cleary, 1980). Stress and coping are connected with the acquisition and cessation of smoking behavior in several ways. In this chapter we employ an integrative, transtheoretical model of change developed from theories of psychotherapy and from research on self-change to examine the connections between stress, coping, and smoking cessation. Presenting data from a 2-year longitudinal study of smokers and exsmokers, we explore coping activity in the self-change of smoking. Finally, we discuss the implications of our analysis for understanding coping and competence in smoking behavior change.

*This work was supported in part by Grant CA 27821 from the National Cancer Institute. The authors thank Lore Feldman and Becky Reyes for their editorial and secretarial assistance.

Model of Stress and Coping

Research on stress has multiplied in recent years. Summarizing almost 30 years of his research in this area, Lazarus (1980) concluded that it is best to view stress as a relational construct and coping as a complex process, not a single act. Stress emerges from an imbalance between the demands on an individual and that individual's assessment of his or her power or resources to meet these demands. If the demands can be met or circumvented, little or no stress is involved. When the person judges that the demands must be addressed, however, and that the resources (internal and external) available to that individual are insufficient to meet the demands, then psychological stress is created. Thus, stress is not a property of either person or situation but results from the transaction or adaptational relationship between them (Lazarus, 1980, p. 36).

Once stress is experienced, a complex operation to evaluate and choose coping options is begun. Two general coping options are available. The first is a problem-solving or instrumental option by which one attempts to change concrete, behavioral aspects of self or situation. The second option, equally important for the maintenance of personal equilibrium, is self-regulation of the emotional stress with more palliative modes of coping (e.g., rationalization, denial, substance use). Despite the emphasis of therapists on problem-solving coping, effective copers can use both types of coping options, and there is often an interaction between the type of problem and the most effective coping options (Cohen & Lazarus, 1973; Lazarus, 1980; Lazarus & Launier, 1978).

As previously stated, cigarette smoking is related to the coping and stress paradigm in several distinct ways. In the initiation and maintenance of the smoking habit, cigarettes represent a palliative coping mechanism that individuals can use to manage distress caused by other life problems. Through a combination of physiological, social, self-image, and habit functions, smoking can increase alertness, reduce feelings of insecurity and perceived threat, enhance relaxation, and help control anxiety, fear, and anger (Gilbert, 1979; Leventhal & Cleary, 1980). For many, smoking becomes a crutch used to regulate emotional responses triggered when stress is created by the demands of work, family, and social relationships.

As often occurs with palliative coping efforts, short-term solutions to problems have consequences that make them problems in their own right. With increasing and overwhelming evidence for links between cigarette smoking and lung cancer, heart disease, and chronic lung disease, smokers experience the demand to rid themselves of this costly and dangerous habit. Again the options available are to change the habit or to use another palliative coping mechanism to reestablish equilibrium between demands and resources. If the problem-solving alternative to modify the smoking habit is chosen, coping becomes involved in yet another way. Successful coping with a firmly embedded though unwanted habit, like cigarette smoking, requires effective action. But the modification of cigarette smoking is a difficult task, and attempts to quit create demands that also produce stress. First, the discomfort created by cessation (for example, craving, loss, and temptation) needs to be addressed. Second, the individual must find other ways to cope with the stress of life problems for which smoking had been an important coping mechanism. Thus, each stage of the initiation and modification of smoking involves psychological stress and coping. This chapter examines the modification of cigarette smoking and coping strategies used at various stages in the process of quitting smoking. Using an integrative, transtheoretical perspective, we explore effective versus ineffective methods for the modification of this troublesome and complex habit.

Cessation Statistics

How successful have individuals been in modifying cigarette smoking? The news is both good and bad. On the positive side, many individuals have successfully coped with cessation. From 1955 to 1978, the percentage of male smokers in the population declined from 52.6 to 37.4% The percentage of female smokers increased during the decade between 1955 and 1966 from 24.5 to 33.7% and then decreased to 30.4% from 1966 to 1978. Former smokers represented 27.4% of the male and 13.9% of the female population in 1978 (U.S. Public Health Service [USPHS], 1979). This represents about 30 million Americans who have quit smoking, with the majority (estimated at 95%) having quit on their own (USPHS, 1979).

On the negative side, 54 million Americans continue to smoke even though most acknowledge health risks and a desire to change. Of current smokers, 70% believe smoking frequently causes disease or death, and the majority (61%) have made at least one serious attempt to stop smoking. Even more surprising is the finding of a survey (Center for Disease Control, 1976) that only 25% of the smokers who have never tried to quit report they would not consider quitting. Thus, many smokers have successfully become former smokers. In addition, most current smokers have judged their habit sufficiently threatening to consider or make an attempt to modify their smoking. Since these attempts have failed for many current smokers, they need to find some other way to reduce the threat created by the habit they now perceive as dangerous but are unable to change. Many smokers have turned to organized treatment programs for help, but results from these programs have been disappointing for most. When treated persons are compared to no-treatment controls and adequate follow-up assessment is done, the success rate seldom exceeds 15 to 25% (Russell, 1977). No uniquely effective intervention method has been discovered, and the critical elements of successful smoking cessation treatment remain largely unknown (Schwartz, 1977; Russell, 1977).

Smoking Cessation and Self-Change

An alternative approach to treatment programs and clinical trials research is to examine the effective elements of self-change. Self-change is the method of most successful quitters and represents the backdrop for any therapy-assisted change. Individuals who present themselves to treatment programs can be viewed as self-change failures. Thus, self-change is the more comprehensive arena for studying coping than studies focusing solely on treatment. Understanding the process of self-change can yield important information about coping in the natural environment and can offer leads for improved interventions.

Initial explorations of the self-change phenomenon for smoking cessation yielded interesting but tentative findings. Self-changers did not appear to differ from treated subjects on smoking history variables (DiClemente & Prochaska, 1982) or on smoking habits, locus of control, and Jackson Personality Inventory measures (Pederson & Lefcoe, 1976). Shiffman (1982) found that both self-changers and treated smokers used similar coping strategies during a relapse crisis, with the successful copers using a combination of cognitive and behavioral coping responses. Perri, Richards, and Schultheis (1977), on the other hand, found with college students that successful self-changers used self-reinforcement procedures significantly more than those who relapsed (see Perri, Chapter 12, this volume). Analyzing retrospective self-reports, Hecht (1978) reported the self-changers tended to quit abruptly without a gradual tapering off (cold-turkey), used few smoking cessation aids or smoking substitutes, and employed distraction or stimulus control methods to prevent relapse. Baer, Foreyt, and Wright (1972) found that the self-changers used multiple quitting techniques which they could not group in any systematic way.

Previous research reveals no comprehensive, integrated picture of the elements or characteristics needed for successful self-change of smoking behavior. We believe that a comprehensive theory of smoking behavior change based on prospective studies would increase our knowledge about the processes that contribute to successful smoking cessation. In our research we addressed these issues by using an eclectic, transtheoretical model of change and a longitudinal research strategy to examine self-changers' coping efforts in the service of smoking cessation.

The Transtheoretical Model

The transtheoretical model was developed both from a systematic examination of psychotherapy theories and research (Prochaska, 1979; Prochaska & DiClemente, 1982) and from initial explorations of smoking cessation (DiClemente & Prochaska, 1982; Prochaska & DiClemente, 1983). From this perspective, change is a function of an individual's coping activity as defined by the processes of change applied in distinct stages of the cessation process.[1] Since smoking is a complex behavior with biological, psychological, and environmental determinants, modification of smoking must be a complex and multidimensional process. The transtheoretical model attempts to isolate and describe basic elements in the complex process of behavior change.

The original version of the model emerged from a comparative analysis of 18 leading therapy systems (Prochaska, 1979) which concluded that the therapy process can be represented as a combination of the nonspecific variables of expectation, attention, and relationship, and the more specific variables called the *processes of change*. These processes represent basic change principles which therapy systems have considered responsible for behavioral change. Originally, five processes were identified which were differentiated along an experiential–environmental dimension that categorizes each change process as operating either at the level of the individual's experience or at the level of his or her environment. The five basic processes were (1) consciousness raising, (2) catharsis, (3) commitment, (4) conditional stimuli, and (5) contingency management. Prior to beginning our longitudinal study, we decided to add a process called cognitive restructuring and to include the helping relationship as a measured process rather than a separate element in the model (Table 13.1).

Considering each level of each basic process as a change process activity, we could now identify 13 separate processes of change that can be examined in any intentional change. These processes represent a wide variety of activities and include the various types of activity relevant to smoking cessation. The processes represent information processing (education, feedback,

---

[1]The transtheoretical model has been expanded to include a construct called the levels of change which attempts to delineate five basic areas of problems: (1) symptom–situational; (2) maladaptive cognitions; (3) interpersonal conflicts; (4) family–system conflicts; and (5) intrapersonal conflicts. The levels were not included in the present research but are an integral component in the latest version of the model (Prochaska & DiClemente, 1984).

Table 13.1

THEORETICAL PROCESSES OF CHANGE AT EXPERIENTIAL (A) AND ENVIRONMENTAL (B) LEVELS

Consciousness raising A. Feedback B. Education	Cognitive restructuring A. Self-reevaluation B. Environment reevaluation
Catharsis A. Corrective emotional experience B. Dramatic relief	Conditioned stimuli A. Counterconditioning B. Stimulus control
Choosing–commitment A. Self-liberation B. Social liberation	Contingency control A. Self-management B. Social management
Helping Relationship	

self-reevaluation); affective elements (corrective emotional experiences, dramatic relief); environmental considerations (social liberation, environmental reevaluation); personal commitment (self-liberation); behavioral strategies (counterconditioning, stimulus control, self-management, social management); and social support (helping relationships). These are basic activities and experiences recognized as coping options available to the smoker seeking to change. Since coping is viewed as a combination of activities, the change processes offer a means of conceptualizing and operationalizing the coping action involved in the modification of smoking behavior.

How individuals utilize these processes is hypothesized to relate to their smoking status, modification efforts, and cessation success. Successful coping to change the habit would involve a coordinated use of these processes. Thus, the processes could be viewed as the repertoire of coping activity available to the smoker. Deficits in coping could result from three different problems with this repertoire. First, an individual could be ignorant of one or more of the processes, which would represent a deficit in knowledge of coping activities and yield a restricted range of options. Second, an individual could be inept at employing one or more of the processes and, hence, would have a deficit in specific coping abilities. Finally, an individual who had both adequate knowledge and ability might inappropriately use the processes at different points in the modification attempt. The deficit here would involve a misapplication of coping mechanisms. The processes of change offer a measurable and comprehensive approach to examining coping activity and coping competence for smoking cessation.

Addictive Behavior Change as a Stage Phenomenon

Change, especially change of an addictive behavior, is not an all-or-nothing phenomenon (Prochaska & DiClemente, 1982). Competence in coping also includes the issue of timing; appropriate action includes not only what to do but also when to do it. Appropriate timing of intervention has been addressed in the therapy literature but has not been as prevalent in discussions of coping and smoking cessation. Recently, much attention has been focused on relapse and maintenance in addictive behavior change (Marlatt & Gordon, 1980; Shiffman, 1982). But maintenance is not the only critical stage in the process.

Our early studies with the transtheoretical model indicated that the processes of change could not be explored accurately without establishing the point in the cycle of change at which these processes were applied (DiClemente & Prochaska, 1982). In a pilot study of 67 smokers who had recently quit, subjects were asked to rate the importance of each process of change in their stopping smoking. Their general response was that it depended on what stage in the course of change we were talking about. In their own language they referred to a series of stages that they had passed through during their course of change. These subjects seemed able to differentiate four stages of change: (1) thinking about stopping smoking, (2) becoming determined to stop, (3) actively modifying their habits and environment, and (4) maintaining their new habit of not smoking. Using this information and including a stage prior to the individual thinking about stopping, we hypothesized five basic stages of change: precontemplation, contemplation, decision-making, active change, and maintenance. We posited that in order to modify an addictive behavior successfully, an individual must negotiate all these stages successfully. Our work assumes that the process of addictive behavior change is often more a cyclical process than a straight line (Prochaska & DiClemente, 1983), a revolving door familiar to treatment personnel of alcoholism, drug abuse, weight reduction, and smoking clinics. Entry into the cycle and exits from the cycle are numerous and can occur quite rapidly. From this perspective, relapse is a frequent and expected element of the cycle. Most smokers make two or three unsuccessful attempts before successfully achieving maintenance.

Since smoking modification appeared to be a stage phenomenon and the processes of change were understood best in the context of the stages of change, we decided to study the self-change of smoking using the stages and processes perspective of the transtheoretical model. We solicited groups of persons who would represent different stages in the process of change. Subjects were followed over a 2-year period to see how they coped with smoking cessation and whether any of the processes of change or other variables we measured would predict movement toward successful cessation.

METHOD

Subjects

Subjects for this longitudinal study were 872 smokers and exsmokers from Rhode Island and Texas who responded to media articles and advertisements. Restrictions on subject selection were that all subjects be currently smoking or have smoked sometime in the past, not be involved in any formal treatment program, and be willing to complete our follow-up questionnaires and participate in periodic interviews for 2 years. Of the total sample 54.7% were married, 23.0% single, 16.5% divorced, and 5.8% separated or widowed; 18.3% had completed high school or less, 41.4% had attended college, 17.8% had bachelor degrees, and 19.3% had some postgraduate education or a graduate degree. Approximately half of the subjects had annual incomes of less than $15,000, while 8% earned more than $30,000 a year.

All subjects were assigned to one of five groups according to their status in the stages-of-change cycle with regard to smoking. Subjects were classified along several dimensions. First, they were divided by smoking status, that is, whether or not they were currently smoking. If they were not smoking, they were subdivided by length of time they maintained nonsmoking. Since 6 months seems to be a cutoff point when the relapse survival curve levels off (Hunt & Bespalec, 1974), *recent quitters* (RQ) were defined as those who quit smoking within the past 6 months, and *long-term quitters* (LTQ) as those who quit more than 6 months prior to filling out the questionnaire. Current smokers were divided along two dimensions. If they had made a quit attempt in the past year but had been unsuccessful in remaining abstinent, they were classified as *relapsers* (R). Smokers who had not made a quit attempt in the past year were further classified by their response to the question, "Are you seriously considering quitting in the next year?" Smokers who responded affirmatively were classified as *contemplators* (C). Smokers who responded negatively were classified as *immotives* (I; unmotivated to change). Although these classifications are somewhat arbitrary, they were considered a theoretically appropriate way to subdivide the population for our study. Thus, subjects were assigned to groups as follows:

1. Long-term quitters (LTQ): These 247 subjects had quit smoking on their own and been abstinent for at least 6 months. Mean duration of

abstinence was 5.9 years and the average age at initiation of smoking was 17.2 years. There were 133 women and 114 men; their mean age was 44 years.

2. Recent quitters (RQ): These 134 subjects had quit smoking on their own within 6 months before entering the study. Mean duration of quitting was 2.2 months; mean age at beginning of smoking was 16.6 years. There were 80 women and 54 men in this group; their mean age was 35 years.

3. Contemplators (C): These 187 subjects had been smoking regularly for the past year with no attempt to quit but were thinking seriously about quitting smoking during the next year. Mean age was 40 years for these 113 women and 74 men. They had begun smoking at a mean age of 17.4 years.

4. Immotives (I): These 108 subjects smoked regularly and reported that they had no intention of quitting during the next year. In this group were 74 women and 34 men whose mean age was 38 years; their average age at initiation was 16.3 years.

5. Relapsers (R): These 196 subjects were smoking currently but had made an attempt to quit smoking in the past year that had lasted at least 24 hours. Mean age was 36 for 129 women and 67 men. Their mean age for beginning smoking was 17.3 years.

The nonsmokers in our study (RQ and LTQ) had smoked for an average of 18 years and during their heaviest smoking period had averaged 32 cigarettes per day. The quitters reported three to four previous attempts to quit and that prior to their most recent attempt to quit, they smoked on the average 28 cigarettes per day. The smokers in our study (I, C, and R) reported smoking about 34 cigarettes per day during their heaviest smoking period, and currently they were smoking approximately 27 cigarettes per day. Smokers also reported an average of three to four previous attempts to quit.

Measures

Assessments relevant to the present study included a Processes of Change Questionnaire (POCQ) which examined the 13 different processes of change related to smoking cessation. Five items measuring each process were rated by subjects on 5-point Likert scales to indicate frequency of occurrence (1, not at all; 5, very often). A smoking history questionnaire examined subjects' current and past smoking patterns and their quitting history. A decisional balance scale based on Janis and Mann's (1977) view of decision making was constructed to measure the perceived importance of the pros (10 items) and cons (10 items) of smoking, each rated on 5-point

Likert scales (Velicer, DiClemente, Prochaska, & Brandenberg, 1985). A self-efficacy measure was also used that consisted of 31 situations that subjects rated for temptation to smoke and their confidence (efficacy) that they would be able to abstain from smoking; temptation and efficacy were rated on separate 5-point scales (DiClemente, Prochaska, & Gibertini, 1985).

Procedure

Subjects were asked to complete an extensive questionnaire and were interviewed at the initiation of the study and at 5–6-month intervals over the next 2 years. Saliva samples were taken to increase the validity of self-report via the bogus pipeline phenomenon (Jones & Sigall, 1971). Subjects received $8 for completing the questionnaire and interview, and they were eligible for 1 of 10 bonus prizes of $50 to $500 to be given every 6 months. Approximately 85% of the original subjects completed the first follow-up. Approximately 70% of the original sample completed questionnaires at the final follow-up.

Processes of Change as Coping Activity

In the theoretical model 13 separate processes of change were assumed to be involved in smoking cessation. The first question we asked of our data was whether our subjects' ratings of the items in the questionnaire would yield separate factors or components that agreed with the theoretical model. A principal components analysis revealed 10 separate processes of change (Table 13.2; see Appendix) each measured by four items in a statistically well-defined and highly reliable manner (Prochaska, DiClemente, Velicer, & Zwick, 1981). Although not all of the processes emerged as separate components, what did happen was very interesting. Feedback and education items combined to form one component which we called Consciousness Raising. Items from the process called corrective emotional experience (emotional upset about smoking) combined with the more cognitive self-reevaluation items to form a component we called Self-reevaluation which included both emotional and cognitive aspects. Subjects did not distinguish between self and social reinforcement items and these combined to form the Reinforcement Management component. The other seven processes emerged as theoretically defined. Thus in their ratings the subjects distinguished 10 separate processes of change. The emergence of these 10 processes, cross-validated in both the Texas and Rhode Island samples, clearly demonstrates the multidimensional nature of smoking cessation coping activity and supports the Processes of Change theory.

Table 13.2

SAMPLE ITEMS AND ALPHA COEFFICIENTS FOR THE 10 PROCESSES OF CHANGE

Process	Alpha[a]	Sample item
Consciousness raising	.88	I look for information related to smoking.
Self-liberation	.89	I tell myself I am able to quit smoking if I want to.
Social liberation	.81	I notice that public places have sections set aside for nonsmokers.
Self-reevaluation	.87	My depending on cigarettes makes me feel disappointed in myself.
Environmental reevaluation	.88	I stop to think that smoking is polluting the environment.
Counterconditioning	.88	I do something else instead of smoking when I need to relax.
Stimulus control	.81	I remove things from my place of work that remind me of smoking.
Reinforcement management	.78	I am rewarded by others if I don't smoke.
Dramatic relief	.91	Warnings about health hazards of smoking move me emotionally.
Helping relationships	.84	I have someone who listens when I need to talk about my smoking.

[a] Alpha coefficients are calculated for each process using the four items that were chosen from the principal component analysis to represent each process. The complete set of items appear in the Appendix.

RESULTS

Coping Strategies in Different Stages of Change

Table 13.3 presents T scores for the 10 change processes, separately for each of the five groups (as classified above) representing the different stages of behavior change.[2] A MANOVA comparing all change process scores across groups was significant, $F(1, 40) = 11.19$, $p < .001$, indicating that there were significant differences on these processes for the different groups of subjects. Separate ANOVAs compared the groups' scores on each of the processes of change. F values and probability levels shown in Table 13.3 demonstrate that there were significant differences between the groups on each of the processes. Newman-Keuls comparisons were then used to deter-

[2] Original scores on each process of change were transformed so that they had a mean of 50 and a standard deviation of 10 (T score). This enabled us to compare processes across groups with a similar measurement system. A higher score indicates more of the named changed process.

Table 13.3
T SCORES OF THE 10 PROCESSES OF CHANGE FOR THE FIVE STAGES OF CHANGE GROUPS

Process	Group					F
	Immotives	Contemplators	Recent quitters	Long-term quitters	Relapsers	
Consciousness raising	45.3	53.1	48.5	48.6	52.2	15.46***
Self-liberation	41.3	48.2	55.9	51.3	50.8	40.82***
Social liberation	51.0	51.4	46.6	50.3	50.1	5.19**
Self-reevaluation	41.5	52.4	51.9	47.8	53.7	38.13***
Environmental reevaluation	44.3	50.8	48.9	51.4	51.4	12.22**
Counterconditioning	42.6	49.3	52.6	52.0	50.4	21.48***
Stimulus control	45.6	48.3	52.5	51.3	50.7	10.28***
Reinforcement management	45.2	49.4	53.8	49.6	51.0	12.41***
Dramatic relief	46.6	51.3	49.0	50.6	51.1	7.21***
Helping relationship	48.5	49.6	51.4	49.2	51.2	2.50*

*$p < .05$. **$p < .001$. ***$p < .0001$.

mine which groups differed on each process. Table 13.4 presents the results of these comparisons with significant differences at the $p < .05$ level. For example, on Consciousness Raising, immotives had the lowest scores and were significantly different from all the other groups; recent quitters and long-term quitters had the next highest scores and differed significantly from the contemplators and relapsers who had the highest mean scores on this process. Differences among groups on the self-efficacy and decisional balance measures are shown in Table 13.5. Significant differences among groups were found in ANOVA comparisons on temptation, confidence, and decisional balance (pros and cons of smoking).

The five groups differ on all of these basic measures with differences not simply attributable to smoker versus nonsmoker distinctions. Among smokers, immotives differ from the other groups of contemplators and relapsers on some measures. Recent and long-term quitters also are not alike on all measures. We explore these differences by examining each stage separately in light of the issues for coping, stress, and smoking modification.

Immotives are individuals who are not motivated to change at present and, thus, they represent the precontemplation stage. They deal with the known dangers of smoking not by considering any action to change the habit but by resigning themselves to continued smoking. In more classical terms they resist change of the detrimental habit and accomodate themselves to smoking by using denial or rationalization (more palliative coping

Table 13.4
GROUP COMPARISONS ON EACH OF THE PROCESSES OF CHANGE

Process	Comparisons of stage-of-change groups[a] Low score → high score
Consciousness raising	I < RQ, LTQ < R, C
Self-liberation	I < C < R, LTQ < RQ
Social liberation	RQ < I, C, LTQ, R
Self-reevaluation	I < LTQ < C, RQ, R
Environmental reevaluation	I < C, RQ, LTQ, R
Counterconditioning	I < C, R < RQ, LTQ
Stimulus control	I < C, R < RQ, LTQ
Reinforcement management	I < C, LTQ, R < RQ
Helping relationship	I, C, LTQ, < R, RQ

[a]I, immotives; C, contemplators; RQ, recent quitters; LTQ, long-term quitters; R, relapsers. < means a significant difference was found at the $p < .05$ level, using Newman-Keuls tests.

mechanisms). These persons' high scores on temptations to smoke and on the perceived importance of positive aspects of smoking (pros) are comparable to those of their smoking counterparts (contemplators and relapsers), but the immotives have the lowest scores of all groups on the perceived negative consequences of smoking and confidence to abstain from smoking.

Table 13.5
GROUP COMPARISONS OF SELF-EFFICACY AND DECISIONAL BALANCE SCORES

Measure	Group					F
	Immotives	Contemplators	Recent quitters	Long-term quitters	Relapsers	
			SELF-EFFICACY			
Temptation						
Mean (SD)	129.6 (20)	119.9 (17)	93.4 (27)	67.3 (32)	118.4 (17)	175**
Confidence						
Mean (SD)	60.5 (23)	61.1 (20)	116.9 (28)	131.1 (32)	68.8 (23)	253**
			DECISIONAL BALANCE			
Pros						
Mean (SD)	26.8 (8)	27.1 (6)	22.5 (7)	18.1 (8)	26.9 (6)	
T score	53	53	48	45	53	35.9*
Cons						
Mean (SD)	26.6 (7)	32.7 (7)	28.8 (8)	23.8 (10)	32.1 (8)	
T score	46	53	50	47	52	24.9*

*$p < .01$. **$p < .001$.

With low self-efficacy and a low estimate of the cons of smoking, they have little motivation to change and are resigned or resolved to smoke. It follows logically that they do little to change the habit. Immotives had significantly lower scores on 8 of the 10 processes of change and clearly do not use problem-solving methods of coping. Only on Social Liberation and Helping Relationship processes are they at all like the other subjects, but they may interpret support they experience in helping relationships as support to smoke rather than support for quitting. As is true for other addictive behaviors, empathy often becomes enabling for individuals who do not want to quit. The fact that their Social Liberation score is as high as that of most other subjects is interesting. Immotives are aware of society's sanctions and the options it offers not to smoke in certain areas. However, they choose not to do anything about it, as their low Self-liberation scores reflect.

Contemplators, on the other hand, are seriously considering taking action at some time in the immediate future. They admit to high levels of temptation and low self-efficacy. They rank both the positive and negative consequences of smoking equally high. This equilibrium in decisional balance may indicate that they are poised for action but still value highly the positive aspects of smoking. While the immotive person experiences little stress from the dangers of smoking and takes little action, the contemplator feels some distress about smoking, at least enough to make him or her consider cessation. Contemplators seem most invested in Consciousness Raising. They are open to information about smoking and quitting. They may be waiting to receive that particular bit of information that will tip their decisional balance toward action. Contemplators also seem engaged in Self-reevaluation in their efforts to move toward action. Environmental considerations, information, and involvement in some emotional and cognitive considerations about the impact of smoking in their lives seem to be the coping activities most used by the contemplators. They are not engaged in the action of behavioral change processes but seem to be generating the information and affective responses that could lead to a decision to take action.

Recent Quitters recently began the process of actively changing or coping with the smoking habit. They have stopped smoking but still have rather high levels of temptation. They rate cons of smoking as more important than the pros, and they have a respectable level of self-efficacy about not smoking. RQs used Self-liberation, the behavioral processes of Reinforcement Management, Counterconditioning, and Stimulus Control as well as Helping Relationships to modify their smoking behavior. RQs seem engaged in self-control and self-management processes. These findings support the retrospective findings of Perri et al. (1977) and Hecht (1978). The period of active change following cessation is a time of increased behavioral activity and commitment to the modification process. Compared to other groups they are quite active copers and appear to be more like the LTQs than any of the smoking groups, except for the relapsers (discussed below).

Long-Term Quitters have negotiated the early stages of change successfully and continue to advance in their efforts to free themselves of the habit. They see the cons of smoking as higher than the pros but give both relatively low scores, which means that smoking may become a nonissue for them. This is reasonable because their temptations are low and their efficacy to abstain from smoking is quite high. Yet they continue to engage in Counterconditioning and Stimulus Control in their efforts to maintain control over their now-dormant smoking habit. Since they have been quit for an extensive period of time, LTQs do not receive as much social support or reinforcement from the environment as the RQs. Yet they continue to engage in some internal (Counterconditioning) and external (Stimulus Control) management processes to avoid relapse. This is, perhaps, the same type of activity engaged in by Shiffman's (1982) subjects who avoided relapse. Unexpected and infrequent situations and temptations to smoke seem to be most dangerous for them. Some level of vigilance is appropriate to insure their continued abstinence.

Relapsers, as a group, at first posed serious problems for us in making sense of the data. They are smokers who made a recent attempt to quit but failed and began smoking again. In their evaluation of the pros and cons of smoking, their temptation levels, and their confidence about not smoking, they resemble the contemplators. In their use of the processes of change they are, however, similar to the contemplators in some respects and to the recent quitters and long-term quitters in others. These individuals seem to continue to engage in Consciousness Raising and Self-liberation as well as Self-reevaluation and Social liberation processes. They also seem to be using Stimulus Control and some Reinforcement Management procedures. Although this seems confusing at first, the data become clearer if we consider the task of the relapsers. Most relapsers are coping with the habit as well as their failure to change successfully; the majority are considering another attempt to change. Approximately 85% of our subjects who made an unsuccessful attempt to quit between the initial assessment and the first follow-up were seriously thinking about quitting again. Thus, in preparing for this, they continue to seek information and to reevaluate themselves and their environment. They have made a recent attempt to quit. They also seem to be keeping active with self-liberation and behavioral processes in attempts to control the habit either in order to keep from relapsing completely to their former level of smoking or to insure that the next attempt will be more successful. On cognitive measures of self-efficacy and decisional balance they seem to be unsure of themselves, realistically in light of the recent failure, but they continue to engage in processes that may help them deal with the relapse experience and future attempts to quit.

Relationship between Stages and Processes of Smoking Cessation

Understanding intra- and intergroup relationships among the processes and stages was only a first step in our research. We really wanted to know whether or not our variables could predict change over time. To test this hypothesis, a predictor set consisting of initial measures of the 10 change processes, smoking temptation, efficacy, and decisional balance was used to predict which subjects would remain in the same groups over time and which would change groups, with data from the 6-month follow-up employed as the criterion. A discriminant function analysis was performed for four of the five initial groups to predict changes in group membership at follow-up. (No analysis was performed for the long-term quitters as very few had changed group membership.) All classification rates were based on an assumption of equal prior probabilities of group membership.

The stepwise discriminant function analysis of the initial contemplators who at the first follow-up became recent quitters ($n = 12$), relapsers ($n = 45$), immotives ($n = 18$), or remained contemplators ($n = 97$) found significant relationships for 7 of the 14 predictor variables. Two functions were statistically significant, accounting for 50.12 and 38.37% of the variance, respectively. The first function (Wilks's lambda = .76, $p = .0002$) distinguished recent quitters from immotives and was defined largely by the cons of smoking (standardized discriminant function coefficient of .84), and Self-reevaluation (.42), Consciousness Raising ($-.48$) and temptation ($-.45$). Contemplators who were recent quitters by follow-up, compared with those who became immotives, tended to have higher cons and Self-reevaluation scores as well as lower Consciousness Raising and temptation levels. The second function (Wilks's lambda = .916, $p = .03$) distinguished between recent quitters and persons who remained contemplators. Although this was not well defined, recent quitters tended to score high in self-efficacy (.51) and cons of smoking (.39), and low in Self-reevaluation ($-.61$), smoking pros ($-.57$), and Social Liberation ($-.44$). Our overall classification accuracy was 46% with most misclassifications occurring in the relapse group. A subsequent classification analysis that excluded this group demonstrated a 77% correct classification.

A stepwise discriminant analysis was also conducted to distinguish among participants who were recent quitters at the initial assessment who were classified 6 months later as long-term quitters ($n = 53$), relapsers ($n =$

36), and those who remained recent quitters ($n = 19$). Only one discriminant function was significant (Wilks's lambda = .86, $p = .01$). This dimension distinguished primarily between subjects who became relapsers and those who became long-term quitters. Only 3 of the 14 predictor variables of the initial assessment contributed significantly to the discrimination among groups: Self-reevaluation ($-.80$), self-efficacy (.63), and Helping Relationships (.45). The continuing recent quitters were about equidistant from relapsers and long-term quitters; continuing recent quitters are an anomalous group that includes people who have relapsed and quit again as well as those who entered the study during the initial assessment period and had only a 4-month follow-up period. In general subjects who relapsed had higher Self-reevaluation and lower self-efficacy and Helping Relationship scores than did those who become long-term quitters. The successful maintainers were less preoccupied with smoking and changing their view of themselves as a smoker, and they were more confident they could abstain. Perhaps, some of this greater confidence was due to relying on or experiencing more support from helping relationships. Classification accuracy based on this function was 51% across all groups, considerably higher than the random classification accuracy of 33%.

Two discriminant functions were significant for distinguishing initial relapsers who became recent quitters ($n = 18$), immotives (n = 26), and contemplators (n = 41), or who remained relapsers ($n = 132$). The first significant function (Wilks's lambda =.77, $p < .0001$) accounted for more than 60% of the variance and distinguished between immotives and relapsers. The function included Social Liberation (.69), Helping Relationship ($-.59$), Self-liberation ($-.47$), Dramatic Relief (.37), Stimulus Control (.35), Counterconditioning ($-.22$), and Self-reevaluation ($-.21$). In general subjects who became immotives had higher Social Liberation, Dramatic Relief, and Stimulus Control scores and lower Helping Relationships, Self-liberation, Counterconditioning, and Self-reevaluation scores than did those who became recent quitters or remained relapsers. The second dimension had a Wilks's lambda of .90 ($p = .04$), accounted for 32% of the variance and distinguished between relapsers and those who became recenter quitters and contemplators. This dimension was clearly defined by Self-reevaluation (.97), Dramatic Relief ($-.84$), Helping Relationship ($-.50$), Counterconditioning ($-.45$), Stimulus Control (.33), Self-liberation (.31), and Social Liberation (.28). Relapsers who gave up tended to have higher Dramatic Relief, Helping Relationship and Counterconditioning scores and lower Self-reevaluation, Stimulus Control, Self-liberation, and Social Liberation scores than did relapsers who became recent quitters or contemplators. Classification accuracy was 43.8%.

Immotives were investigated with a discriminant analysis conducted on two groups: those who remained immotives ($n = 73$) and those who changed status in any way ($n = 31$). The discriminant function had a Wilks's lambda of .78, $p = .0004$ and retained six variables: Social Liberation (−.58), Self-reevaluation (.71), Reinforcement Management (.33), the cons (.64) and pros (−.67) of smoking and temptation (.25). Immotives who changed tended to have high Self-reevaluation and con scores, and low Social Liberation and pro scores. Classification accuracy was 74% on predicted group memberships.

Summary of Discriminant Analysis Results

Summarizing these functions is complex. Because of the small numbers of subjects in some of the predicted groups, caution should be used in interpreting results and replication is needed for any substantial generalization. But the initial results are intriguing. All the predictor variables are activities or cognitive self-evaluations of current attitudes which can change over time and which in fact differ between groups in the various stages of change.

What variables seem to be associated with movement through the stages of change? First, of the 14 predictor variables entered, 13 contributed to at least one function. The variables in each function varied greatly, however, in their contribution to prediction. Second, variables had both positive and negative loadings, so that doing something was not simply better than doing nothing. Using some processes was detrimental in some cases. For example, recent quitters who relapsed tended to have higher Self-reevaluation scores and lower scores on Helping Relationship. Continuing the Self-reevaluation process with little social support seems to be a sign of a short-term quitter who is overly preoccupied with smoking and headed for relapse. Too much self-reevaluation for quitting subjects is predictive of relapse. However, low levels of self-reevaluation in the immotives and relapsers lead to more entrenched smoking, while greater self-reevaluation tends to predict progress for contemplators. Although self-reevaluation seems to be a critical activity, optimal use depends on the stage of change.

Other processes, particularly Dramatic Relief and Social Liberation, tended to predict no change or regression. More frequent use of these processes seemed predictive for contemplators remaining contemplators, immotives remaining immotives, and relapsers becoming immotives. Being very aware of dramatic messages about the dangers of smoking and society's efforts to control smoking and promote nonsmoking may either mobilize smokers' rebelliousness about being told what to do or indicate that these smokers are so preoccupied with smoking that taking action is quite problematic. An alternative explanation could be that excessive use of some processes, especially those oriented to environmental events, may indicate individuals who are so focused outward that they lack the inner directedness necessary for change. Previous retrospective research lends some support for this alternative explanation. Relapsers reported relying more on environmental processes of change, whereas long-term quitters reported relying more on experiential processes (Prochaska, Crimi, Lapsanski, Martel, & Reid, 1982).

The cognitive variables showed more consistency for prediction. Higher levels of self-efficacy contribute to active change and maintenance. Lower levels of temptation are related to movement toward action possibly because they are associated with a greater sense of control over smoking and with more self-reevaluation of the habit. Decisional-balance variables also are related to movement toward change. Greater perceived importance of the cons and less emphasis on the pros is predictive of quitting smoking. The lower the importance of cons compared to pros, the more likely is the smoker to resist change.

CONCLUSIONS

If we combine the cross-sectional and longitudinal studies, a preliminary picture of the self-change of smoking begins to emerge. The results from our study are consistent in most respects with the theoretical model of self-change described previously. Smoking modification certainly seems best characterized as a cycle of change, with smokers entering and exiting the cycle at different points in time and spending varying lengths of time in the separate stages. Immotives appear quite attached to their habit and almost committed not to engage in any cognitive or behavioral activity to modify their smoking. Approximately 60% of the immotives who entered our study had not taken action to quit smoking for the 2-year duration of the study. If immotives are going to become active, they need to engage in self-reevaluation to become upset enough with themselves and the habit to reverse their evaluations of the importance of the positive and negative aspects of smoking. Contemplators, on the other hand, seem already engaged in consciousness raising and other cognitive activities. The dilemma for them is whether and when to take action. Individuals in contemplation often spend a long time in contemplation. Contemplators in our study spent an average of at least 12 months contemplating before they took action. It is not clear what moves the contemplators to action. However, some increase in the perceived negative consequences of smoking and some growing sense of efficacy to control their smoking seems an important outcome of their cognitive change process activity that would lead to action.

Cessation and the initial stages of maintenance seem marked by a lessening of cognitive preoccupation about smoking, a growing sense of self-efficacy and social support to help deal with the distress of quitting and the distressing emotions (anger, anxiety, frustration, depression) that trigger relapse. The role of social support in maintenance seems to be an important one that is receiving more attention recently (Mermelstein, Lichtenstein, & McIntyre, 1983). The view that smoking cessation is a very individualistic endeavor dependent on the amount of willpower employed needs to be reexamined. Relapse, on the other hand, may not be as negative a consequence as has been thought. Relapsers are a very active group, often moving back into contemplating another serious attempt to quit and continuing modification activities. At the end of our 2-year study, 27% of the relapsers who entered the study were not smoking, whereas only 11.5% of the contemplators were not smoking. Although the amount and type of activity they engage in is confusing, they seem to need to continue to reevaluate themselves as smokers and possibly reevaluate the relapse experience in order to make a more successful attempt to modify their smoking.

Implications for Treatment and Research

The processes of change offer a valuable means of identifying and isolating active coping mechanisms. The processes investigated are activities engaged in by the individual instead of the more stable personality or dispositional characteristics which traditionally have been examined in smoking cessation research (Spielberger & Jacobs, 1982). Our research shows little indication to date that the processes are influenced by personality characteristics. The 10 processes had very low and nonsignificant correlations with measures of persistence (Jackson Personality Inventory), social desirability, assertiveness, and internal–external locus of control. Coping activity for smoking cessation appears rather independent of these trait measures, at least in these correlational analyses.

At the level of theory, the processes of change offer an organized and integrated view of coping. In previous retrospective research, activities related to the successful self-change of smoking behavior have been identified, but no coherent patterns for the activities have been found that would direct intervention efforts. The processes we describe represent a middle level of abstraction between theory and isolated techniques or activities. As such, they have the potential for examining modification of smoking behavior systematically. In addition, the processes offer a meaningful way of organizing coping activities for smoking cessation as well as for other problems, such as alcoholism, sexual dysfunction, psychic distress, and personality disorders (Prochaska & DiClemente, 1984).

Finally, the processes of change represent coping activities open to intervention and capable of being brought under self-control. If our research continues to demonstrate relationships between the processes and movement through the stages of change, intervention should become more process- and stage-specific. Programs could be designed to influence certain processes of change and program impact could be measured by increases or decreases in the level of certain processes as well as by self-evaluations of temptation, efficacy, and decision-making variables. Program evaluation should include an assessment of these variables along with the more traditional outcome measures.

Change as a Stage Phenomenon

Previous divisions of the population into smokers and nonsmokers appear too simplistic. Since change is a stage phenomenon, the stages of change offer a valuable way of subdividing the population of smokers and nonsmokers in relation to amounts and types of coping activity—a unique view of smoking modification. Our initial analyses indicated that the stages require and involve different coping skills and strategies. Moreover, outcome of smoking modification involves more than substance-abuse behavior change. Using only smoking cessation as an outcome measure can make the move from precontemplation to maintenance seem more like magic than intentional change. Researchers and clinicians need a sophisticated and differentiated view. The stages of change provide both a differentiation and a series of intermediate steps that are accurate and useful for tracking the process of smoking modification. For example, we need to distinguish whether media smoking control programs are designed to address immotives or contemplators. Action may be an appropriate outcome for the latter but not the former. A program that can get immotives to seriously consider quitting or to engage in self-reevaluation is a success even if it does not get anyone to quit smoking for the present.

The stages are not only sequential but also cyclical in nature. The frustrating quality of addictive behavior change is integrally related to this cyclical nature. Once through the cycle is not enough for most individuals struggling with smoking cessation. Relapsers in our study seemed to be a confused and confusing group, continuing action and contemplation processes while they resumed the smoking habit. Most want to make another attempt to change. Relapse is a significant event; how individuals handle it affects their future modification efforts. Smoking cessation programs that offer a view of cessation that includes few negative consequences or repercussions may contribute to a distorted view of smoking modification among smokers. Instead of seeing relapse as failure, smoking control programs should help relapsers consolidate and direct their coping efforts toward reentry into the cycle of change. Perhaps smoking control programs could help relapsers explore what they learned from their recent attempt to quit smoking and focus on the positive aspects of their attempt (see Marlatt & Gordon, 1980). Programs could develop more adaptive self-statements about the relapse experience that reinforce the effort, not the failure. If we can see the relapsers as quitters in the making, we could promote their self-efficacy and reduce their view of being hopelessly locked into the smoking habit.

Further Research

The stages and processes of change help us to understand and to investigate further the critical questions in the process of smoking cessation. Although the initial findings of our research are exciting, our conclusions are tentative. Replication and more research are needed. Our results raise many more questions than they answer. How can immotives become more invested and active in contemplating change? What are the critical processes that initiate contemplation? Is there an optimal time period or amount of coping activity for individuals in contemplation, active change, or maintenance? What processes influence decisonal balance considerations? What are the differences between chronic contemplators and those who take precipitous action or those who take responsible, successful action? What coping activity increases self-efficacy? What keeps active changers preoccupied with self-reevaluation? Are there ways to capitalize on relapse as a learning experience? Continued research with longitudinal data will address these questions. We believe that the assessment instruments and the concepts of the transtheoretical approach can enrich clinical and research endeavors to understand coping and competence in the modification of smoking and other addictive substance use problems.

APPENDIX: PROCESSES OF CHANGE QUESTIONNAIRE

Consciousness Raising
  1. I recall articles dealing with the problems of quitting smoking.
  2. I think about information from articles and advertisements on how to stop smoking.
  3. I recall information people have personally given me on how to stop smoking.
  4. I recall information people have personally given me on the benefits of quitting smoking.

Self-liberation
  1. I tell myself I can choose to smoke or not.
  2. I tell myself I am able to quit smoking if I want to.

3. I tell myself that if I try hard enough I can keep from smoking.
   4. I make commitments not to smoke.

Social liberation
   1. I see "No Smoking" signs in public buildings.
   2. I notice that public places have sections set aside for smokers.
   3. I find society changing in ways that make it easier for the nonsmoker.
   4. I notice that nonsmokers are asserting their rights.

Self-reevaluation
   1. My dependency on cigarettes makes me feel disappointed in myself.
   2. I get upset when I think about my smoking.
   3. I reassess the fact that being content with myself includes changing the smoking habit.
   4. I consciously struggle with the issue that smoking contradicts my view of myself as a caring and responsible person.

Environmental reevaluation
   1. I am considering the belief that people quitting smoking will help to improve the world.
   2. I stop to think that smoking is polluting the environment.
   3. I consider the view that smoking can be harmful to the environment.
   4. I am considering the idea that the world around me would be a better place without my smoking.

Counterconditioning
   1. Instead of smoking I engage in some physical activity.
   2. I find that doing other things with my hands is a good substitute for smoking.
   3. When I am tempted to smoke, I think about something else.
   4. I do something else instead of smoking when I need to relax or deal with tension.

Stimulus control
   1. I remove things from my home that remind me of smoking.
   2. I keep things around my place of work that remind me not to smoke.
   3. I remove things from my place of work that remind me of smoking.
   4. I put things around my home that remind me not to smoke.

Reinforcement management
   1. I can expect to be rewarded by other if I don't smoke.
   2. I am rewarded by others if I don't smoke.
   3. Other people in my daily life try to make me feel good when I don't smoke.
   4. I reward myself when I don't smoke.

Dramatic relief
   1. Warnings about health hazards of smoking move me emotionally.
   2. Dramatic portrayals of the evils of smoking effect me emotionally.
   3. I react emotionally to warnings about smoking cigarettes.
   4. Remembering studies about illnesses caused by smoking upsets me.

Helping relationships
   1. I can be open with at least one special person about my experience with smoking.
   2. I have someone who listens when I need to talk about my smoking.
   3. I have someone whom I can count on when I'm having problems with smoking.
   4. Special people in my life accept me the same whether I smoke or not.

REFERENCES

Baer, P. E., Foreyt, J. P., & Wright, S. (1977). Self-directed termination of excessive cigarette use among untreated smokers. *Journal of Behavior Therapy and Experimental Psychiatry, 8,* 71–74.

Benfari, R. C., Eaker, E. D., Ockene, J., & McIntyre, K. M. (1982). Hyperstress and outcomes in a long-term smoking intervention program. *Psychosomatic Medicine, 44*(3), 227–235.

Center for Disease Control & National Cancer Institute. (1976). *Adult Use of Tobacco—1975.* (Contract No. CDC 21-74-520). Washington, DC: Author.

Cohen, F., & Lazarus, R. S. (1973). Active coping processes, coping dispositions, and recovery from surgery. *Psychosomatic Medicine, 35,* 375–389.

DiClemente, C. C., & Prochaska, J. O. (1982). Self-change and therapy change of smoking behavior: A comparison of processes of change in cessation and maintenance. *Addictive Behaviors, 7,* 133–144.

DiClemente, C. C., Prochaska, J. O., & Gibertini, M. (1985). Self-efficacy and the stages of change of smoking cessation. *Cognitive Therapy and Research, 9,* 181–200.

Gilbert, D. G. (1979). Paradoxical tranquilizing and emotion-reducing effects of nicotine. *Psychological Bulletin, 86,* 643–661.

Hecht, E. (1978). *A retrospective study of successful quitters.* Paper presented at the annual meeting of the American Psychological Association, Toronto, Canada.

Hunt, W. A., & Bespalec, D. A. (1974). An evaluation of current methods of modifying smoking behavior. *Journal of Clinical Psychology, 30,* 431–438.

Janis, I. L., & Mann, L. (1977). *Decision-making. A psychological analysis of conflict, choice and commitment.* New York: The Free Press.

Jones, E. E., & Sigall, H. (1971). The bogus pipeline: A new paradigm for measuring affect and attitude. *Psychological Bulletin, 76,* 349–364.

Lando, H. A. (1977). Successful treatment of smokers with a broad-spectrum behavioral approach. *Journal of Consulting and Clinical Psychology, 45,* 361–366.

Lazarus, R. S. (1980). The stress and coping paradigm. In L. A. Bond & J. C. Rosen (Eds.), *Competence and coping during adulthood.* Hanover, NH: University Press of New England.

Lazarus, R. S., and Launier, R. (1978). Stress-related transactions between person and environment. In L. Pervin & M. Lewis (Eds.), *Perspective in interactional psychology.* New York: Plenum Press.

Leventhal, H., & Cleary, P. D. (1980). The smoking problem: A review of the research and theory in behavioral risk modification. *Psychological Bulletin, 88,* 370–405.

Marlatt, G. A., & Gordon, J. R. (1980). Determinants of relapse: Implications for the maintenance of behavior change. In P. O. Davidson & S. M. Davidson (Eds.), *Behavioral medicine: Changing health lifestyles.* New York: Brunner/Mazel.

Mermelstein, R., Lichenstein, E., & McIntyre, K. (1983). Partner support and relapse in smoking-cessation programs. *Journal of Consulting and Clinical Psychology, 51,* 465–466.

Pederson, L. L., & Lefcoe, N. M. (1976). A psychological and behavioral comparison of ex-smokers and smokers. *Journal of Chronic Diseases, 29,* 431–434.

Perri, M. G., Richards, S. C., & Schulteis, K. R. (1977). Behavioral self-control and smoking reduction: A study of self-initiated attempts to reduce smoking. *Behavior Therapy, 8,* 360–365.

Prochaska, J. O. (1979). *Systems of psychotherapy: A transtheoretical analysis.* Homewood, IL: Dorsey Press.

Prochaska, J. O., Crimi, P., Lapsanski, D., Martel, L., & Reid, P. (1982). Self-change processes, self-efficacy and self-concept in relapse and maintenance of cessation of smoking. *Pschological Reports, 51*, 983–990.

Prochaska, J. O., & DiClemente, C. C. (1982). Transtheoretical therapy: Toward a more integrative model of change. *Psychotherapy: Theory, Research and Practice, 19*, 276–288.

Prochaska, J. O., & DiClemente, C. C. (1983). Stages processes of self-change of smoking: Toward an integrative model of change. *Journal of Consulting and Clinical Psychology, 51*, 390–395.

Prochaska, J. O., & DiClemente, C. C. (1984). *The transtheoretical approach: Crossing traditional boundaries of therapy.* Homewood, IL: Dow Jones-Irwin.

Prochaska, J. O., DiClemente, C. C., Velicer, W. F., & Zwick, W. (1981). *Measuring the processes of change.* Paper presented at the annual meeting of the International Council of Psychologists, Los Angeles.

Russell, M. A. H. (1977). Smoking problems: An overview. In M. E. Jarvik, J. W. Cullen, E. R. Gritz, T. M. Vogt, & L. J. West (Eds), *Research on smoking behavior* (DHEW Publication No. ADM 78-581). Washington, DC: U.S. Government Printing Office.

Schwartz, J. L. (1977). Smoking cures: Ways to kick an unhealthy habit. In M. E. Jarvik, J. W. Cullen, E. R. Gritz, T. M. Vogt, & L. J. West (Eds.), *Research in smoking behavior* (DHEW Publication No. ADM 78-581). Washington, DC: U.S. Government Printing Office.

Shiffman, S. (1982). Relapse following smoking cessation: a situational analysis. *Journal of Consulting and Clinical Psychology, 50*, 71–86.

Spielberger, C. D., & Jacobs, G. A. (1982). Personality and smoking behavior. *Journal of Personality Assessment, 46*, 396–403.

U.S. Public Health Service. *Smoking and health: A report of the Surgeon General* (DHEW Publication No. PHS 79-50066). Washington, DC: U.S. Government Office.

Velicer, W. F., DiClemente, C. C., Prochaska, J. O., & Brandenberg, N. (1985). A decisional balance measure for assessing and predicting smoking status. *Journal of Personality and Social Psychology, 48*, 1279–1289.

Chapter 14

Common Processes of Self-Change in Smoking, Weight Control, and Psychological Distress*

JAMES O. PROCHASKA
CARLO C. DICLEMENTE

INTRODUCTION

The search for common processes of change has been called the most important new trend in psychotherapy (Bergin, 1982). The search for such processes is occurring not only with clients who seek professional treatment but also for persons attempting to cope on their own with problems such as substance abuse. In Chapter (13) we discuss the processes and stages of change for individuals coping with addictions to cigarette smoking. The processes of change offer a means of identifying active coping mechanisms. The stages of change enable us to subdivide the population of smokers and nonsmokers in a manner meaningful for intervention or for self-change. However, an important question remains unanswered. Are these processes unique to smoking cessation or are they relevant in the assessment of coping activities for other problems related to substance abuse? Using the same constructs of the stages and processes of change, in this chapter we investigate and compare the self-change processes used by individuals to cope with such problems as smoking, weight control, and psychological distress.

Psychological distress (e.g., depression and anxiety) is important not only as a problem in its own right but also because it contributes to problems such as substance abuse. Emotional distress is one of the most common reasons why people relapse in their attempts to overcome addictive behaviors (Chaney and Roszell, Chapter 11, this volume; DiClemente, Gordon, &

*This research was supported by Grant CA 27821 from the National Cancer Institute.

Gibertini, 1983; DiClemente, Prochaska, & Gibertini, 1985; Marlatt & Gordon, 1980). When people are emotionally distressed they are tempted to turn to alcohol, food, tobacco, or other substances in order to cope with their distress. If more effective processes can be identified for coping with distress, substance abuse could be reduced by relieving the need to rely on drugs as a means of coping with distress.

The search for common processes of change for distress, smoking, and weight control addresses the critical theoretical question of whether there are general principles of coping or whether all coping is specific to a particular problem. If a common set of change processes can be discovered for coping with diverse problems such as psychological distress, overeating, and smoking, we will be closer to developing a comprehensive model of change. A more comprehensive model of change could lead to more integrative intervention programs for helping people to overcome a variety of addictive behaviors and to cope with problems of emotional distress that may contribute to substance abuse.

How individuals cope with distress has important implications for initiation and cessation of substance abuse. Before examining the common processes of change in smoking, weight control, and distress, we discuss the extent and nature of psychological distress. Many people do not realize how prevalent is the problem of psychological distress. Research shows, however, that over the course of their lives, most adults are troubled by at least one episode of psychological distress, characterized by anxiety, depression, cognitive impairment, and a sense of helplessness. Even among a sample of college students, 80% had already been troubled by psychological distress (Prochaska, Norcross, & Hambrecht, 1983). A national survey of 405 psychotherapists found that 83% had themselves been troubled by at least one episode of psychological distress. At the same time, almost all of the psychotherapists (98%) treat clients for such distress (Prochaska & Norcross, 1982). In a household survey in Philadelphia, 20% of the women were found to have suffered from such high distress during the past year that psychiatric interviewers agreed that they were in need of psychiatric treatment (Mellinger et al., 1983).

The manifestations of psychological distress—depression, anxiety, cognitive impairment, and sense of hopelessness—are strikingly similar to what other investigators have called the Nonspecific Psychological Distress Syndrome (Dohrenwend, Shrout, Egri, & Mendelsohn, 1980; Vernon & Roberts, 1981), Emotional Distress Syndrome (President's Commission on Mental Health, 1978), demoralization (Frank, 1973), and the MMPI 2-7-0 profile (Marks & Seeman, 1963; Strupp & Bloxom, 1975; Strupp & Hadley, 1979). The President's Commission on Mental Health (1978) estimated that at any given time as much as 25% of the adult population suffers intensely from the Emotional Distress Syndrome. National household surveys have indicated that more than a third of the women (34%) and nearly a fifth of the men (19%) were troubled by psychological distress in the past 12 months. This general condition has been observed in a wide variety of circumstances, such as in combat soldiers (Eastwood, 1975) and psychiatric patients (Dohrenwend & Crandell, 1970; Langner, 1962). As "the fever of mental health," psychological distress is a prevalent, highly recognizable, and debilitating clinical syndrome.

It is important to note that the majority of distressed individuals do not take their problems to mental health professionals. Rather, they overcome their difficulties through their own adaptive capabilities or with the help of friends, clergy, or others who may provide counsel (Cowen, 1982; Strupp, 1982; Veroff, Kulka, & Douvan, 1981). Although approximately 15% of the U.S. population may have diagnosable mental disorders each year, only 3% of the population receives specialized mental health services in any given year (Regier, Goldberg, & Taube, 1978). In summarizing 11 epidemiological studies, the Presidents Commission on Mental Health (1978) concluded that "only about one-fourth of those suffering from a clinically significant disorder have been in treatment" (p. 16). Similarly, while psychological distress is one of the most common reasons for seeking psychotherapy, the vast majority of distressed individuals struggle with their problems on their own (Mellinger, Balter, Manheimer, Cisin, & Parry, 1978). At present, too little is known about the processes involved in reducing psychological distress among persons who change without benefit of mental health services.

As indicated by Wills and Shiffman in Chapter 1, psychoactive medications, and other substances with physiological or psychological properties, represent one important mechanism used to cope with psychic distress. The National Household Survey provided important data on the use of psychotherapeutic medications as means of coping with psychological distress (Mellinger et al., 1978). This survey indicated that of women with high distress, 34% used psychotherapeutic medications at least once in the past year and 14% used such medications regularly (daily or almost daily for 2 months or longer). Of the highly distressed men, 23% had used a psychotherapeutic medication (tranquilizer, daytime sedative, or antidepressant) at least once and 10% used it regularly. Unfortunately, this investigation raised rather than answered the question of what most people do to overcome high distress, if only a small minority use medication regularly.

A survey of a representative sample of adults in Oakland, California, went beyond the use of just psychotherapeutic medications for coping with psychological problems (Uhlenhuth, Balter, & Lipman, 1978). Of the women who sought help for a target problem, 67% visited a physician, 8% visited a therapist, 10% increased alcohol intake, and 63% talked with family or friends. The survey also found that the vast majority of subjects reported habitual consumption of nonmedicinals, such as snacks, alcohol, coffee, tea, and tobacco, whether they reported a target problem or not. The majority of subjects also reported using over-the-counter drugs during the past year. Although this study reflects the range of procedures that people use for coping with problems, it had several deficiencies. First, it did not specifically connect psychological distress or any other target problem with specific methods of change. Second, it did not specifically relate the habitual consumption of nonmedicinals and nonprescription drugs to attempts to overcome target problems.

Substance use in the community does not necessarily parallel what pharmacological research would recommend. Alcohol use for self-treatment of depression and anxiety appears more common than use of antidepressants or antianxiety agents, even though misuse of alcohol can produce depression and anxiety (Aneshensel & Huba, 1983; Uhlenhuth et al., 1978). Of distressed subjects classified as major depressives on the basis of the Hopkins Symptom Checklist, only 11% used an antidepressant while 23% used antianxiety agents (Uhlenhuth & Balter, 1981). Of distressed subjects classified as agoraphobic with panic only 7% used an antidepressant, the substance that research recommends, while most took antianxiety drugs (Uhlenhuth & Balter, 1981). Of psychically distressed subjects in the community, most cope with their anxiety and/or depression without the use of prescription psychotherapeutic medications (Uhlenhuth & Balter, 1981). Again the question arises as to what processes the majority of people use to cope with anxiety and depression.

Not only is little known about how people overcome psychological distress on their own, little is known about how people change other common problems like smoking and overeating. The change processes used to cope with these three common problems were investigated within the 2-year longitudinal study of self-change approaches to smoking that we report in Chapter 13. Smokers and exsmokers were assessed every 6 months on change processes and other variables related to quitting smoking. Because many of these subjects had reported problems with weight control and psychological distress, they provided a convenient sample for studying the processes of change that were common to three different problem behaviors.

METHOD

Measures

In Chapter 13 we identify the change processes that people used during different stages of changing smoking behavior. These 10 processes serve here as the foundation for a comparative analysis of people coping with three different problems. In addition to the 10 processes already described (DiClemente & Prochaska, Chapter 13, this volume), two additional processes were tested: Substance Use and Interpersonal Systems Control. These two processes had been identified in research on how psychotherapists treat themselves and their clients for psychological distress (Prochaska & Norcross, 1983). Substance use involves the intake of physical substances in order to help overcome a problem. Substances include alcohol, tranquilizers, and other medications, as well as diet aids, substances containing nicotine, caffeine, or other stimulants. The Substance Use scale does not differentiate between professionally prescribed medications and self-medication. Interpersonal systems control involves either avoiding people who contribute to a problem or seeking out people who decrease the problem. This process involves the selective use of social stimulus controls to assist in self-control. In contrast, Helping Relationships rely on empathy and openess rather than social pressure to facilitate change.

Our research, then, was designed to assess which of the following 12 processes of change were common across three different problems:

1. Consciousness raising
2. Self-liberation
3. Social liberation
4. Self-reevaluation
5. Environmental reevaluation
6. Counterconditioning
7. Stimulus control
8. Reinforcement management
9. Dramatic relief
10. Helping relationship
11. Substance use
12. Interpersonal systems control

Separate forms of the Processes of Change Questionnaires (POCQ) were created for smoking, weight control, and psychological distress. The three questionnaires were included at different points in our 2-year longitudinal study of self-change. All subjects received all of the questionnaires. The expanded version of the smoking questionnaire reported here was given at the 12-month follow-up, the weight control questionnaire at 18 months, and psychological distress questionnaire at 24 months. Each of the three questionnaires had 50 items that were worded consistently across the three problem areas. Each of the questionnaires used 5-point Likert scales ranging from never to repeatedly using the process. These 50 items represented the 12 change processes and were used in the statistical analyses. Table 14.1

Table 14.1
SAMPLE ITEMS FOR THE CHANGE PROCESSES FOR SMOKING, OVEREATING, AND DISTRESS

Process	Smoking item	Overeating item	Distress item
Consciousness raising	I look for information related to smoking.	I look for information related to overeating.	I look for information related to distress.
Self-liberation	I tell myself I can choose to smoke or not.	I tell myself I can choose to overeat or not.	I tell myself I can choose to change or not.
Reinforcement management	I am rewarded by others if I don't smoke.	I am rewarded by others if I don't overeat.	I am rewarded by others if I don't get distressed.
Helping relationship	I can be open with at least one special person about my smoking experiences.	I can be open with at least one special person about my overeating experiences.	I can be open with at least one special person about my experience with distress.
Dramatic relief	Dramatic portrayals about smoking effect me emotionally.	Dramatic portrayals about overeating effect me emotionally.	Dramatic portrayals about distress effect me emotionally.
Stimulus control	I put things around my home that remind me not to smoke.	I put things around my home that remind me not to overeat.	I put things around my home that remind me not to get distressed.
Social liberation	I find society changing in ways that make it easier for the nonsmoker.	I find society changing in ways that make it more supportive of thin people.	I find society changing in ways that make it easier for distressed people.
Environmental reevaluation	I am considering the view my friends and family deserve a smoke-free environment in which to live.	I am considering the view my friends and family deserve a healthier environment in which to live.	I am considering the view my friends and family deserve a distress-free environment in which to live.
Substance use	I use stop smoking aids.	I use diet aids to lose weight.	I take some type of drugs for my distress.
Counterconditioning	Instead of smoking, I engage in some physical activity.	Instead of eating I engage in some physical activity.	I engage in some physical activity when I am beginning to feel distressed.
Interpersonal systems control	I leave places where people are smoking.	I leave places where people are eating a lot.	I leave places where other people are adding to my distress.

provides sample items for each of the processes across the three problem areas.

Subjects

Participants in this research were from Rhode Island and Texas. In response to newspaper articles and advertisements, they had volunteered to participate in a study on self-change in smoking. This was basically a smoking cessation sample, and the questionnaires on weight control and psychological distress were included as secondary foci of the study. Subjects were informed that the study would last 2 years and that they would be asked to complete a questionnaire every 6 months. In return they would be paid $4 for completing each questionnaire and would be eligible to win 1 of 10 bonus prizes ranging from $25 to $250.

The sample was composed predominantly of middle-aged and middle-class adults, 62% of whom were women. The mean age was 40 years and the median was 37 years. Approximately half of the participants reported income of less than $15,000 and 8% earned more than $30,000. Of the total sample, 62% were married, 27% single, 15.5% divorced, and 5.8% separated or widowed. Nearly one-fifth (19.3%) of the sample completed high school or less, 41.7% had attended some college classes, 17.8% had college degrees, and 19.7% had some postgraduate education. The sample was primarily Caucasian (93.4%). Subjects were assigned to groups based on self-reports of problem behaviors.

At the 12-month assessment there were 605 subjects who currently or in the past had been regular smokers. At the 18-month assessment there were 420 subjects who currently or in the past had been at least 10% over their ideal weight. At the 24-month assessment there were 320 subjects who currently or in the past had had at least one episode of psychological distress.

Principal Component Analysis

Each time a change processes questionnaire was administered for a particular problem, subjects were asked a series of questions about the problem and their attitudes toward changing the problem. Individuals who were smoking, were 10% overweight, or reported high psychological distress were considered to have a problem in the respective area. Subjects then were asked if they were actively involved in trying to change these problems (action), were seriously considering change in the next year (contemplation), or had successfully coped with these problems and were attempting to maintain these changes (maintenance). Subjects' responses to these questions were used to classify them as to their stage of change: Action, Contemplation, or Maintenance. Subjects reported taking action about weight ($n = 195$) and distress ($n = 129$) problems more frequently than with smoking ($n = 24$). On the other hand, more smokers were contemplating change ($n = 156$) than were overweight individuals ($n = 10$). Because of printing errors on the distress questionnaire, we were not able to assess the contemplation and maintenance stages for psychic distress. Only individuals in the action stage for distress were used in this analysis.

A principal component analysis (PCA) for the Smoking POCQ was completed on the 605 subjects who had been regular smokers. Similarly, the PCA for the Weight Control POCQ was performed on the 420 subjects who reported past or present weight control problems. The three PCAs were used to identify the component structure within each problem area and to assess consistency in structures across problem areas.

Smoking Processes of Change. The PCA yielded 11 components accounting for 67.2% of the total variance. On the 50 items, 49 items loaded .40 or greater on a single component. Internal consistency (alpha) coefficients were calculated for each change process defined by this solution. Coefficient alphas ranged from .77 to .88. These analyses indicated that there were 11 processes of change used in changing smoking behavior. Of the original 12 processes that were hypothesized, only self-reevaluation did not emerge as a separate process. Self-reevaluation items loaded with self-liberation items. Although these processes emerged as separate components in our original analysis reported in Chapter 13, they are interrelated both theoretically and statistically. In the original analysis self-liberation and self-reevaluation were significantly correlated ($r = .50$).

Weight Processes of Change. The PCA on the weight control items yielded 11 components accounting for 70.2% of the total variance. Again 45 of the 50 items loaded .40 or greater on a single component. Coefficient alphas ranged from .68 to .96 with a mean alpha of .81. These analyses indicated that there were 11 change processes used in weight control. Of the original 12 processes only self-reevaluation did not emerge as a separate process. Again self-reevaluation items loaded with self-liberation items.

Distress Processes of Change. The PCA of the distress items also yielded 11 components accounting for 68.9% of the total variance. Once again 49 of the 50 items loaded .40 or greater on a single component. Coefficient alphas ranged from .67 to .91 with a mean alpha of .87. Of the original 12 processes hypothesized, only self-reevaluation failed to emerge as a separate process. The self-reevaluation items loaded primarily with environmental reevaluation items.

14. COMMON PROCESSES OF SELF-CHANGE

In summary, within each of the three problem areas a stable component structure emerged, as evidenced by well-defined components displaying high internal consistency and accounting for a substantial percentage of the total variance. Across three diverse problem areas the clear identification of common processes of change emerged. Of the 12 theoretical change processes, 11 were replicable across problems with smoking, weight, and psychological distress. The fact that very similar structures emerged for each of the processes of change instruments suggests that our basic model of change processes has considerable generalizability across a diversity of problems.

RESULTS

The results of this research were used to address the following questions. Do individuals use particular processes of change more often when coping with weight problems than with smoking or distress? Are there similarities across problem areas with respect to how frequently each process of change is used? Do people in comparable stages of change for each problem use the processes of change with the same frequency even though they are coping with different problems? Do the same people use particular processes of change more frequently when they are coping with different problems?

In order to address these questions we limited our comparisons only to change processes defined by the same items across distress. That is, six of the change processes (Consciousness Raising, Self-liberation, Reinforcement Management, Helping Relationship, Dramatic Relief, and Stimulus Control) are measured by the same items with only the name of the problem (smoking, weight, or distress) being different. With five of the processes, however, some of the items themselves had to be different. With substance use, for example, comparable items for each problem are: "I use stop-smoking aids," "I take diet aids to lose weight," and "I take some type of drugs for my distress." To compare processes directly that are defined by different items would confound item differences and problem differences. When comparing processes across different problem areas, then, we make direct statistical comparisons only of the six change processes that are defined by the same items. Table 14.1 presents a sample item for each of the change processes across each of the three target problems.

Table 14.2 shows how frequently different groups of people in the Action stage for each problem used the 11 change processes for coping with smoking, weight control, and psychological distress. Table 14.2 divides the processes into the six with comparable items and the five with somewhat different items. The rank order for the means of the six comparable processes is also presented in Table 14.2. Informal comparisons indicate that the ranks

Table 14.2
USE OF CHANGE PROCESSES FOR SMOKING, WEIGHT, AND DISTRESS BY PEOPLE IN ACTION[a]

Process	Smoking (S) n = 24			Weight (W) n = 195			Distress (D) n = 129			Significant group differences	Group differences
	M	SD	Rank	M	SD	Rank	M	SD	Rank	F(2, 345)	
Consciousness raising	2.2	1.0	3	3.2	0.9	3	2.8	0.8	3	18.1**	W > D > S
Self-liberation	3.3	1.2	2	3.8	0.8	1	3.2	0.9	2	17.0**	W > S, D
Reinforcement management	2.1	1.0	5	2.1	1.0	5	2.3	1.1	5	1.1	None
Helping relationship	3.5	1.3	1	3.4	0.9	2	3.7	1.0	1	3.4*	D > W
Dramatic relief	2.2	0.9	4	2.3	1.0	4	2.4	1.0	4	0.5	None
Stimulus control	1.8	1.0	6	2.0	0.8	6	1.8	0.9	6	4.1*	W > D
Social liberation	2.8	1.0		3.8	0.9		2.2	0.9			
Environmental reevaluation	2.2	1.0		1.5	0.6		2.2	0.9			
Substance use	1.4	0.7		1.5	1.0		1.5	1.0			
Counterconditioning	2.7	1.0		2.9	0.8		3.1	0.8			
Interpersonal systems control	1.8	0.9		2.2	1.0		3.5	0.8			

[a] The 5-point Likert scales assessed frequency of use from 1, never, to 5, repeatedly. The first six items are comparable processes.
*$p < .01$. **$p < .001$.

for the six processes are nearly identical across the three problem areas. Thus, subjects seem to use a similar pattern of processes in taking action with these problem areas.

People in the Contemplation and Maintenance stages were clearly identified only for smoking and weight. Results for the Contemplation and Maintenance stages yielded a similar pattern of change process use. For subjects in the Contemplation stage, the rank orders for how frequently they used each of six processes were identical to the ranks for the people in the Action stage. For smokers in the Maintenance stage, rank orders were nearly identical except that Helping Relationships and Self-liberation were tied for first. Ranks for weight control subjects in Maintenance were also very similar, with Self-liberation and Helping Relationships tied for first and Reinforcement Management ranked sixth rather than fifth.

Similarity in the rank ordering of six different processes of change across three different problem areas and three different stages of change, implies remarkable similarity in the frequency with which people apply these processes of change to different problems. For our subjects there appears a general pattern of coping activity that is employed to cope with problems of smoking, weight, and psychological distress.

In spite of nearly identical rank orders, important differences do exist in the absolute level of using particular change processes for coping with three different problems. Table 14.2 indicates, for example, that in the Action stage, Consciousness Raising is relied on more frequently by people coping with weight problems than in coping with distress. Consciousness Raising is used more frequently, however, in coping with distress than with smoking. Self-liberation is also relied on more by people coping with weight problems than by people dealing with distress or smoking. On the other hand, Helping Relationships are called on more by distressed people than by overweight people. Stimulus control techniques are used more to control weight than to control distress, even though this process is used least for all three problems. Similar data are reported by Perri in Chapter 12 of this volume.

Three significant differences were found between overweight individuals and smokers who were contemplating taking action on their problems. In each case, overweight individuals used specific processes of change more than smokers. Similar results were found for people in the Maintenance stage. Weight-control subjects relied on Consciousness Raising and Stimulus Control techniques significantly more than did former smokers.

These results suggest that when it comes to losing weight people read more articles and books, think more about feedback they have received, make more commitments to change, and modify stimuli in their environment more than people who intend to quit smoking. Distressed individuals, on the other hand, turn more to helping relationships to overcome distress than do people who are trying to lose weight (Wills, 1982, 1983). Psychological distress seems to elicit more affiliative coping mechanisms, whereas weight control elicits more coping efforts involving information and control of cues related to eating.

Within-Subjects Comparisons

It is possible that these differences in how frequently particular processes are used with particular problems are due to subject differences rather than problem differences. After all, we have been comparing the processes of change used by different groups of people who have different problems. What would happen if we compared the same subjects who are in the same stage of change but are coping with different problems?

Table 14.3 shows how frequently 15 subjects used the six comparable processes when contemplating losing weight versus quitting smoking. These results are nearly identical to what was found when 156 smokers were compared to 70 overweight individuals who were in the contemplation stage. That is, the overweight subjects relied much more on Consciousness Raising, Self-liberation, and Stimulus Control than did smokers.

Table 14.3 indicates the same pattern of results for subjects who are in the maintenance stage with both smoking and weight. These subjects rely significantly more on Consciousness Raising, Self-liberation, and Stimulus Control when they are maintaining weight loss compared to maintaining smoking cessation.

Table 14.4 indicates a similar pattern of results for subjects who are taking action to lose weight and to overcome psychological distress.[1] These subjects rely significantly more on Consciousness Raising, Self-liberation, and Stimulus Control to lose weight than to overcome distress.

Obviously there are some limitations to these comparisons. We have isolated processes and stages but do not include data on successful or unsuccessful change of problem behavior. In Chapter 13, particular processes are found to be relevant for certain stages and are related to successful smoking cessation. Our current analysis does not include outcome data for these subjects. Also, the same group of subjects was used in the analyses of weight, smoking, and distress problems. Different populations need to be sampled and replication of these results is imperative. Although we have included more processes of change than have been examined previously, we make no claim that we have isolated all the possible processes of change. Keeping these limitations in mind, these results suggest that coping with

[1]Because there were too few smokers taking action, within-subjects comparisons could not be made for smoking.

Table 14.3

COMPARISONS OF THE SAME SUBJECTS IN CONTEMPLATION AND MAINTENANCE ON SIX PROCESSES FOR COPING WITH SMOKING AND WEIGHT

Process	Smoking		Weight		$F(1, 14)$
	M	SD	M	SD	
	CONTEMPLATION				
	$n = 15$				
Consciousness raising	2.4	0.78	3.1	0.88	20.96***
Self-liberation	2.9	0.83	3.4	0.81	6.36*
Reinforcement management	2.0	0.90	1.9	0.94	ns
Helping relationship	3.2	0.69	3.7	0.66	ns
Dramatic relief	2.5	0.97	2.2	0.96	ns
Stimulus control	1.3	0.37	1.9	0.75	10.79**
	MAINTENANCE				
	$n = 21$				
					$F(1, 20)$
Consciousness raising	2.1	0.86	2.6	1.05	15.50***
Self-liberation	2.1	1.39	3.0	1.01	5.96**
Reinforcement management	1.7	1.20	1.8	0.91	ns
Helping relationships	2.4	1.02	2.8	0.95	ns
Dramatic relief	1.9	1.13	1.8	1.22	ns
Stimulus control	1.3	0.69	1.9	1.93	10.34**

*$p < .05$. **$p < .01$. ***$p < .001$.

Table 14.4

COMPARISON OF SAME SUBJECTS IN ACTION ON SIX PROCESSES FOR COPING WITH WEIGHT AND DISTRESS

Process	Weight		Distress		$F(1, 17)$
	M	SD	M	SD	
	ACTION				
	$n = 18$				
Consciousness raising	3.2	0.83	2.8	0.84	5.86*
Self-liberation	3.7	0.77	3.1	0.97	11.78**
Reinforcement management	2.3	1.00	2.4	1.18	ns
Helping relationship	3.3	0.89	3.7	1.14	ns
Dramatic relief	2.5	0.87	2.6	1.03	ns
Stimulus control	2.0	0.73	1.6	0.67	6.93*

*$p < .05$. **$p < .01$.

substance abuse and psychological distress involves a common set of change processes that are applied in a distinct pattern across problems.

DISCUSSION

The results of these comparisons of processes of change with different problems both within and across subjects indicate that similar processes or coping mechanisms can be identified and measured. Moreover, a distinct pattern of coping activities emerged with Helping Relationships, Self-liberation, and Consciousness Raising being used most frequently across different problems. Pattern similarity, however, is not equivalent to equivalence in absolute frequency across problems. We found that subjects use some processes more for certain problems than for others. These similarities and differences are intriguing.

If this type of comparative research continues to demonstrate that there is a small set of common change processes that people use to cope with a diversity of problems, then the task for interveners could be greatly simplified. Currently there are more than 250 therapies competing for attention on the therapeutic marketplace (Henrik, 1980). Clinicians who prefer to take a more comprehensive approach to helping clients with substance abuse and other problems face a difficult task in just naming, let alone learning, 250 different therapies. To master 10 or 12 processes of change, however, is a much more realistic task.

Once we understand how various processes contribute to successful change, therapists would have to assess which change processes they overemphasize with clients and which processes they underutilize. Therapists trained in a single therapeutic system would probably have to add certain processes to their therapeutic repertoire. Almost all systems of therapy emphasize only 2 or 3 processes of change rather than 10 or 12 processes (Prochaska, 1984). Aversive therapies for alcohol or tobacco abuse, for example, rely primarily on such processes as contingency control and/or counterconditioning. Unless aversive approaches are applied in conjunction with other therapies, the use of all other coping processes would be left to the individual substance abuser, who may or may not be effective in applying other processes. Many self-changers may actually use more change processes than are in the armament of some traditional therapists. Most therapists, however, are quite skilled with particular change processes and could build on these strengths as they become more complete clinicians.

Therapists would also have to assess which processes clients may be overemphasizing, such as an excessive use of substances in coping with distress, and which processes clients are underemphasizing compared to self-changers. Therapists may have to teach certain substance abusers about a process like counterconditioning, while other clients have already discovered innovative ways of using this process. If we conceptualize therapy as a cooperative endeavor between a therapist's efforts to influence change and the client's efforts at self-change, then therapists need to be able to count on clients doing at least their fair share of the therapeutic work. Clients who sit passively and dependently waiting to be magically changed by a therapist can spend long and frustrating years in therapy "waiting for Godot."

Research indicates that an estimated two-thirds of the variance in therapy outcome is due to the clients' efforts and only one-third is due to the therapists' efforts (Prochaska & Norcross, 1982). Furthermore, an average of 1 hour of therapy per week represents less than 1% of the clients waking week. Effective intervention with problems like substance abuse, therefore, needs to facilitate clients becoming active changers both inside and outside the therapy setting. It is important for clinicians to assess which change processes substance abusers are actively applying outside of therapy. As the Processes of Change Questionnaire becomes better developed with norms for different types of substance abuse, it could serve as a means of assessing the frequency with which outpatients are using each of the change processes to cope with substance abuse problems from week to week. Intervention programs could also begin to assess if they are indeed modifying the change processes that they are designed to affect. In collaboration with researchers at Brown University, we are examining the extent to which a behaviorally based program for problem drinkers impacts upon behavioral change processes. In this problem drinkers program, patients are taught to apply functional analysis to their alcohol abuse. In didactic group and individual sessions they learn concepts and techniques for applying such processes as Counterconditioning, Reinforcement Management, and Stimulus Control to help control their drinking. This research will also assess the extent to which clients continue to use these newly learned coping processes after they leave the intensive 2-week program.

Teaching clients how to use 10 or 12 processes of change is easier if the clients recognize that they are learning a more comprehensive model of change that can be applied to a diversity of problems. Individuals who are intending to quit smoking, for example, are frequently concerned about gaining weight. People becoming free from an excessive reliance on alcohol frequently fear they will not be able to cope with psychological distress without alcohol. Psychologically distressed patients may fail to comply with medical prescriptions because of fears of becoming dependent on chemical substances. If clients are mastering a model of change that is relevant not only to the immediate problem they are facing but also to future problems that inevitably arise, their self-efficacy should be enhanced not just for their most pressing problem but for coping with problems in general.

With substance abuse problems like smoking and overeating, a majority of abusers may not be willing to participate in formal intervention programs even when they are available at the work site (Abrams & Follick, 1983; McAlister, 1975). A majority of these substance abusers, however, would probably use self-help materials if effective materials were available. Over 70% of smokers, for example, report that they would take advantage of effective self-help manuals even though they would not attend formal smoking cessation programs (McAlister, 1975). A major thrust in our laboratory is to develop for smokers self-help materials that are based on data and models of self-change approaches to smoking cessation. These manuals are designed to teach smokers how to cope with specific issues that arise at each of the stages of change and how to use particular change processes to progress from one stage of change to the next. These manuals also show how the general processes of change can be used to cope with weight-control problems and emotional distress problems that can lead to relapse. A first-generation manual has been compared to the leading manual for smoking cessation with rather encouraging results. Data-based self-help materials such as these could also serve as important adjuncts to therapy. Such materials could help clients to be more effective in their own efforts to cope with substance abuse problems.

Theoretically, the research reported here supports our assumption that there is a general structure of self-change processes that is common across a diversity of substance abuse and other psychological problems. Specialists working with different types of substance abuse have all too often been content-oriented. Thus, we have specialists in alcohol abuse, drug abuse, smoking abuse, and food abuse. As clinicians, however, we are primarily specialists in change. If we can indeed validate a structure to change that is common to a range of substance abuse problems, our challenge shall be a more shared mission of helping individuals to change regardless of which substance is creating problems in living. Our research suggests that the structure of change involves the systematic implementation of a general set of coping processes across a series of stages of change.

Of course, much more research is needed to identify the most effective techniques for operationalizing each process of change. With Consciousness Raising, for example, traditional techniques in therapy have included observation (Bowen, 1978), clarification, confrontation, and interpretation (Greenson, 1967). Which of these techniques is the most effective remains to be determined. More research is also needed on how particular change processes can be misapplied both by self-changers and by professional interveners. We previously indicated that many self-changers can mismedicate themselves for psychological distress by an excessive reliance on alcohol, even though alcohol can have a delayed effect of increasing anxiety and/or depression (Uhlenhuth et al., 1978). Similarly, professionals can recommend the wrong substance for certain forms of distress, such as the reliance on antianxiety rather than antidepressant medications for treating panic reactions (Uhlenhuth & Balter, 1981).

There are some striking parallels between how frequently self-changers use particular processes of change and how frequently such processes are used in formal therapy. Among self-changers, a helping relationship is the first or second most frequently used approach for coping with smoking, weight, and emotional distress problems. By comparison, in previous research with experienced therapists, the therapeutic relationship was the most frequent process used to help clients with psychological distress (Prochaska & Norcross, 1983). In fact, therapists rely on a helping relationship more when treating clients than when treating themselves for psychological distress. It should not be surprising that a helping relationship is the most commonly used process for coping if we remember that the therapeutic relationship has consistently been one of the most important variables related to successful therapy outcome (Frank, 1973; Goldfried, 1980; Lambert, 1983; Strupp & Hadley, 1979).

A contrasting example concerns substance use as a coping or change mechanism. Substance use as a change process is applied as a direct action approach. When applied effectively, the substance is chosen because it is believed to be effective in overcoming a specific target problem, such as diet aids for weight control, Nicoban for smoking, or tricyclates for depression. Such use of substances as change agents contrasts with the palliative use of substances to cope with stress (Wills & Shiffman, Chapter 1, this volume). Substances, such as alcohol, food, and tobacco, can be used to provide some immediate relief from stress, even though the substances have no direct or long-term effects on the problem the individual is coping with.

Although surveys report increased consumption of alcohol and other nonprescription drugs to deal with psychological problems, substance use is one of the least frequently applied processes for self-changers coping with smoking, weight, and psychological distress problems. Similarly, experienced therapists with doctoral degrees report substance use as the least frequently applied process in treating their own distress. In treating clients, however, therapists recommend specific substances significantly more often than when they treat themselves (Prochaska & Norcross, 1983). Furthermore, psychologists in medical settings recommend substance use significantly more often than psychologists practicing in nonmedical settings. Given how readily chemical substances can be abused, lay people as self-changers and therapists as self-changers may be functioning most wisely by keeping to a minimum the use of substances as a means of coping with a diversity of problems.

The research reported here suggests that no single process is likely to be a panacea for any particular problem with substance abuse or with psychological problems in general. Our research on self-changers does suggest, however, that a small set of common processes may represent the methods that people use to cope with a range of problems like psychological distress and substance abuse. This commonality of processes opens a new way of thinking about intervention as well as a new area of research examining coping mechanisms for substance abuse and psychological distress.

REFERENCES

Abrams, D., & Follick, M. (1983). Behavioral weight-loss intervention at the worksite: Feasibility and maintenance. *Journal of Consulting and Clinical Psychology, 51,* 226–233.

Anehensel, C., & Huba, G. (1983). Depression, alcohol use, and smoking over one year: A four-wave longitudinal causal model. *Journal of Abnormal Psychology, 92,* 134–150.

Bergin, A. (1982). Comment on *Converging themes in psychotherapy*. In M. Goldfried (ed.). *Converging themes in psychotherapy.* New York: Springer.

Bowen, M. (1978). *Family therapy in clinical practice.* New York: Jason Aronsen.

Cowen, E. L. (1982). Help is where you find it: Four informal helping groups. *American Psychologist, 37,* 385–395.

DiClemente, C., Gordon, J., & Gibertini, M. (1983, August). *Self efficacy and the determinants of relapse in alcoholism.* Paper presented at the annual meeting of the American Psychological Association, Anaheim, CA.

DiClemente, C. C., Prochaska, J. O., & Gibertini, M. (1985). Self-efficacy and the stages of self change of smoking. *Cognitive Therapy and Research, 9,* 181–200.

Dohrenwend, B. P., & Crandell, D. L. (1970). Psychiatric symptoms in community, clinic, and mental hospital groups. *American Journal of Psychiatry, 126,* 1611–1621.

Dohrenwend, B. P., Shrout, P. E., Egri, G., & Mendelsohn, F. S. (1980). Nonspecific psychological distress and other dimensions of psychopathology. *Archives of General Psychiatry, 37,* 1229–1236.

Eastwood, M. R. (1975). *The relation between physical and mental illness.* Toronto: University of Toronto Press.

Frank, J. D. (1973). *Persuasion and healing.* Baltimore: John Hopkins Press.

Greenson, R. (1967). *The technique and practice of psychoanalysis.* New York: International Universities Press.

Goldfried, M. R. (Ed.). (1980). Some views on effective principles of psychotherapy. *Cognitive Therapy and Research, 4,* 269–306.

Henrik, R. (1980). *The psychotherapy handbook: The A to Z guide to more than 250 different therapies in use today.* New York: Meridan Book, New American Library.

Lambert, M. (1983). *Psychotherapy and patient relationships.* Homewood, IL: Dow-Jones-Irwin.

Langner, T. S. (1962) A 22-item screening score of psychiatric symptoms indicating impairment. *Journal of Health and Human Behavior, 3,* 269–272.

McAlister, A. (1975). Helping people quit smoking: Current progress. In A. Enelow & J. Henderson (Eds.), *Applying behavioral science to cardiovascular risk.* New York: American Association.

Marks, P. A., & Seeman, W. (1963). *The acturial description of abnormal personality: An atlas for use with the MMPI*. Baltimore: Williams & Wilkins.

Marlatt, A., & Gordon, J. (1980). Determinants of relapse: Implications for the maintenance of behavior change. In P. O. Davidson & S. M. Davidson (Eds.), *Behavioral medicine: Changing health lifestyles*. New York: Brunner/Mazel.

Mellinger, G. D., Balter, M. B., Manheimer, D. I., Cisin, I. H., & Parry, H. J. (1978). Psychic distress, life crisis, and use of psychotherapeutic medications: National household survey data. *Archives of General Psychiatry, 35,* 1045–1052.

Mellinger, G. D., Balter, M. B., Uhlenhuth, E. H., Cisin, I. H., Manhiemer, D. I., & Rickels, K. (1983). Evaluating a household survey measure of psychic distress: II. Improving levels of agreement between survey and clinic measures. *Psychological Medicine, 13,* 607–621.

President's Commission on Mental Health. (1978). Mental health: Nature and scope of the program. *Task panel reports to the President's commission on mental health* (Vol. 2). Washington, DC: U.S. Government Printing Office.

Prochaska, J. O. (1984). *Systems of psychotherapy: A transtheoretical analysis*. Homewood, IL: Dorsey Press.

Prochaska, J., & Norcross, J. (1982). The future of psychotherapy: A Delphi poll. *Professional Psychology, 5,* 620–627.

Prochaska, J., & Norcross, J. (1983). Psychotherapists' perspectives on treating themselves and their clients for psychic distress. *Professional Psychology: Research and Practice, 14,* 642–655.

Prochaska, J. O., Norcross, J. C., & Hambrecht, M. (1983). *Patterns of psychic distress in college students*. Unpublished manuscript.

Regier, D., Goldberg, I., & Taube, C. (1978). The *de facto* U.S. mental health services system: A public health perspective. *Archives of General Psychiatry, 35,* 685–693.

Strupp, H. H. (1982). The outcome problem in psychotherapy: Contemporary perspectives. In J. H. Harvey & M. M. Parks (Eds.), *The Master lecture series* (Vol. 1). Washington DC: American Psychological Association.

Strupp, H. H., & Bloxom, A. L. (1975). An approach to the problem of defining a patient population in psychotherapy research. *Journal of Counseling Psychology, 22,* 231–237.

Strupp, H. H., & Hadley, S. W. (1979). Specific vs. nonspecific factors in psychotherapy: A controlled study of outcome. *Archives of General Psychiatry, 36,* 1125–1136.

Uhlenhuth, I., & Balter, M. (1981, December). Use of psychotherapeutic drugs by the American public. Paper presented at the annual meeting of the American College of Neuropsychopharmacology, San Diego, CA.

Uhlenhuth, I., Balter, M., & Lipman, R. (1978). Minor tranquilizers: Clinical correlates of use in an urban population. *Archives of General Psychiatry, 35,* 650–655.

Vernon, S. W., & Roberts, R. E. (1981). Measuring nonspecific psychological distress and other dimensions of psychopathology. *Archives of General Psychiatry, 38,* 1239–1247.

Veroff, J., Kulka, R., & Douvan, E. (1981). *Mental health in America: Patterns of help-seeking from 1957 to 1976*. New York: Basic Books.

Wills, T. (1982). *Basic processes in helping relationships*. New York: Academic Press.

Wills, T. (1983). *Social comparison in coping and help-seeking*. New York: Academic Press.

Part V

SUMMARY AND INTEGRATION

Chapter 15

Coping and Substance Abuse: Implications for Research, Prevention, and Treatment

G. ALAN MARLATT

INTRODUCTION

Taken as a whole, the chapters in this book represent an emerging paradigm shift in the addictions field. Basically the shift involves a movement away from understanding addiction primarily as a biologically based disorder (addiction as disease) toward a model that construes addictive behavior as an habitual maladaptive means of coping with stress. In this concluding chapter, I attempt to summarize some of the main points in this paradigm shift, from both theoretical and practical perspectives, and to outline issues and questions for future research in this area. Following a section on theoretical issues, this chapter contains sections on both stress and coping, followed by a final discussion of issues for future research.

THEORETICAL PERSPECTIVES

Traditional theories of addiction (Lettieri, Sayers, & Pearson, 1980) have focused on pharmacological properties of drugs and their physiological effects. Although individual differences such as genetic predisposition and "addictive personality" traits are considered important from the biological perspective, the primary emphasis is on uncontrollable, endogenous biological processes as the basis of addiction. Exposure to the drug and the development of physical dependency are considered the primary determinants of addiction, a position that views the addicted individual as a helpless pawn of forces beyond volitional control. Addiction is thus defined in terms of increased physical tolerance to drug effects and the presence of somatic withdrawal symptoms upon cessation of drug use. In a recent theoretical paper on the nature of opiate addiction (cited several times in previous chapters), Alexander and Hadaway (1982) refer to this traditional definition of addiction as an "exposure orientation"—positing that biological exposure to drugs is the primary basis of addiction. An important corollary of this definition is that the addicted individual cannot change his or her habitual use of drugs without external intervention or treatment, since loss of control (and volitional attempts to change) is often considered a pathognomonic symptom of addictive disease (see Jellinek, 1960).

The alternative to the exposure orientation as defined by Alexander and Hadaway (1982) is the "adaptive orientation," "the view that opiate addiction is an attempt to adapt to chronic distress of any sort through habitual use of opiate drugs" (p. 367). The adaptive model views the individual as an active agent of change rather than a helpless victim of uncontrollable forces. As Alexander and Hadaway have noted:

> The two orientations also differ in their underlying psychological assumptions. The exposure orientation is essentially deterministic, depicting addiction as caused by exposure to opiate drugs. On the other hand, the adaptive orientation assumes a purposive organism that may choose to change its addictive behavior when more efficacious possibilities become evident. (p. 368)

The thrust of the material in this volume can be considered an attempt to extend the adaptive orientation to a wide range of addictive behaviors in addition to opiate drug use.

The adaptive orientation to addiction has had a long history, despite its recent emergence as an alternative to the exposure model. In his foreword to this volume, Moos (himself a pioneer of the adaptive orientation) describes four historical roots of this approach: stress and coping theory (studies of adaptation to various life crises), psychoanalytic theory (with its emphasis on ego defense mechanisms as attempts to cope with stress), evolutionary theory and behavior modification (coping as survival-based adaptation and the study of cognitive and behavioral coping mechanisms), and the study of life cycle perspectives (e.g., Erikson's work). Beyond these I place additional emphasis on recent developments in social learning theory (e.g., Bandura, 1977) and cognitive-behavioral therapy (e.g., Beck, 1976; Meichenbaum, 1977). Both of these fields have made significant contributions with an emphasis on cognitive processes (expectancies, attributions, self-efficacy) and on situational determinants of behavior (as an alternative to trait-like dispositional constructs).

The adaptive orientation does not negate the significance of biological or drug factors in addiction. It does not assume, for example, that addiction is founded exclusively on psychological as compared to physiological processes. To define addiction in such either/or terminology would soon lead to enmeshment in the philosophical trap of mind–body dualism. Rather, the emphasis is on the *interaction* of psychological and physiological factors in addiction and on the role of the individual as a purposive (vs. reactive) organism who uses or abuses drugs as a means of attempting to cope with stress. The source of stress includes both psychological stressors and physical distress, the latter often arising from physiological drug effects (including those mediated by tolerance and withdrawal). From the adaptive orientation, it is still important to examine such factors as physical dependency (e.g., Skinner & Allen, 1982) and to search for possible biological commonalities underlying the addiction (as described in Chapter 2 by Grunberg & Baum). Yet the emphasis shifts from the study of such factors as primary determinants of addiction (exposure orientation) to an attempt to discover how such physical factors influence the individual's cognitions (beliefs and expectancies) and attempts to change (coping and relapse). A key assumption of this approach is that the individual is capable of change, including self-initiated change, and that psychological and learning factors play a paramount role in the change process. Perhaps addiction, as viewed from the adaptive orientation, is best described as a psychosomatic condition, since both mind and body are intimately intermeshed in the problem.

In the present volume, many authors emphasize that the adaptive orientation represents a theoretical approach characterized by reciprocal determinism and homeostatic mechanisms of change. Echoing the statements of such theorists as Bandura (1982) and Lazarus (1966), most chapter authors adopt the position that stress and coping are reciprocally interacting processes, each influencing the other, and that stress is best defined as a transaction (or adaptational relationship) between the person and the situation or stressor. As Wills and Shiffman state in their conceptual framework (Chapter 1), stress results from an imbalance of environmental demands and available resources; the individual attempts to cope as a means of restoring balance or equilibrium. Homeostasis thus plays a key motivational role in the coping process, whether or not drugs are used as an attempt to cope with stress. The interactive homeostatic approach cited by several authors (e.g., Wills & Shiffman, Chapters 1, 3, and 9; Pentz, Chapter 5; DiClemente & Prochaska, Chapters 13 and 14) has come to replace the linear causation model epitomized by the tension-reduction theory of addiction.

According to tension-reduction theory, addictive behavior is reinforced in direct proportion to the degree of tension-reduction afforded by the pharmacological properties of the drug (e.g., Cappell, 1975; George & Marlatt, 1983; Marlatt, 1976). Empirical support for the tension-reduction model is mixed at best, partly due to a failure to include important mediating variables such as dose level, set (psychological expectancies), and setting. This approach is also limited by its exclusive emphasis on negative reinforcement or drive-reduction as the primary determinant of addiction (i.e., that drug use is reinforced by tension reduction. As indicated by several authors in this volume, drug use is also strongly influenced by positive reinforcement (e.g., feelings of euphoria or getting "high") or by the belief that this is an important outcome in drug use.

STAGES OF CHANGE IN SUBSTANCE USE

Another significant theoretical contribution advanced by several authors is the notion of *stages of change* in the addictive process. As Moos notes in his foreword, the field is moving away from an emphasis on outcome (e.g., Did the child end up smoking or not?; Did the patient relapse or remain abstinent?) to an emphasis on *process of change*. In addition, as Shiffman points out in Chapter 9, there is a shift of attention from individual outcomes (e.g., who relapses) to the study of how the process of relapse occurs both within and between individuals. The new focus on process has led several investigators to postulate discrete stages in both the initial development and subsequent attempts to change an addictive habit. In Chapter 1, Wills and Shiffman note three stages in involvement in drug use: initiation, regular use, and cessation of use. Biglan, Weissman, and Severson (Chapter 4) add that different learning factors may be involved in each stage and that factors associated with the onset of drug use may be independent from factors associated with the maintenance of regular use (e.g., that negative reinforcement may play a greater role in maintenance than it does in initiation or onset of drug use).

Perhaps the most comprehensive theory of stages of change as applied to the cessation of drug use is that described by Prochaska and DiClemente (Chapters 13 and 14). These authors delineate five discrete stages in the change process: precontemplation, contemplation, decision making, active change, and maintenance of change. If we add initiation of use and the maintenance of regular ongoing use (similar to the precontemplation stage), we are left with a six-stage model: initiation, regular use–precontemplation, contemplation, decision making (some would argue that these latter two could be combined into a single stage of contemplation and commitment), active change, and maintenance. In our own work on the process of relapse (Marlatt & Gordon, 1985), we argued that different learning processes may be involved in initial cessation of drug use and maintenance of these changes over time. The stages of change model is proving to be a very useful heuristic device in the study of addiction.

It is important to highlight the distinction between the initial development (etiology) of an addictive behavior and factors associated with changing these behaviors. In contrast with the disease model and its concern with uncontrollable endogenous factors in the etiology of addiction, social learning theorists have noted that the person is capable of exercising control and assuming personal responsibility for the process of changing an addictive habit. This approach endorses a proactive stance in the habit–change process, in sharp contrast with the more passive, reactive position of personal powerlessness inherent in the disease model. Does accepting responsibility for change mean that the individual is to be held personally responsible for the initial development of the problem, thereby suggesting a throwback to the discredited moral model of addiction (in which drug use is viewed as a moral weakness or deficit in self-control or willpower)?

The distinction between attribution of responsibility for the development of a problem (who is to blame for a past event) and attribution of responsibility for a solution (who controls future events) has been developed in an excellent paper by Brickman et al. (1982). These authors derive four general models specifying the form people's behavior will take when they try either to help others or to help themselves. The essence of their models is as follows:

> In the first (called the moral model because of past usage of this term), actors are held responsible for both problems and solutions and are believed to need only proper motivation. In the compensatory model, people are seen as not responsible for problems but responsible for solutions, and are believed to need power. In the medical model, individuals are seen as responsible for neither problems nor solutions and are believed to need treatment. In the enlightenment model, actors are seen as responsible for problems but as unable or unwilling to provide solutions, and are believed to need discipline. (p. 368)

All four models can be found in the addiction field. The moral model can still be found in fundamental religious beliefs about the nature of addiction (addiction as a sinful act committed by those lacking in moral fiber or willpower to resist temptation). It has been supplanted largely by the disease model in recent years; the disease model exonerates the addicted person from personal responsibility for the problem (it is due instead to genetic or biological forces beyond volitional control) and recommends external treatment for the condition. The enlightenment model, which Brickman and his colleagues identify with such approaches as Alcoholics Anonymous, Narcotics Anonymous, and some therapeutic communities (such as Synanon for opiate addiction), the emphasis is on "enlightening" participants as to the true nature of their problem and the need to "surrender personal control" as a means of changing the behavior in favor of accepting the influence of a "higher power" (religious doctrine and/or the power of a self-help fellowship).

The final model, one that embodies the principles endorsed in this volume, is the compensatory model. Here people are not considered responsible for the development of problems (e.g., becoming trapped in an addictive behavior pattern by the combined influence of stress, positive and negative reinforcement, classical conditioning, social modeling), but are able to compensate for their difficulties by assuming responsibility for changing their behavior—even in the face of apparent setbacks. Programs based on this philosophy, even though they are often identified as a kind of behavioral "treatment" approach, differ from most externally based treatment programs in that they teach the client to become eventually the agent of change. Here one is reminded of the classic adage attributed to Maimonides: "Give a man a fish and he eats for a day; teach a man to fish and he eats for a lifetime." Giving him a fish may provide a temporary solution to the problem, but teaching him how to fish is clearly the best long-term solution. As Brickman and his coauthors (1982) conclude:

> Finally, we are inclined to see cognitive behavior therapy as embodying the assumptions of the compensatory model. The role of the therapist is the limited but critical one of teaching clients how to alter maladaptive cognitive processes and environmental contingencies. Once taught how to recognize and control these contingencies, clients are expected to set their own standards, monitor their own performance, and reward or reinforce themselves appropriately. (pp. 379–380)

STRESS, TEMPTATION, AND HIGH-RISK SITUATIONS

One of the central assumptions that runs through many chapters in this book is that drugs are often used as an attempt to cope with stress. Although stress itself (as experienced by the individual) is the result of an interaction among biological factors, situational stressors, and the individual's capacity to cope, a number of relatively common stress situations have been identified by various chapter authors. These situations have been referred to collectively as "high-risk situations" (Marlatt & Gordon, 1980), or situations associated with an increased probability of drug use as an attempt to cope with stress. High-risk situations appear to play a role in the initiation of drug use in adolescence (see Chapters 3, 4, and 5), in the maintenance of problematic substance use (see Chapters 6 and 7), and in relapse following a period of abstinence (see Chapters 9, 10, and 11).

Although recent research has focused primarily on stress and coping as determinants of relapse, a similar approach to the *initiation phase* of substance use (experimentation with drugs and the early stages of use) holds considerable promise for the development of effective primary prevention programs for adolescent populations. Initiation of drug use may occur in response to generalized stressors, including peer pressure and the stress of adolescent adjustment to the demands of increasing adult responsibilities. Compared with research on the prevention of relapse in former drug users (tertiary prevention), studies applying the stress and coping approach to primary prevention (e.g., the chapters in this volume on the primary prevention of smoking) are sometimes more difficult to evaluate because of inherent methodological problems. Unlike clinical intervention studies, in which subjects receive extensive, individual attention, primary prevention research is geared toward all subjects (whether or not they are likely to use the substance in question), who differ in motivation and baseline level of substance use. Also, since the assessment of outcome may take many months or even years in primary prevention studies, the results of this research may appear less powerful than client-focused clinical research.

High-risk situations associated with relapse can be divided into two main categories. The first category consists of situations associated with prior drug use, including attempts to cope with physical withdrawal and responses to drug-related cues. Although physical withdrawal may play a relatively minor role with certain drugs such as marijuana, cocaine, or tobacco (Shiffman reports in Chapter 9 that less than half of the smokers he studied reported physical withdrawal in association with relapse), it appears to exert more influence with the opiates and other substances in which physical dependency is more easily developed (see Chapters 6 and 11). Similarly, drug cues (e.g., running across a previously hidden drug supply) may elicit conditioned responses (e.g., conditioned craving) that increase the probability of relapse.

Most relapses reported in this book, however, fall in the second category, consisting of high-risk situations that act as stressors in their own right, independent of physical withdrawal or exposure to conditioned drug stimuli. These situations include experiences of negative emotional states (e.g., anger, boredom, interpersonal conflict), social pressure, and other stressful situations (see Chapters in Part IV). Many of these situations appear to be associated with prior drug use, presumably as an attempt to cope with the stress evoked by such situations (e.g., smoking as an attempt to quell feelings of anger). When these same situations arise after the person has discontinued drug use, the resultant stress may trigger a lapse unless the individual has developed an alternative coping response.

It seems likely that these two categories of high-risk situations are often confused with each other. An individual may experience stress in a high-risk situation (e.g., an argument with one's spouse) that is then attributed to physical withdrawal, since both include the experience of negative affect. The consequences of such a misattribution might lead to a relapse if the person believes that only drug use would alleviate the distress. A correct attribution, on the other hand (i.e., that the anger arises from a specific interpersonal incident rather than from generalized withdrawal symptoms), may motivate the individual to develop more effective coping responses (e.g., communication or assertive skills).

Stress can also be studied at different levels of analysis, ranging from the impact of distal major life events (e.g., divorce, unemployment, illness) to proximal day-to-day upsets and hassles, as indicated by Wills and Shiffman in Chapter 1. In terms of the first level of analysis, both Tucker (Chapter 6) and Timmer, Veroff, and Colten (Chapter 7) provide some support for the notion that general life-style issues and stressful life events (e.g., economic, marital, and work-associated stress) are associated with increased drug use. Such broad-level assessments of major sources of stress, often obtained via population surveys and questionnaires, make it difficult to ascertain specific causal relationships between stress and drug use (e.g., does stress increase drug use as an attempt to cope, and/or does excessive drug use exacerbate stress levels or contribute to such major life events as divorce or physical illness?).

A more fine-grained approach is to assess stressful events and associated coping responses on a day-to-day basis. Stone, Lennox, and Neale (Chapter 8) report a study of this type in which they attempted to relate ongoing daily problems to alcohol use. Despite the many strengths of this study, the authors found significant but weak relationships between coping with such day-to-day problems and the use of alcohol. One potential reason for these generally weak results may be that the drinking level was assessed retrospectively for the year preceding the analysis of daily problems and that subjects were assigned to drinking categories (e.g., light or heavy drinkers) on this basis. In addition, the authors fail to assess alcohol use as an explicit item on their coping inventory. Future research on drug use as a means of coping with stress on a day-to-day level might consider the use of an inventory of daily hassles (e.g., specific stressful events that crop up daily, such as unpaid bills, headaches, family arguments), rather than focusing on the single most bothersome problem of the day. Some recent studies have shown a higher correlation between daily hassles and psychological and physical symptoms compared to the relatively weak association found for major life events and these symptoms (Delongis, Coyne, Dakof, Folkman, & Lazarus, 1982; Kanner, Coyne, Schaefer, & Lazarus, 1981).

EXPECTANCIES AND DECISION MAKING

Stressful situations may lead to drug use (initiation or relapse) to the extent that the individual harbors positive outcome expectancies about the drug and its effects as a means of countering or reducing stress (see Marlatt, 1984). Outcome expectancies can be shaped by both experiences of positive reinforcement (e.g., the euphoric rush or initial high caused by the drug) and by negative reinforcement (e.g., relief of tension or anxiety). In their conceptual framework, Wills and Shiffman (Chapter 1) argue convincingly that positive and negative states of affect represent independent dimensions (statistically uncorrelated) and that positive affect is not simply the absence of negative affect. This is an important point that needs further investigation in terms of outcome expectancies for drug use, since it implies that individuals may expect a drug to independently produce feelings of euphoria (increase in positive affect) and feelings of tension reduction (decrease in negative affect). Perhaps different outcome expectancies are generated depending on the type of situation involved (e.g., smoking to calm one's nerves prior to an exam vs. smoking in a celebratory party setting). Individual differences in substance use, such as gender of user, may also be mediated by differential outcome expectancies (as noted in Chapters 6 and 8).

Research on outcome expectancies in alcohol use reveals a significant relation between self-reported positive expectancies (e.g., that alcohol will transform negative moods into positive ones) and degree of alcohol use and problem drinking (e.g., Brown, Goldman, Inn, & Anderson, 1980; Southwick, Steele, Marlatt, & Lindell, 1981). Future studies may reveal a similar pattern of results for drugs other than alcohol. The study of outcome expectancies for drug effects is consistent with a "behavioral economic" theory of drug use (Ainslie, 1975). In this approach, drug use is considered a function of the rewards and costs involved for either use or abstention from use. The perceived *payoff matrix* for deciding to use drugs or not is a promising area for future research. Outcome expectancies and perceived payoffs may be assessed in terms of subjective expected utilities for various outcomes (e.g., to smoke or refrain from smoking). Although these methods have been used in the study of decision making in various areas (Beach & Beach, 1982), they have yet to be applied systematically to the study of drug use.

Theories of decision making and choice behavior appear to have important implications for the study of both initiation of drug use and relapse following cessation of use (see Chapter 3 and 12). The results of such an analysis may be helpful in assisting individuals to better appraise and cope with high-risk situations. Such appraisal-based coping may provide valuable assistance in helping clients anticipate and plan for such high-risk situations in terms of developing alternatives to drug use that lead to similar payoffs (e.g., choosing to exercise or meditate as a means of reducing tension). Individuals may come to realize that there is more than one way to obtain a sought-after outcome and that the long-range positive payoffs of a "positive addiction," such as exercise or meditation, outweigh the short-term payoffs (immediate gratification) associated with "negative addictions" such as drug use (see Glasser, 1976).

In terms of the high-risk stressors described by various authors in this volume, one common element seems to stand out from the others: the *affective tone* of the situation. As Shiffman points out in Chapter 9, for example, the affective tone of the situation emerges as the single most critical element in classifying relapse crises. Drugs have many effects, but chief among them are changes in affect or emotional state; the physiological underpinnings of such hedonic change are described by Grunberg and Baum in Chapter 2. Research also suggests that the affective response to psychoactive drugs is often biphasic in nature—the initial high or state of excitation and positive physical sensations is often followed by a delayed reaction that is opposite in hedonic quality (see Solomon, 1980; Siegel, 1979).

Several important implications arise from an analysis of biphasic drug effects. The first is that the user's positive outcome expectancies may be focused on the initial high phase of the biphasic response, and that the delayed secondary effects (e.g., fatigue, depression, incipient withdrawal) play a less significant role because of their delayed status (temporal gradient of reinforcement). The second implication is that drug use may be viewed as a more positive choice in situations characterized by prior negative emotional states. Prior to drug use, the individual may be experiencing dysphoric feelings arising from a stressful life situation and/or from the delayed effects of heavy prior use. The functional utility of drug use in this situation may be very positive compared to nonuse to the extent that the individual expects that the drug will transform the negative feelings into more positive feelings. Although this transformation of affect from negative to positive may occur in the short-run (i.e., during the initial phase of the biphasic response), in the long-run the user may find himself or herself caught in a vicious circle as he or she attempts to cope with the negative aftereffects of drug use (the second, "downer" phase of the biphasic response) by increasing drug use (Marlatt, 1984; Marlatt & Gordon, 1985). Further study of both high-risk situations and associated outcome expectancies should provide valuable new knowledge with direct applications for substance abuse treatment and prevention.

COPING, SELF-EFFICACY, AND MOTIVATION FOR CHANGE

One of the central issues in this volume is the extent to which coping is consistent within individuals across situations (cross-situational consistency of coping) or is specific to the situation (situation-specific coping). As Shiffman notes (Chapter 9), this issue is similar to the trait versus state controversy in personality theory: Is coping a trait-like disposition (the individual uses more or less the same coping strategies in all situations) or does the situational state account for most of the variance in coping differences? Another variation on this theme is to consider whether certain coping responses apply across multiple situations, regardless of the person using them, and whether other coping responses apply only to specific kinds of situations. In Chapter 1, Wills and Shiffman propose such a distinction in their discussion of *generalized* coping skills that can be used to cope with a variety of life stressors (e.g., general problem solving) as distinct from *specific* coping skills for unique situations (e.g., drink refusal skills in social pressure situations).

Chapter authors vary considerably on the question of generalized versus specific coping. In his study of coping with smoking relapse crises, Shiffman concludes that all coping strategies reported by his subjects were equally effective (70% survival rate) compared to the absence of coping (except for less effective willpower coping and the use of self-punitive thoughts). As Shiffman notes, it may be the fact of coping rather than its specific character that determines outcome (Chapter 9). Shiffman also notes, however, that coping appears to be situation-specific and that there is little evidence of cross-situational consistency of coping within the same individuals. In terms of classifying coping responses, Shiffman analyzes both behavioral and cognitive coping and concludes that either type is relatively effective when used alone (60% survial rate for both) and most effective when used in combination (82% survival rate). Along with Chaney and Roszell (Chapter 11), Shiffman suggests that coping speed (latency to respond) may also be a critical factor in coping effectiveness.

Along these same lines, Pentz (Chapter 5) argues that training in general interpersonal skills to enhance personal competency is central to the prevention of substance abuse in adolescents. The prevention program described by Pentz did not target skill training to specific temptation situations and is therefore an example of a generalized coping skill approach. DiClemente and Prochaska (Chapters 13 and 14) propose a common set of change processes (coping strategies) and argue that these "problem-solving coping options" are used across a wide variety of areas of change, from smoking cessation to coping with psychological distress (Chapter 14). Other authors caution against positing such a transsituational commonality in coping. In his study of self-initiated change in smoking, weight control, and drinking, Perri (Chapter 12) reports that coping strategies differ in their effectiveness in terms of the target area of change (e.g., use of self-reinforcement or stimulus control) and warns against premature acceptance of a "uniformity myth" in the study of common elements of change.

Other investigators have found that coping responses are sometimes specific to the high-risk situation encountered. Although we (Curry & Marlatt,

Chapter 10) note that different coping strategies reported by subjects who attempted to quit smoking on their own appear to be equally effective compared to no coping attempts (a finding also reported by Shiffman in Chapter 9), we also found that specific coping responses were employed more often in certain situations. Although self-instruction was the coping response most often reported across situations, behavioral avoidance was reported more often as a means of coping with general urges and interpersonal conflict situations, whereas cognitive coping was used most often in intrapersonal negative emotional states. Chaney and Roszell (Chapter 11) also report some interesting data on situational differences related to self-efficacy ratings and coping responses. Despite these differences, these authors fail to find a relationship between different methods of coping and treatment outcome in their study of heroin addicts; Chaney and Roszell conclude that one type of coping is not necessarily superior to another but rather it is how well the chosen coping method is executed that is important (Chapter 11).

The controversy over coping as a situation-specific or generalized process appears to be based in large part on how coping is assessed by the investigator. Typologies of coping responses can be derived either on the basis of the investigator's theoretical predilections (in which categories are generated deductively from the theory) or on the basis of what subjects tell us through self-reports and other measures (in which categories are inductively generated from available data). An example of the deductive method is DiClemente and Prochaska's (Chapter 13) transtheoretical model of change, in which categories of change were initially deduced from a comparative study of systems of psychotherapy and then applied to the study of habit change (e.g., smoking). Here the coping categories are derived from a general theory of change and not from an ecological assessment of what subjects actually do to cope in the smoking cessation process. In contrast, other investigators begin by asking subjects what they do to cope with problems and then inductively derive coping categories on this basis. Stone and his colleagues (Chapter 8), as an example of this approach, asked subjects to sort a wide variety of potential coping responses into conceptually unique categories. In the Daily Coping Inventory used by these authors, subjects are asked about a significant problem during the day and whether or not coping was attempted; if so, subjects were then asked to specify the particular thought or action employed as a coping response. The advantage of involving subjects directly in the development of coping categories is that the inductive procedure taps into the subjects' own perceptions of coping and avoids possible omissions or misperceptions that might occur when the investigators develop their own coding system on an a priori theoretical basis.

STAGES OF COPING

The assessment and categorization of coping response may benefit from an analysis of coping stages, as several authors indicate in the present volume. Wills and Shiffman (Chapter 1), for example, speak of three temporal stages in coping: anticipatory coping (prestressful event), immediate coping (in the stressful situation itself), and restorative coping (poststress event). The advantage of this system is that coping can be conceptualized as three discrete temporal stages: coping prior to the stressor situation, coping in high-risk situations as they occur, and coping after the situation passes. Similarly, Stone et al. (Chapter 8) note that drug use can be viewed either as an attempt to cope directly with a problematic situation (primary coping) or as a result of unsuccessful attempts to cope with the problem (secondary coping). A similar analysis is employed by Chaney and Roszell (Chapter 11), who adopt a stage-level analysis of coping developed by Moos and Billings (1982). In the Moos and Billings system, based on the theoretical model of stress and coping developed by Richard Lazarus (1966), coping is classified into three main foci or areas of application: (1) appraisal-based coping, including the coping responses of logical analysis, cognitive redefinition, and cognitive avoidance; (2) problem-focused coping, including seeking information or advice, taking action, and the use of alternative rewards; and (3) emotion-focused coping. Substance use as a means to cope can occur at any of these stages, as can more adaptive coping strategies.

If a stage model of coping is utilized in the assessment and categorization of coping responses, it is necessary to specify the stage in which the situation occurs along with details about the type of situation involved. The same logic applies to self-efficacy ratings in which subjects rate their ability to cope with specific situations. For pretreatment assessment of coping and efficacy, situations could be described in each of the three stages (appraisal-based, problem-focused, and emotion-focused). Situations could be presented in written form or via audio- or videotape, as suggested by Biglan et al. (the "taped situations test" described in Chapter 4) and by Chaney and Roszell (the "situational competency test" described in Chapter 11).

A final issue addressed in this section is the question of *determinants of coping:* Can coping be predicted, and what factors are involved? Several chapter authors address this question, and these contributions are briefly reviewed. In their conceptual model of stress and coping, Wills and Shiffman (Chapter 1) outline five general factors that may influence selection of a coping response: severity of the stressor, perceived changeability of the stressor, whether coping is targeted toward the temptation situation itself or to the underlying cause of the temptation, the difficulty and perceived cost of coping, and personality and individual differences. In terms of demographic factors and other individual differences, Tucker (Chapter 6) reports that sex differences may be an important factor in coping (some data indicate that men are better in coping with some types of situations than women). Shiffman (Chapter 9) examines a variety of coping determinants for smoking cessation, including the impact of prior treatment (those with prior smoking treatment reported use of more behavioral coping), the passage of time (less coping occurs over time since cessation), prior familiarity with the high-risk situation (expected vs. unexpected situations), and other environmental factors (e.g., prior use of alcohol). In an interesting analysis, Shiffman provides a "risk profile" of factors that could inhibit behavioral coping (see Figure 9.2, Chapter 9), although he concludes that cognitive coping is less affected by such risk factors.

In our study of self-initiated smoking cessation (Curry & Marlatt, Chapter 10), we report that personal beliefs about smoking and the process of cessation both influence coping (e.g., those who believed that quitting smoking was more a matter of learning than willpower were more likely to use behavioral coping). Several authors focus on social support as an important mediator of coping (social support as a coping resource and/or stress buffer). In terms of personality factors, DiClemente and Prochaska (Chapter 13) fail to find any effect of the personality dimensions they studied (locus of control and social desirability) on the utilization of coping processes. It may be that future research will show that some individual differences (e.g., intelligence, self-esteem) play a critical role in the coping process.

MOTIVATION AND COPING

Perhaps the most important determinant of coping, one rarely touched on by the various authors of this book, is motivation and intentionality. Only a few points concerning the potential role of motivational factors in coping are discussed in the text, but the implications of these may prove to be significant in future research. Biglan et al. (Chapter 4) report in their analysis of smoking onset in adolescents that subjects who smoked the most were more likely to come to the first smoking initiation experience with a *prior intention* to smoke. Along similar lines, Chaney and Roszell (Chapter 11) report that the majority of relapses among their heroin addicts were *premeditated*, and that although most patients recalled thinking about coping prior to the relapse, only 38% actually attempted to cope. In Perri's study of self-initiated habit change (Chapter 12), successful subjects rated themselves as more motivated and committed to personal change (and that they were more motivated by the negative consequences of the habit) as compared to unsuccessful subjects.

15. IMPLICATIONS FOR RESEARCH AND INTERVENTION   381

Although the role of motivation as a factor in the coping process is not yet well understood, I suspect that it plays a very important role and that future studies should include assessment of motivational states. The influence of motivation on self-efficacy also needs further investigation. One possible role of motivation is that it provides the energy or drive for a commitment to change and that one's intentions to cope are strongly influenced by this process. Motivation itself is probably not sufficient to bring about lasting change, however, since it fails to provide a *means* of carrying out the intentional goal. Motivation without associated coping capacity may be what subjects refer to as willpower. As Shiffman points out (Chapter 9), willpower can be defined as the global application of intent in the absence of specific coping skills; willpower alone was an ineffective method of quitting smoking in Shiffman's study. Without motivation to change, however, merely instructing a person in coping skills may have little results in the change process. Both motivation (the will) and skills (the way) must be considered crucial elements of the change process: Where there's a will, there's a way, but without either, one is lost. If motivation is lacking, it may be necessary to return to the contemplation and decision-making stages of the behavior change process (DiClemente & Prochaska, Chapters 13 and 14) before going on with coping skill training.

ISSUES FOR FUTURE RESEARCH

The application of the stress and coping model to substance abuse is still in its infancy. Despite the relative newness of this approach, research and treatment applications of this model are becoming more numerous and extensive, as evidenced by the wide range of investigations reported in this volume. It is also refreshing to find, particularly in the controversy-laden field of addiction, a data-based theoretical orientation in the stress and coping model. If this approach continues to characterize the current paradigm shift in the study of substance abuse, the emerging paradigm will be based on empirical findings rather than on the untested dogma and clinical lore that are so often associated with the more traditional disease models of addiction. Despite advances that already have been made, many of them documented in the preceding chapters, a number of empirical questions remain to be resolved. Since the stress and coping model is heuristically rich, only a few such points are addressed here. Careful readers will find a gold mine of additional ideas and questions for future study throughout the volume.

One important area for future study is the relation of coping with specific high-risk situations to long-term outcome, a point that Moos also makes in his foreword. What are the long-range consequences of successful coping, in terms of primary and secondary prevention of substance abuse and for relapse prevention (tertiary prevention)? Since most of the chapters in this volume focus upon the effectiveness of short-term coping (i.e., whether coping can prevent a lapse in a particular high-risk situation), we still need longitudinal studies of both treatment effectiveness (or self-initiated habit change) and the overall effectiveness of prevention programs based on the stress and coping model. Are some forms of coping more effective in the short-run than the long-run and vice versa? Several authors make a distinction between coping responses that are specific to the high-risk situation (e.g., refusal responses in peer pressure situations) and other more generalized coping skills that relate to global life stressors (e.g., general problem solving or relaxation skills). Research is needed to determine whether specific and general coping skills are additive in their effectiveness or whether specific skills are more effective in the early stages of intervention compared to the long-range usefulness of more global coping techniques.

In our own program of relapse prevention (Marlatt & Gordon, 1985), we advocate that therapists combine specific skill training for high-risk situations with more global coping aimed toward decreasing anxiety, heightening self-esteem, and increasing the individual's sense of perceived efficacy across a variety of risk situations. The global coping strategies we have studied in the area of alcohol use, as an illustration, have included general problem solving (Chaney, O'Leary, & Marlatt, 1978), meditation and relaxation training (Marlatt & Marques, 1977), and aerobic exercise (Murphy, Pagano, & Marlatt, 1984).

Several authors included religion (prayer, religious beliefs, etc.) as a coping strategy in stressful situations. What is the relative effectiveness of more passive forms of coping (religious beliefs, meditation, deep-muscle relaxation, biofeedback, etc.) as compared to more active forms of coping? Is "surrender of control" and acceptance of a "higher power" (as in Alcoholics Anonymous and other related groups) an effective form of passive coping for some individuals? To what extent do religious values preclude substance abuse in adolescence?

Another area ripe for investigation is the relationship between coping, self-efficacy, and attributions. Although research reported in this volume and elsewhere supports the notion that self-efficacy ratings (personal judgements of how well one is likely to cope in a given high-risk situation) are predictive of outcome and subsequent coping, we need to learn more about determinants of self-efficacy and how they can be enhanced in substance abuse prevention and treatment programs. The role of motivation as it affects self-efficacy is still unclear. Along similar lines, we know very little as yet about the role of attributions for coping (or the failure to cope) and their impact on subsequent coping and ratings of self-efficacy. In our own work on relapse (Marlatt & Gordon, 1985), we postulated an attributional reaction called the abstinence violation effect (AVE) that may play a mediating role in determining whether or not an initial slip is followed by a total relapse in the self-regulation of addictive behavior change. We postulated that attributions of the cause of a slip (the first drink, cigarette, or other substance following a period of voluntary abstinence) to internal, uncontrollable factors such as lack of willpower or an underlying addictive disease make it less likely that the individual will cope in an attempt to regain control. Attributions of a slip to external (situational) factors that are controllable (via learning new coping responses), on the other hand, may facilitate coping as a means of preventing the lapse from escalating into a relapse. Along similar lines, Chaney and Roszell (Chapter 11) make a distinction between self-efficacy ratings for relapse prevention (prevention of the initial lapse) and for relapse termination (stopping use once a lapse occurs) and report significant differences between these two efficacy ratings in different risk situations. Future research that includes assessment of both self-efficacy and attributions for coping should prove valuable in providing answers to some of these questions.

Another key issue that arises in the present text is whether treatment differs from self-initiated attempts to change. Several authors studied the process of self-initiated habit change, including Shiffman (Chapter 9), Curry and Marlatt (Chapter 10), Perri (Chapter 12), and DiClemente and Prochaska (Chapters 13 and 14). Although the primary focus in these chapters is on smoking, Perri (Chapter 12) extended his analysis to weight loss and changing drinking patterns. Although few studies made a direct comparison between self-initiated change and treatment-mediated change, it is of interest theoretically to speculate about such comparisons. One would expect significant differences in motivation and the use of coping skills between individuals who have attempted to change on their own and those who have sought professional treatment for their problem.

One important consideration in this regard is the way in which the change process is perceived by self-quitters versus treatment-quitters. Perhaps those who have received external treatment (e.g., medication, aversion, hypnosis, skill training) believe that treatment is most effective in its early stages but that, in the long run, the effects wear off over time. People who hold this belief may feel they are in greater danger of relapse as the time since treatment termination increases. Relapse curves should show short-term positive benefits of treatment (lower relapse rates), followed by higher relapse rates in the long-term if treatment is considered to be of maximal effectiveness closer to the time of its administration. Self-quitters, on the other hand, may make several attempts or trials before they can master the skills required to cope with temptations. The relapse rates for self-quitters may therefore resemble a trial-and-error learning curve (as the new skills are mastered) in which higher initial rates of relapse are followed by a stabilization effect with fewer errors or lapses occurring in the long run (see Schachter, 1982). Clearly, we can learn much from future research that compares the process of habit change with and without external treatment.

There are a number of important methodological problems that must be taken into account in future research on stress and coping in substance abuse. Despite the common topics covered in the text, there is still a wide variation evident in methodological approaches used by various investigators. Retrospective cross-sectional studies of relapse and of the initiation of substance abuse are still commonly used, despite the advantages of prospective, longitudinal studies with long-term follow-up periods. Further work is also needed to improve our understanding of high-risk situations and their psychometric properties (e.g., relative frequency of occurrence over time, duration, intensity of temptation). Questionnaire and survey studies that depend on global definitions of stress and temptation should be augmented with assessment of specific situations specified on a day-to-day basis.

Similarly, we are still in the early stages of developing a reliable assessment procedure for categorizing and measuring coping responses. Although we make distinctions, say, between cognitive and behavioral coping responses, such distinctions remain somewhat arbitrary. It is difficult, for example, to conceive of a behavioral coping response that was not preceded by cognitive appraisal and decision making that dictates the choice of a specific coping response, be it behavioral or cognitive. Coping categories based on temporal and problem-focused stages of coping seem to offer the greatest promise in this regard. Greater attention also must be paid to general life-style factors as potential mediators of stress and coping, including the role of social support, socioeconomic and demographic status, basic religious and other beliefs, and the use of exercise and relaxation.

Finally, despite our initial success with the psychosocial approach to the study of stress and coping, we must begin to integrate these findings with the biology of substance abuse, as indicated by Grunberg and Baum (Chapter 2). Clearly, substance abuse is influenced strongly by both psychosocial and biobehavioral determinants. Any complete account of the problem of addiction must include both these perspectives. In the past, traditional theories of addiction have placed too much emphasis on the pharmacology and physiology of addictive *drugs,* and only recently has progress been made in bringing back the *person* into the picture. Future research based on an integrative approach that shows how the psychosocial and biobehavioral facets of the problem interact and are reciprocally determined will provide the greatest payoff for both understanding addiction and the development of effective prevention and treatment programs.

REFERENCES

Ainslie, G. (1975). Specious reward: A behavioral theory of impulsiveness and impulse control. *Psychological Bulletin, 82,* 463–496.

Alexander, B. K., & Hadaway, P. F. (1982). Opiate addiction: The case for adaptive orientation. *Psychological Bulletin, 92,* 367–381.

Bandura, A. (1977). *Social learning theory.* Englewood Cliffs, NJ: Prentice-Hall.

Bandura, A. (1982). Self-efficacy mechanism in human agency. *American Psychologist, 37,* 122–147.

Beach, B. H., & Beach, L. R. (1982). Expectancy-based decision schemes: Sidesteps toward applications. In N. T. Feather (Ed.), *Expectations and actions: Expectancy-value models in psychology.* Hillsdale, NJ: Erlbaum.

Beck, A. T. (1976). *Cognitive therapy and the emotional disorders.* New York: International Universities Press.

Brickman, P., Rabinowitz, V. C., Karuza, J., Coates, D., Cohn, E., & Kidder, L. (1982). Models of helping and coping. *American Psychologist, 37,* 368–384.

Brown, S. A., Goldman, M. S., Inn, A., & Anderson, L. R. (1980). Expectations of reinforcement from alcohol: Their domain and relation to drinking patterns. *Journal of Consulting and Clinical Psychology, 48,* 419–426.

Cappell, H. (1975). An evaluation of tension models of alcohol consumption. In Y. Gibbins, H. Israel, & R. E. Kalant (Eds.), *Research advances in alcohol and drug problems* (Vol. 2). New York: Wiley.

Chaney, E. F., O'Leary, M. R., & Marlatt, G. A. (1978). Skill training with alcoholics. *Journal of Consulting and Clinical Psychology, 46,* 1092–1104.

DeLongis, A., Coyne, J. C., Dakof, G., Folkman, S., & Lazarus, R. S. (1982). Relationship of daily hassles, uplifts, and major life events to health status. *Health Psychology, 1,* 119–136.

George, W. H., & Marlatt, G. A. (1983). Alcoholism: The evolution of a behavioral perspective. In M. Galanter (Ed.), *Recent developments in alcoholism* (Vol. 1). New York: Plenum Press.

Glasser, W. (1976). *Positive addiction.* New York: Harper & Row.

Jellinek, E. M. (1960). *The disease concept in alcoholism.* New Brunswick, NJ: Hill House Press.

Kanner, A. D., Coyne, J. C., Schaefer, C., & Lazarus, R. S. (1981). Comparison of two modes of stress measurement: Daily hassles and uplifts vs. major life events. *Behavioral Medicine, 4,* 1–39.

Lazarus, R. S. (1966). *Psychological stress and the coping process.* New York: McGraw-Hill.

Lettieri, D. J., Sayers, M., & Pearson, H. W. (Eds.). (1980). *Theories on drug abuse: Selected contemporary perspectives* (NIDA Research Monograph #30). Washington, DC: U.S. Government Printing Office.

Marlatt, G. A. (1976). Alcohol, stress, and cognitive control. In I. G. Sarason & C. D. Spielberger (Eds.), *Stress and anxiety* (Vol. 3). Washington, DC: Hemisphere.

Marlatt, G. A. (1984, March). *Alcohol, the magic elixir: Stress, expectancy, and the transformation of emotional states.* Paper presented at the annual Coatesville Jefferson Conference, Stress, Alcohol, and Drug Interactions, Coatesville, PA.

Marlatt, G. A., & Gordon, J. R. (1980). Determinants of relapse: Implications for the maintenance of behavior change. In P. O. Davidson & S. M. Davidson (Eds.), *Behavioral medicine: Changing health lifestyles*. New York: Brunner/Mazel.

Marlatt, G. A., & Gordon, J. R. (1985). *Relapse prevention: Maintenance strategies in the treatment of addictive behaviors*. New York: Guilford Press.

Marlatt, G. A., & Marques, J. K. (1977). Meditation, self-control and alcohol use. In R. B. Stuart (Ed.), *Behavioral self-management: Strategies, techniques and outcomes*. New York: Brunner/Mazel.

Meichenbaum, D. (1977). *Cognitive-behavior modification*. New York: Plenum Press.

Moos, R. H., & Billings, A. G. (1982). Conceptualizing and measuring coping resources and processes. In L. Goldberger & S. Breznitz (Eds.), *Handbook of stress: Theoretical and clinical aspects*. New York: Macmillan.

Murphy, T., Pagano, R. R., & Marlatt, G. A. (1984). *Lifestyle modification with heavy alcohol drinkers: Effects of aerobic exercise and meditation*. Manuscript submitted for publication.

Schachter, S. (1982). Recidivism and self-cure of smoking and obesity. *American Psychologist, 37,* 436–444.

Siegel, S. (1979). The role of conditioning in drug tolerance and addiction. In J. D. Keehn (Ed.), *Psychopathology in animals: Research and treatment implications*. New York: Academic Press.

Skinner, H. A., & Allen, B. A. (1982). Alcohol dependence syndrome: Measurement and validation. *Journal of Abnormal Psychology, 91,* 199–209.

Solomon, R. L. (1980). The opponent-process theory of acquired motivation: The costs of pleasure and the benefits of pain. *American Psychologist, 35,* 691–712.

Southwick, L., Steele, C., Marlatt, A., & Lindell, M. (1981). Alcohol-related expectancies: Defined by phase of intoxication and drinking experience. *Journal of Consulting and Clinical Psychology, 49,* 713–721.

Author Index

Numbers in italics refer to the pages on which the complete references are cited.

A

Abelson, H. I., 74, 92
Abrams, D. B., 13, 15, 20, 21, 67, 92, 173, 174, 196, 197, 198, 199, 219, 360
Adams, R. D., 40, 61
Adkins, D., 20, 24
Agnati, L. F., 46, 47, 55
Aiken, P. A., 3, 22
Ainslie, G., 375, 385
Albee, G., 118, 139
Alexander, B. K., 3, 21, 149, 166, 168, 168, 227, 240, 267, 268, 289, 291, 368, 385
Allegrante, J. P., 114
Allen, B. A., 369, 386
Altman, F., 267, 284, 291
Altshuler, H. L., 49, 54
Amenson, C. S., 4, 23, 69, 93
Amér, B., 30, 55
Amér, I., 30, 55
Amir, S., 30, 54
Amit, Z., 30, 54
Anderson, L., 173, 196, 197, 375, 385
Aneshensel, C. S., 119, 120, 126, 139, 272, 291, 348, 362
Antonovsky, A., 167, 168
Antonucci, T. C., 174, 175, 197
Appel, P. W., 271, 291
Archer, E., 139
Arkowitz, H., 108, 115, 310, 316
Armor, D. J., 295, 302, 309, 315, 317
Arnon, D., 151, 169
Arundell, R., 139
Ary, D. V., 97, 99, 100, 103, 109, 114, 116
Ashton, H., 18, 21
Austin, G. A., 147, 168
Averill, J. R., 128, 141
Avis, N., 13, 23

B

Bachman, J. G., 17, 22, 121, 140
Baeder, D. H., 32, 60
Baer, P. E., 237, 240, 322, 342
Bahna, G., 149, 168
Bain, G., 33, 34, 50, 58
Baizman, E. R., 39, 43, 47, 48, 50, 53, 55
Bajusz, E., 32, 60
Baker, E., 82, 93
Balter, M., 175, 182, 198, 271, 272, 292, 346, 347, 348, 361, 363
Bandura, A., 118, 120, 123, 126, 127, 139, 296, 300, 312, 315, 368, 369, 385
Bane, A. L., 96, 109, 115
Barnes, G. M., 209, 219
Barnett, L. W., 295, 316
Barrett, J. E., 26, 37, 52, 54
Baucom, D. H., 3, 22
Baum, A., 15, 26, 29, 54, 384
Bauman, K. E., 96, 114
Bavry, J., 95, 100, 114, 116
Beach, B. H., 375, 385
Beach, L. R., 375, 385
Beard, E. L., 32, 54
Beck, A. T., 205, 219, 368, 385
Becker, M. H., 128, 142
Belenko, S., 154, 161, 168
Bellack, A. S., 103, 104, 105, 114, 312, 317
Benfari, R. C., 262, 265, 319, 342
Benner, P., 120, 126, 142
Benson, J. A., Jr., 31, 56
Bentler, P. M., 67, 92, 121, 122, 124, 126, 127, 138, 139, 140
Berger, L. H., 148, 169
Bergin, A., 345, 362
Bernstein, A., 3, 19, 22, 196, 197
Berstein, D. A., 300, 315
Bespalec, D. A., 326, 342

Best, J. A., 14, 22, 102, *115*
Bethune, J. E., 28, *54*
Bhargava, H. N., 46, *54*
Bianchine, J. R., 49, *56*
Bigelow, G. E., 34, 36, 38, 42, 52, *56*, 237, *240*
Biglan, A., 15, 17, 91, *93*, *95*, *96*, *97*, *99*, 100, 102, 103, 105, 108, 109, 113, 114, *115*, *116*, 370, 379, 380
Billings, A. G., 8, 10, *24*, 148, 151, 156, 167, *169*, 201, *219*, 239, *241*, 269, 274, 281, *292*, 379, *386*
Bliss, F., 302, *315*
Bloom, F. E., 26, 46, 47, 48, 50, *54*
Bloxom, A. L., 346, *363*
Blum, K., 49, *54*
Bodnar, R. J., 31, *54*
Bohus, B., 30, *54*
Bolme, P., 46, 47, *55*
Border, J. R., 32, *55*
Borgers, D., 74, *92*
Borman, A., 32, *57*
Borowski, E., 50, *61*
Botvin, G. J., 15, 22, 63, *65*, 67, 82, 90, *92*, *93*, *96*, *115*, 118, 128, 139, *139*
Bosquet, W. F., 32, *55*, *60*
Bowen, M., 360, *362*
Bradley, R., 46, 47, *55*
Brady, J. V., 33, 36, *55*
Braiker, H. B., 295, 302, 309, *317*
Branch, L. G., 295, *316*
Brandenberg, N., 328, *343*
Brecher, E. M., 38, *55*
Brehm, S. S., 310, *315*
Breuer, C., 32, *57*
Brickman, P., 118, 139, *139*, 371, 372, *385*
Bromet, E., 302, *315*
Brooks, G. W., 30, *58*
Broste, S. K., 223, *241*
Brotman, R., 150, *170*
Brown, B. S., 267, 284, *291*
Brown, C. H., 119, *141*
Brown, S., 173, 196, *197*, 375, *385*
Brown, Z. A., 30, *54*
Brownell, K. D., 313, 314, *315*
Brutus, M., 31, *54*
Bry, B., 130, *139*
Bryant, F., 178, 179, *197*, *198*
Bugen, L. A., 69, *92*
Bunnell, B. N., 29, 47, *58*
Burling, T. A., 237, *240*
Burt, M., 148, 149, *168*
Butler, L., 118, *141*
Butt, N. M., 47, *55*

C

Cafferata, G. L., 3, 19, 22, 196, *197*
Cahalan, D., 209, *219*, 295, 309, *315*
Campbell, F., 29, *55*
Cannon, W. B., 27, 31, *55*
Cappell, H., 36, *55*, 369, *385*
Carroll, E. E., 147, *168*
Carroll, G. F., 32, *54*
Carroll, L. J., 312, *315*
Cartensen, H., 30, *55*
Caryn, M. A., 74, *93*
Cavanaugh, J., 42, *56*
Center for Disease Control & National Cancer Institute, 295, *315*, 321, *342*
Chamberlain, K., 3, *23*
Chan, D. A., 268, *292*
Chaney, E. F., 7, 20, 22, 236, 270, 275, 276, 279, 290, *291*, 345, 377, 378, 379, 380, 382, 383, *385*
Chaplin, J. P., 32, *60*
Chase, J. A., 18, *23*, 68, *93*
Chassin, L., 17, 22, 96, 98, *115*, *116*, 137, *139*, *140*
Chavkin, C., 30, *55*
Chelune, G. J., 271, *291*
Christiansen, B. A., 14, 22
Cisin, I., 74, *92*, 175, 182, *198*, 209, *219*, 271, 272, *292*, 346, 347, *363*
Clark, C. P., *115*
Clark, R., 49, *55*
Cleary, P. D., 13, 14, 15, *23*, 63, *65*, 67, *93*, *96*, *116*, 181, *197*, 295, 313, *316*, 319, 320, *342*
Co, C., 50, *61*
Coates, D., 118, 139, *139*, 371, 372, *385*
Coates, T. J., 67, *92*
Cobb, S., 30, *58*
Cohen, F., 201, *219*, 320, *342*
Cohen, J., 76, 82, *92*, *115*, 234, *240*
Cohen, P., 76, 82, *92*, *115*
Cohen, S., 19, 20, *22*, *23*, 68, 82, 84, *92*
Cohn, E., 118, 139, *139*, 371, 372, *385*
Colletti, G., 314, *315*
Collier, H. O. J., 47, *55*

Collins, L. M., 98, *115*
Colten, M. E., 10, 12, 144, 147, 149, 150, 155, 166, *168*, 217, 374
Condiotte, M., 237, *240*, 286, *291*, 300, *315*
Conway, T. L., 19, 22
Cooper, J. R., 267, 284, *291*
Cooperstock, R., 148, *169*
Corbit, J. D., 35, *61*
Corty, E., 22, 138, *140*
Cosgrove, J., 102, *115*
Cowen, E. L., 347, *362*
Cox, B. M., 30, 39, 43, 46, 47, 48, 50, 53, 54, *55*
Coyne, J. C., 4, 6, 11, 22, 172, *197*, 200, 201, *219*, 374, *385*
Crandell, D. L., 347, *362*
Crimi, P., 337, *342*
Cronkite, R. C., 20, 22, 268, *291*
Cross, D. G., 308, *315*
Crossley, H. M., 209, *219*
Crowell, C. R., 36, *55*
Cullen, M. H., 49, *57*
Cummings, C., 224, 236, *240*, 276, 279, *291*
Cunningham, C. L., 36, *58*, *59*
Cunningham, W. R., 138, *140*
Curry, S., 20, 21, 224, 237, 269, 286, 290, 380, 383
Curzon, G., 32, *56*
Cuskey, W. R., 148, *169*
Cuthbert, N. J., 47, *55*
Czechowicz, D., 267, 284, *291*

D

Dakof, G., 4, 22, 374, *385*
Danaher, B., 118, *141*
Danos, G. T., 32, *54*
d'Avernas, J. R., 102, *115*
Davis, D. H., 37, *60*
Davis, V. E., 49, *55*
Davis, W. N., 173, 196, *198*
Deardorff, C. M., 173, 174, *197*
Deci, E. L., 310, *315*
DeLongis, A., 4, 22, 374, *385*
Demone, H. W., 209, *220*
Densen-Gerber, J., 148, *169*
Dent, C. W., 96, *114*
Depner, C. E., 174, 175, 180, *197*, *198*

DeVellis, R., 70, 81, *93*
DeWied, D., 30, *54*, *55*
Dews, P. B., 37, *56*
DiClemente, C. C., 11, 15, 17, 19, 22, 222, 322, 323, 325, 328, 338, *342*, *343*, 345, 346, 349, *362*, 369, 370, 377, 378, 380, 381, 383
Diener, E., 13, *22*
Dill, C. A., 96, 102, *115*
Dillman, T. E., 128, *142*
Doell, S. R., 3, 22
Doerfler, L. A., 312, *315*
Dohrenwend, B. P., 4, 22, 143, *145*, 179, *197*, 205, *219*, 346, 347, *362*
Dohrenwend, B. S., 4, 22, 143, *145*
Donegan, N. H., 39, 40, 41, 49, *55*
Donovan, D. M., 290, *291*
Donovan, J. E., 18, *23*, 68, *93*
Douvan, E., 177, 178, 179, 180, 183, *198*, 347, *363*
Dow, M. G., 108, 113, *115*
Driever, C. W., 32, *55*
Dunnette, M., 128, *140*
D'Zurilla, T. J., 237, *240*, 314, *315*

E

Eaker, E. D., 319, *342*
Eastwood, M. R., 347, *362*
Eggers, J., 104, 111, 112, *115*
Egri, G., 179, *197*, 346, *362*
Ehrman, R., 36, *60*
Eiser, J. R., 20, *23*, 236, *240*, 269, 284, *292*
Eisinger, R. A., 262, *265*
Eisler, R. M., 101, 103, *115*
Ekehammar, B., 291, *292*
Eldred, A. E., 158, 165, *169*
Elmadjian, F., 28, *55*
Emrich, H. M., 30, 31, *59*
Endó, J., 50, *61*
Eng, A., 90, *92*, 118, 128, 139, *139*
Epstein, S., *140*, 239, *240*
Erbaugh, J., 205, *219*
Esposito, R. U., 34, *55*
Eubanks, J. D., 49, *54*
Euker, J. S., 30, *56*
Evans, R. I., 69, *92*, 95, 96, 97, 102, 109, *115*

F

Falk, J. L., 26, 37, 56
Faller, C., 99, 102, 103, 105, 109, *114*
Farkas, M. I., 154, *169*
Feinhandler, D. A., 49, *54*
Fendler, K., 30, *56*
Fertel, R. H., 49, *56*
Festinger, L., 101, *115*
Fidell, L. S., *169*
Finney, J. W., 268, *292*
Fishburne, P. M., 74, *92*
Fishman, A. P., 31, *61*
Fishman, J., 39, *56*
Flay, B. R., 102, *115*
Fleming, J. P., 119, *141*
Fleming, J. S., 82, *93*
Florin, P., 126, *142*
Folkman, S., 4, 10, *22*, 151, *169*, 201, *219*, *239*, *240*, 374, *385*
Follick, M. J., 360
Ford, M. E., 119, *140*
Foreyt, J. P., 237, *240*, 322, *342*
Francis, D. L., 47, *55*
Frank, J. D., 346, 361, *362*
Frankenhaeuser, M., 29, *56*
Frederikson, L. W., *115*
Freeman, M. E., 50, *61*
Friedman, L. S., 91, *93*, 96, 99, 103, 105, *114*, *115*
Frith, C. D., 14, *22*
Froman, T., 138, *140*
Fuchs, C. Z., 312, *315*, *317*
Furner, R. L., 32, *61*
Fuxe, K., 46, 47, *55*

G

Gallison, C., 109, *114*
Gallo, E., 32, *55*
Gambrill, E. S., 70, *93*
Garber, J., 173, *197*
Gardner, E., 129, 130, *140*
Garrow, J. S., 313, *315*
George, F. E., 130, *139*
George, W. H., 369, *385*
Gershaw, N. J., 119, 128, 131, *140*
Gerstein, D. R., 154, *169*
Gibertini, M., 15, *22*, 328, *342*, 346, *362*
Gibson, A., 30, 31, *56*
Gilbert, D. G., 6, 14, *22*, 236, *240*, 320, *342*

Gilchrist, L. O., 118, 119, 127, 128, *140*, *142*
Ginsburg, M., 30, 31, *56*
Gispen, W. H., 30, *54*
Glaser, S. R., 108, 113, *115*
Glasgow, R., 108, 109, *114*, *115*
Glasser, W., 375, *385*
Glauser, E. M., 41, *56*
Glauser, S. C., 41, *56*
Glusman, M., 31, *54*
Glynn, K., 91, *93*
Glynn, T. J., 148, 149, *168*
Goldberg, D. P., 205, *219*
Goldberg, I., 347, *363*
Goldberg, S. R., 37, *56*
Goldfried, M. R., 237, *240*, 314, *315*, 361, *362*
Goldman, M. S., 14, *22*, 173, 196, *197*, 375, *385*
Goldstein, A., 30, *55*
Goldstein, A. P., 119, 128, 131, *140*
Goldstein, J. M., 46, 47, 48, *58*
Goldstein, S., 11, 12, 244, 262, *265*, 310, *315*
Gomberg, E. S. L., 147, *169*
Gordon, J. R., 15, *22*, 224, 236, *240*, 243, 244, *265*, 268, 270, 274, 276, 280, 288, *292*, 310, *316*, 325, 340, *342*, 345, 346, *362*, *363*, 370, 372, 376, 382, 383, *386*
Gordon, N. B., 149, *168*
Gordon, N. P., 63, *65*
Gore, S., 153, *169*
Gottlieb, N., 209, *220*
Gottlieb, N. H., 13, *23*
Gottman, J. M., 138, *141*
Gourash, N., 174, *197*
Grabowski, J., 36, *60*
Graham, J. W., 98, *115*
Gray, J. J., 312, *315*
Gray, S. J., 31, *56*
Green, A. R., 32, *56*
Green, D. E., 13, *23*, 74, *93*, 228, *240*
Greene, N. M., 42, *60*
Greenson, R., 360, *362*
Greenwald, J. E., 49, *56*
Griffith, J. D., 42, *56*
Griffiths, C. T., 128, 138, *142*
Griffiths, R. R., 34, 36, 38, 42, 52, *56*
Grinder, R. E., 139, *140*
Gritz, E., 243, *265*

AUTHOR INDEX 391

Groza, P., 32, 56
Grunberg, N. E., 15, 26, 29, 41, 51, 52, 56, 384
Gruson, L., 118, *141*
Gunn, R. C., 20, *23*
Guthrie, T. J., 96, 102, *115*

H

Hadaway, P. F., 3, *21*, 149, 166, 168, *168*, 227, *240*, 267, 268, 289, *291*, 368, 385
Hadley, S. W., 346, 361, *363*
Haertzen, C. A., 39, *56*
Hakstian, A. R., 14, *22*
Haley, N. J., 74, *93*
Hall, M., 30, 31, *56*
Hall, S. M., 295, *315*
Ham, J. M., 32, *56*
Hambrecht, M., 346, *363*
Hannon, J. R., 271, *292*
Hansen, W. B., 69, *92*, 96, 97, 98, 109, *115*
Harding, J. S., 143, *145*
Hart, S. L., 30, 31, *56*
Harvey, S. C., 42, *56*
Hastings, A. G., 49, *57*
Hatsukami, D., 236, *240*
Hauss, W. H., 32, *56*
Havis, J., 96, 109, *115*
Hawkins, R. C., 3, *22*, 69, 70, *92*
Hecht, E., 322, 332, *342*
Hedges, S. M., 205, *219*
Heffernan, T., 315, *315*
Held, J., 42, *56*
Heller, K., 128, *140*
Helzer, J. E., 37, *60*
Henderson, A. H., 96, 102, *115*
Henningfield, J. E., 34, 36, 38, 42, 52, 56, *57*
Henrik, R., 358, *362*
Herbert, M., 49, *57*
Herman, C. P., 52, *60*
Hersen, M., 15, *24*, 104, *114*, 271, *293*
Hess, S., 34, 49, *58*
Hilf, R., 32, *57*
Hill, P. C., 96, 102, *115*
Hillier, V. F., 205, *219*
Hinson, R. E., 36, *61*
Hirschman, R. S., 91, *93*
Hoberman, H., 84, *92*

Holaday, J. W., 28, 39, 46, 47, 48, 51, *57*
Holbrook, J. M., 41, 42, 43, 44, 45, *57*
Holmes, T. H., 201, 205, *219*, 220, 273, *291*
Hooks, N. T., 39, *56*
Hops, H., 99, 102, 103, 105, *114*, *115*
Horan, J. J., 104, *115*
Horn, D. A., 13, *23*, 228, *240*
Horvath, W. J., 128, *142*
Hout, C. N., 173, 174, *197*
Huba, G. J., 119, 120, 121, 122, 124, 125, 126, 127, *139*, *140*, *141*, 272, *291*, 348, *362*
Hubert, L. J., 138, *140*
Hughes, J., 47, *58*
Hughes, J. R., 236, *240*
Hung, L. H., 46, *61*
Hunt, W. A., 221, 222, 223, *240*, 295, *315*, 326, *342*
Hurd, P. D., 118, *140*
Hurwitz, I., 262, *265*
Husaini, B. A., 14, *24*, *198*, 201, 216, *219*
Hymowitz, N., 223, *241*

I

Ikard, F. F., 13, *23*, 228, *240*
Ilfeld, F. W., Jr., 82, *93*, 268, *291*
Ingle, D. J., 28, *57*
Inhelder, B., 119, *142*
Inn, A., 14, *22*, 173, 196, *197*, 375, *385*

J

Jackson, D. N., 205, *219*
Jacobs, D. R., 118, *140*
Jacobs, G. A., 338, *343*
Jaffe, J. H., 33, 34, 35, 38, 39, 40, 41, 42, 43, 44, 45, 52, *57*
Jandorf, L., 205, *219*
Janis, I. L., 327, *342*
Jarvik, M. E., 41, *57*, 237, *241*, 244, 259, 263, *265*
Jasinski, D. R., 36, 39, *56*, *59*
Jeffcoate, W. J., 49, *57*
Jeffery, R. W., 296, *316*
Jellinek, E. M., 368, *385*
Jenkins, C. D., 26, *57*
Jessor, R., 18, *23*, 68, *93*, 118, 120, 127, 128, 136, *140*, 174, *197*
Jessor, S. L., 118, 120, 127, *140*, 174, *197*
Jhamandas, K., 50, *57*

Johnson, B. D., 147, *168, 169*
Johnson, C. A., 90, *93,* 97, 99, *116,* 118, 128, *140, 141*
Johnson, P. B., 188, *197*
Johnson, T., 20, *24,* 224, 238, *241*
Johnston, L. D., 17, *22,* 121, *140*
Jones, C., 271, *293*
Jones, E. E., 328, *342*
Jones, S. L., 270, *291*
Jöreskog, K. G., 124, *140*
Judd, C. M., 98, *116*
Judd, I. L., 154, *169*
Junge, B., 74, *92*
Jurani, M., 32, *60*

K

Kaestner, E., 271, *291*
Kahle, L. R., 126, *140*
Kahn, J. A., 308, *315*
Kahn, R. L., 174, *197*
Kalant, H., 36, *58*
Kalant, O. J., 147, *169*
Kalin, R., 173, *196, 197*
Kandel, D. B., 17, 18, *23,* 63, *65,* 68, *93,* 119, 122, *141*
Kanfer, F. H., 296, 297, 300, 312, *316*
Kanfer, R., 270, *291*
Kanner, A. D., 374, *385*
Kant, G. J., 29, 30, 47, *58*
Kaplan, H. B., 18, *23*
Karoly, P., 296, 297, 312, *316*
Karuza, J., 118, 139, *139,* 371, 372, *385*
Kasl, S. V., 30, *58*
Kasper, J., 3, 19, *22,* 196, *197*
Kazdin, A. E., 123, 124, 129, 130, *141*
Kellam, S. G., 119, *141*
Kelly, D. D., 30, 31, *54, 58*
Kelly, J. G., 119, *141*
Kerlinger, F. N., 134, *141*
Kern, J. M., 104, 111, 112, *115*
Kersell, M. A., 102, *115*
Kessler, R. C., 17, 18, *23,* 68, *93,* 119, *141,* 181, *197*
Khantzian, E. J., 149, *169*
Kidder, L., 118, 139, *139,* 371, 372, *385*
Killen, J., 67, *92,* 118, *141*
Kim, S., 128, 138, *141*
Kirschenbaum, D. S., 295, 296, 301, 310, 312, *316*

Kirschner, L. B., 31, *58*
Kissin, B., 151, *168*
Kleber, H. D., 271, 272, 273, *291, 293*
Klee, W. A., 47, *58*
Klein, P., 119, 128, 131, *140*
Kleinman, M., 151, *168*
Klingel, D. M., 126, *140*
Kniskern, J., 100, *116*
Knox, W. E., 32, *58*
Kohrs, M. B., 300, 314, *316*
Konturek, S. J., 39, *58*
Kopel, S., 310, *316*
Kopin, I. J., 32, *58*
Kornblith, S. J., 312, *317*
Kornetsky, C., 33, 34, 50, *58*
Kosten, T. R., 272, 273, *291*
Kosterlitz, H. W., 47, *58*
Kozak, C., 117, 119, 128, 138, *141*
Kozlowski, L. T., 52, *60*
Krank, M. D., 36, *61*
Krasnegor, N., 28, *59*
Krosnick, J. A., 98, *116*
Krueger, D. W., 20, *23,* 273, *291*
Kruskal, J. B., 277, 278, *291*
Kulka, R. A., 126, *140,* 177, 178, 179, 180, 183, *198,* 347, *363*
Kvetnansky, R., 32, *58*

L

Lambert, M., 361, *362*
Lamparski, D., 104, *114*
Lando, H. A., *342*
Lane, J. D., 50, *61*
Langner, T. S., 7, *24,* 143, *145,* 347, *362*
Lanyon, R. I., 270, *291*
Lapsanski, D., 337, *342*
Lasagna, L., 35, *58*
Launier, R., 320, *342*
Law, P.-Y., 51, *57*
Lawson, T. R., 273, *293*
Lazarus, R. S., 4, 6, 8, 10, 11, 22, *23,* 33, 48, *58,* 120, 126, 128, *141, 142,* 151, *169,* 173, *197,* 200, 201, *219,* 239, 240, 290, 292, 320, *342,* 369, 374, 379, *385*
Lefcoe, N. M., 322, *342*
Leighton, D. C., 143, *145*
Lennox, S., 6, 11, 374
Lenox, R. H., 29, 47, *58*

AUTHOR INDEX

Leon, G. R., 3, *23*
Leong, C., 131, *141*
Lettieri, D. J., 33, *58*, 147, 165, *168, 169*, 267, *291*, 367, *385*
Levenson, R. W., 138, *141*
Leventhal, H., 13, 14, 15, *23*, 63, *65*, 67, 91, *93*, 96, *116*, 295, 313, *315*, 319, 320, *342*
Levine, A. S., 34, 47, 48, 49, 50, 51, 52, *58*
Levine, E., 117, 119, 128, 138, *141*
Levison, P. K., 33, *58*
Lewinsohn, P. M., 4, *23*, 69, *93*, 212, *219*
Lewyckj, R., 278, *293*
Li, C. H., 46, 51, *57, 61*
Libet, J., 212, *219*
Lichtenstein, E., 11, 20, 21, *23*, 24, 91, *93*, 96, 100, 105, 109, *114, 115, 116*, 223, 237, *240*, 243, *265*, 286, *291*, 296, 300, 310, 313, 314, *315, 316*, 338, *342*
Liebling, B., 52, *60*
Lin, B. C., 46, *61*
Lin, C. S., 46, *61*
Lin, S.-H., 46, *61*
Lindell, M., 14, *24*, 375, *386*
Lindenthal, J. J., 205, *219*
Lipman, R., 347, 348, 361, *363*
Litman, G. K., 20, *23*, 236, *240*, 269, 284, *291*
Locke, H. J., 205, *219*
Loh, H. H., 39, 46, 48, 51, *57, 61*
Ludwig, W. W., 314, *317*
Luepker, R. V., 90, *93*, 97, 99, 102, *116*, 118, 128, *140, 141*
Lungu, D., 32, *56*
Lutz, R. N., 300, 314, *316*

M

McAdoo, W. G., 314, *316, 317*
McAlister, A., 15, *22*, 63, *65*, 67, 92, 96, 102, *115, 116*, 119, 139, *141*, 360, *362*
McAllister, D. A., 310, *315*
McClearn, G. E., 26, *59*
McClelland, D. C., 173, 180, 196, *198*
Maccoby, N., 102, *116*, 119, 139, *141*
McConnell, S., 95, 100, *114*
McCully, J., 36, *61*

McIntyre, K., *24*, 310, 314, *316*, 319, 338, *342*
Mack, J. F., 149, *169*
McKearney, J. W., 37, *58*
McKennell, A. C., 13, 18, *23*, 86, *93*
MacMahon, B., 96, *116*
MacMahon, H. E., 31, *58*
Macklin, D. B., 143, *145*
McReynolds, W. T., 300, 314, *316*
Magnusson, D., 291, *292*
Mahoney, M. J., 298, *317*
Malick, J. B., 46, 47, 48, *58*
Maltese, J., 237, *241*, 263, *265*
Manheimer, D., 175, 182, *198*, 346, 347, *363*
Mann, L., 327, *342*
Mansfield, J. G., 36, *59*
Margulies, R. Z., 17, 18, *23*, 68, *93*, 119, *141*
Marks, P. A., 346, *363*
Marlatt, G. A., 11, 12, 14, 15, 20, 21, 22, *23*, 24, 171, 174, 175, 176, 187, *195, 198*, 224, 236, 237, *240*, *241*, 243, 244, 254, 262, 263, *265*, 268, 269, 270, 274, 275, 276, 280, 286, 288, 290, *291, 292*, 310, 314, *315, 316*, 325, 340, *342*, 346, *363*, 369, 370, 372, 374, 375, 376, 380, 382, 383, *385, 386*
Marques, J. K., 236, *240*, 382, *386*
Marsh, J. C., 149, *169*
Martel, L., 337, *342*
Martin, S. S., 18, *23*
Martin, W. R., 38, 39, *57, 59*
Mason, J. W., 26, 29, 30, *59*
Masterpasqua, F., 127, *141*
Masuda, M., 205, *220*
Matarazzo, J. E., 221, *240*
Mathews, C. O., 310, *316*
Maxwell, S. E., 96, 102, 109, *115*
Mechanic, D., *219*
Mehrabian, A., 6, 15, *24*
Mehren, B., 302, *316*
Meichenbaum, D., 10, *23*, 88, *93*, 118, *141*, 368, *386*
Meites, J., 30, *56*
Melges, F. T., 173, 174, *197*
Mellinger, G., 175, 182, *198*, 346, 347, *363*
Mello, N. K., 37, 40, *59*
Mendelsohn, F. S., 179, *197*, 346, *362*

Mendelson, J. H., 37, 40, 59
Mendelson, M., 205, 219
Mermelstein, R., 11, 20, 21, 23, 24, 310, 314, 316, 338, 342
Mettlin, C., 95, 116
Meyeroff, J. L., 29, 30, 47, 58
Michael, S. T., 143, 145
Millan, M. J., 30, 31, 59
Miller, C., 104, 111, 112, 115
Miller, W. R., 314, 316
Milliones, J., 15, 24, 271, 293
Mischel, W., 270, 292
Mittelmark, M. B., 69, 92, 96, 97, 99, 109, 115, 116
Miya, T. S., 32, 60
Mock, J., 205, 219
Moon, V. H., 31, 59
Moos, B. S., 302, 317
Moos, R. H., 8, 10, 20, 22, 24, 148, 151, 156, 167, 169, 201, 219, 239, 241, 268, 269, 274, 281, 291, 292, 302, 315, 317, 379, 386
Mordkoff, A. M., 32, 59
Morley, J. E., 34, 47, 48, 49, 50, 51, 52, 58, 59
Morris, D. P., 32, 59
Morrison, R. L., 103, 104, 105, 114
Morse, D. E., 52, 56
Mougey, E. H., 30, 58
Murphy, T., 382, 386
Murray, D. M., 90, 93, 97, 99, 116, 119, 128, 141, 142
Myers, J. K., 205, 219

N

Natelson, B. H., 28, 59
National Institute on Drug Abuse, 148, 155, 169
National Research Council, 26, 59
Nautel, C. L., 99, 102, 103, 105, 114, 115
Neale, J. M., 6, 11, 70, 93, 144, 202, 203, 206, 214, 220, 374
Neff, J. A., 14, 24, 198, 201, 216, 219
Neill, J. D., 30, 59
Nelson, R. O., 103, 116
Nemeth, S., 32, 60
Newlin, D. B., 314, 316
Nishi, S. M., 147, 169
Nomura, J., 32, 60

Norcross, J., 346, 349, 359, 361, 363
Novelly, R. A., 271, 293
Nowlis, V., 205, 220
Nurco, D. N., 271, 272, 292
Nuttall, R. L., 262, 265

O

Oates, J. A., 42, 56
O'Brien, C. P., 36, 39, 40, 41, 49, 60, 227, 240
Ockene, I. S., 262, 265
Ockene, J. K., 223, 241, 262, 265, 319, 342
Oehler, G., 32, 60
O'Leary, M. R., 20, 22, 270, 275, 291, 382, 385
Olshavsky, R. W., 17, 22, 116, 137, 140
Olsson, G., 20, 24, 273, 293
O'Malley, P. M., 17, 22, 121, 140
Opler, M. K., 143, 145
Oppenheim, A. N., 20, 23, 236, 240, 269, 284, 292
Opton, E. M., Jr., 128, 141
Ordman, A. M., 310, 312, 316
O'Rourke, T. W., 114

P

Pagano, R. R., 382, 386
Pallenon, U., 116
Parker, J. B., 271, 291
Parkes, C. M., 119, 141
Parks, G. A., 310, 314, 316
Parry, H. J., 175, 182, 198, 347, 363
Paulhus, D., 82, 93
Paulsen, B. K., 300, 314, 316
Pearlin, L. I., 4, 8, 14, 19, 24, 148, 150, 167, 169, 195, 198, 201, 216, 217, 220, 239, 240
Pearson, H. W., 33, 58, 147, 169, 267, 291, 367, 385
Pechacek, T. F., 90, 93, 97, 99, 116, 118, 128, 140, 141, 236, 241
Pederson, L. L., 322, 342
Pedhazur, E. J., 134, 141
Peleg, M., 269, 292
Penick, S. B., 295, 317
Pennington, L. L., 30, 58
Pentz, M. A., 118, 119, 122, 123, 124, 125,

127, 128, 129, 130, 131, 132, 139, 140, *141*, 369, 377
Pepper, M. P., 205, *219*
Perlick, D., 52, *60*
Perri, M. G., 11, 20, 296, 297, 298, 314, 316, 322, 332, *342*, 355, 377, 380, 383
Perry, C., 67, *92*, 102, *116*, 118, 119, 139, *141*, *142*
Perry, W., 34, *55*
Perschuck, M., 20, *24*
Persson, L. O., 3, *24*
Peterson, G. L., *115*
Phillips, P. E., 49, *54*
Piaget, J., 119, *142*
Pilowsky, I., 205, 212, *220*
Pirie, P. L., *116*
Platt, J. J., 271, *292*
Polich, J. M., 295, 302, 309, *315*, *317*
Polish, E., 49, *55*
Pomerleau, O. F., 20, *24*, 41, *60*, 313, *317*
Poulos, C. X., 36, *55*
Prather, J. E., 148, 149, 150, *169*
President's Commission on Mental Health, 346, *363*
Presson, C. C., 17, *22*, 98, *116*, 137, *140*
Price, R. H., 128, *140*
Prochaska, J. O., 11, 17, 19, 222, 322, 323, 325, 328, 337, 338, *342*, *343*, 345, 349, 358, 359, 361, *362*, *363*, 369, 370, 377, 378, 380, 381, 383
Prosser, C. L., 31, *58*
Prusoff, B., 273, *292*

Q

Quastler, H., 31, *58*
Quay, H. C., 117, 130, *142*
Quay, L. C., 117, 130, *142*

R

Raab, W., 32, *60*
Rabinowitz, V. C., 118, 139, *139*, 371, 372, *385*
Radabaugh, C. W., 14, 19, *24*, 195, *198*, 216
Radius, S. M., 128, *142*
Rahe, R. H., 19, 22, 201, *219*, 273, *291*
Raines, B. E., 95, *115*
Rakoczi, I., 30, *56*

Ramirez, S., 87, *93*
Ramsey, C., 31, *56*
Rapkin, D., 237, *241*, 263, *265*
Rawson, N. S. B., 20, *23*, 236, *240*, 269, 284, *292*
Read, L., 237, *241*, 263, *265*
Redfield, J., 202, *220*
Regier, D., 347, *363*
Rehm, L. P., 212, *220*, 312, *315*, *317*
Reid, P., 337, *342*
Reidenberg, M. M., 41, *56*
Reifenstein, R. W., 31, *56*
Reiss, A. J., Jr., 205, *220*
Rennie, T. A. C., 143, *145*
Rhoads, D. L., 20, *24*, 150, *169*
Richards, C. S., 296, 297, 298, 312, 314, 315, *315*, *316*, *317*, 322, 332, *342*
Richey, C., 70, *93*
Rickels, K., 346, *363*
Riedl, M., 34, *58*
Riegle, G. D., 30, *56*
Riordan, C., 273, *292*
Ritchie, J. M., 40, 42, *60*
Roach, C., 36, *55*
Robbins, C., 18, *23*
Roberts, R. E., 346, *363*
Robins, L. N., 37, *60*
Rochefort, G. J., 28, *60*
Rodin, J., 39, 40, 41, 49, 51, *55*, *62*
Rohsenhow, D. J., 236, *241*
Roka, L., 32, *60*
Romano, J. M., 312, *317*
Room, R., 295, 309, *315*
Rosenberg, H. S., 20, *24*, 270, *292*
Rosenberg, M., 82, *93*
Rosenberger, J., 28, *60*
Rosenstock, I. M., 128, *142*
Rosenthal, T., 118, 127, *142*
Roskies, E., 290, *292*
Roszell, D. K., 7, 236, 276, 279, *291*, 345, 377, 378, 379, 380, 383
Roth, D. M., 312, *317*
Rounsaville, B. J., 271, 272, 273, *291*, *293*
Rovner, S. A., 154, *169*
Rowland, N. E., 51, *59*
Rozelle, R. M., 96, 102, 109, *115*
Rozensky, R. H., 312, *317*
Rupe, B. D., 32, *60*
Russ, N. W., 237, *240*
Russel, M., 209, *219*

Russell, H. A., 6, 15, *24*
Russell, M. A. H., 322, *343*
Rusy, B. R., 41, *56*
Ryan, K. B., 102, *115*
Ryser, P. E., 150, *169*

S

Saeed, S. A., 47, *55*
Saffran, M., 28, *60*
Salber, E. J., 96, *116*
Samsonowitz, V., 224, 238, *241*
Sanchez-Craig, B. M., 127, *142*, 269, *293*
Savage, D. J., 173, 174, *197*
Sayers, M., 33, *58*, 147, *169*, 267, *291*, 367, *385*
Schachter, S., 35, 38, 49, 52, 53, *60*, 222, 222, 243, 265, 296, 300, *317*, 384, *386*
Schaefer, C., 374, *385*
Schatzberg, A. F., 149, *169*
Schayer, R. W., 32, *60*
Schenk, W. G., 32, *55*
Schinke, S. P., 118, 128, *142*
Schmahl, F. W., 32, *60*
Scholomskos, D., 273, *292*
Schooler, C., 4, 8, *24*, 148, 150, 167, *169*, 201, 217, 220, 239, *241*
Schultheis, K. R., 296, *317*, 322, 332, *342*
Schultz, J. M., 97, 99, *116*
Schuster, C. R., 37, *56*
Schwartz, J. L., 322, *343*
Schwarz, R. D., 49, *56*
Schwertner, H. H., 49, *54*
Scura, W. C., 271, *292*
Seeman, W., 346, *363*
Seifter, J., 32, *60*
Seligman, M. E. P., 173, *197*
Selye, H., 26, 27, 28, 31, *60*
Severson, H. H., 15, 17, *95*, 99, 100, 102, 103, 105, 109, *114*, *115*, 370
Sexton, M., 223, *241*
Shapiro, R. M., 314, *317*
Sheehan, P. W., 308, *315*
Sher, K. J., 128, *140*
Sherman, S. J., 17, 22, 98, *116*, *140*
Shiffman, S. M., 7, 11, 13, 14, 20, *24*, 41, *60*, 67, 81, 85, 86, 217, 226, 228, 230, 236, 237, *241*, 244, 252, 259, 262, 263, 264, *265*, 279, 280, 286, 290, 300, 310, 311, *317*, 322, 325, 333, *342*, 361, 369, 374, 375, 377, 378, 379, 380, 381, 383
Shrout, P. E., 179, *197*, 346, *362*
Siegel, S., 36, *61*, *241*, 279, *293*, 376, *386*
Sigall, H., 328, *342*
Silverstein, B., 52, *60*
Silvis, S. E., 47, *59*
Simon, E. J., 46, 54, *61*
Singer, G., 29, *55*
Singer, J. E., 26, 29, 38, 53, *54*, *60*
Sjöberg, L., 3, 20, *24*, 224, 238, *241*, 273, *293*
Skinner, H. A., 369, *386*
Slack, W. W., 32, *56*, 57
Slinkard, L. A., 67, 92, 118, *141*
Smith, G. M., 223, *241*
Smith, J. E., 50, *61*
Smythies, J., 46, 47, *55*
Sobell, M. B., 11, *24*
Solomon, R. L., 6, *24*, 35, 39, 40, 41, 49, *61*, 279, *293*, 376, *386*
Southwick, L., 14, *24*, 375, *386*
Sowder, B., 148, 149, *168*
Spealman, R. D., 37, *56*
Speckart, G., 67, *92*, 126, 138, *139*
Spevak, P. A., 314, *316*
Spiaggia, A., 31, *54*
Spielberger, C. D., 338, *343*
Spitzhoff, D., 87, *93*
Sprafkin, R. P., 119, 128, 131, *140*
Srole, L., 143, *145*
Stambul, H. B., 302, *315*
Stapleton, J., 269, *292*
Starke, K., 50, *61*
Steele, C., 14, *24*, 375, *386*
Stepney, R., 18, *21*
Stitzel, R. E., 32, *61*
Stitzer, M. L., 237, *240*
Stone, A. A., 6, 11, 70, *93*, 144, 202, 203, 205, 206, 212, 214, *219*, 220, 374, 378, 379
Strakova, A., 32, *60*
Strupp, H. H., 346, 347, 361, *363*
Stuart, R. B., 314, *317*
Stunkard, A. J., 295, *317*
Su, C.-Y., 46, *61*
Suffett, F., 150, *170*
Sutak, M., 50, *57*
Szidon, J. P., 31, *61*

AUTHOR INDEX

T

Takane, Y., 278, *293*
Tallarida, R. J., 41, *56*
Taube, C., 347, *363*
Taube, H. D., 50, *61*
Taylor, P., 40, 41, *61*
Telch, M., 118, *141*
Tellegen, A., 69, 78, *94*
Ternes, J. W., 36, *60*
Theis, H. E., 128, 138, *142*
Thomas, R. K., 18, *23*, 86, *93*
Thompson, E. L., 102, *116*
Thompson, G., 129, 130, *140*
Thompson, R. F., 26, 47, 48, 49, 50, *62*, 99, 109, *114*
Thompson, T., 37, *61*
Thompson, W. D., 273, *292*
Thoresen, C. E., 298, *317*
Tilton, K. A., 74, *93*
Timmer, S. G., 10, 12, 19, 144, 178, *198*, 217, 374
Tolan, P., 127, *141*
Tomarken, A. J., 295, 296, 301, 310, 312, *316*
Tseng, L.-F., 46, *61*
Tucker, J. A., 11, *24*
Tucker, M. B., 8, 12, 19, 143, 147, 148, 149, 150, 151, 152, 157, 165, 167, *169*, 170, 217, 374, 380
Tuncalp, S., *114*
Twentyman, C. T., 314, *317*

U

Uhlenhuth, E. H., 346, 347, 348, 361, *363*
United States Department of Health and Human Services, 41, *61*, 95, 99, *116*
United States Department of Health, Education, and Welfare, 41, *61*
U.S. Public Health Service, 321, *343*

V

Vaillant, G. E., 295, 310, *317*
Van Hasselt, V. B., 15, *24*, 271, *293*
Vaughan, R., 79, 87, *93*
Velicer, W. F., 328, *342*, *343*
Velten, E., 237, *241*
Verbrugge, L. M., 148, 150, *170*, 206, *220*
Vernon, S. W., 346, *363*
Veroff, J., 10, 12, 144, 177, 178, 179, 180, 183, *197*, *198*, 217, 347, *363*, 374
Vickers, R. R., Jr., 19, *22*
Victor, M., 40, *61*
Vigas, M., 32, *60*
Volkart, E. H., *219*
Vourakis, C., 45, *61*
Vuchinich, R. E., 11, *24*

W

Wack, J. T., 41, 51, *62*
Wahlstrom, G., 50, *62*
Walder, C. P., *57*
Waldorf, D., 271, 272, 274, *293*
Walker, K., 269, *293*
Wallace, J. E., 49, *54*
Wallace, K. M., 205, *219*
Wallston, B. S., 70, 81, *93*
Wallston, K. A., 70, 81, *93*
Walsh, M. J., 49, *55*
Wandersman, A., 126, *142*
Wang, Y.-T., 46, *61*
Wanner, E., 173, 196, *198*
Ward, C. H., 205, *219*
Ward, H., 19, *22*
Warren, D. T., 174, *198*
Warshawsky, A., 174, *198*
Washington, M. N., 158, 165, *169*
Watts, W. A., 82, *93*
Way, E. I., 33, *62*
Wei, E., 46, *57*
Weiner, N., 41, *62*
Weissman, W., 15, 17, 99, 102, 103, 105, *114*, *115*, 370
Weisz, D. J., 26, 47, 48, 49, 50, *62*
Weschler, H., 209, *220*
Whitehead, C. C., 49, *62*
Whitworth, H., 273, *293*
Wide, L., 30, *55*
Wikler, A., 35, *62*, 227, *242*
Wille, R., 271, *293*
Williams, C., 118, 128, 139, *139*
Williams, J. M., 104, *115*
Wills, T. A., 5, 6, 12, 17, 18, 19, *22*, *24*, 67, 68, 79, 81, 82, 85, 86, 87, *93*, *94*, 96, 97, 111, 156, 174, *198*, 217, 225, 228, *242*, 264, 279, 280, 356, 361, *363*, 369, 374, 375, 377, 379
Wilson, G. T., 173, 174, *198*

Wimersma Griedanus, T., 30, *55*
Winfree, L. T., 128, 138, *142*
Wing, R. R., 296, *316*
Winstead, D. K., 273, *293*
Winter, D., 180, *198*
Wish, M., 277, 278, *291*
Wishart, D., *293*
Witkin, J. M., 26, 37, *54*
Wolf, H., 32, *60*
Wolpe, J., 119, *142*
Wong, L. K., 49, *56*
Woolf, D. S., 38, 39, 40, *62*
Wright, S., 237, *240*, 332, *342*

Wrubel, J., 120, 126, *142*
Wuthmann, C., 302, *315*
Wyler, A. R., 205, *220*

Y

Yates, B. T., 312, *315*
Young, F. W., 278, *293*

Z

Zamfir, V., 32, *56*
Zevon, M. A., 69, 78, *93*
Zibotics, H., 30, *56*
Zwick, W., 328, *343*

Subject Index

A

Adaptive orientation, 267–268, 368–369, see also Exposure orientation
Addiction, see Dependence
Addictive personality, 367
Adolescence
 and aggression as behavioral style, 129
 intervention programs, 87–92, 101–110, 129–131
 substance use in, 74–78, 99–101
Adrenal gland, 27–28
Affect, see also Depression; Negative affect; Positive affect
 Affect Balance Scale, 69
 management of, 5, 10, 14, 227, 236
 measures, 205
 motivation for substance use, 33
 precipitant of relapse, 224, 227–228, 236, 244, 279, 288
 substance use prediction, 84, 86, 217
Age, as predictor of substance use, 172, 175–176, 188–196, 212, 216
Aggression, as predictor of substance use, 81
Alcohol and alcohol use, see also Substance use
 amount of drinking, 208–213
 availability, 172
 cessation, 269–270, 301–315
 and cognitive management, 271
 and coping, 143–144, 171–197, 199–200, 203, 213, 217–218
 and economic stress, 189–191
 and endogenous opioid peptides, 49
 expectation of effect, 14
 initiation, 74–92, 119–136, 300
 and job stress, 193–194
 and marital stress, 192
 measures, 208–209
 motivation for use, 14–15
 ongoing use, 172–197, 199–219
 pharmacologic effects, 40
 predictors of use, 76–82, 91
 problem drinking, 300
 and resources, 171, 185–188
 role in smoking relapse, 232, 238
 and self-change, 301–315
 severity of problem, 304
 and social support, 154
 and stress, 3–5, 48–53, 67–92, 143–144, 152–155, 171–197, 199–219
 and tension-reduction, see Tension reduction hypothesis
 tolerance, 40
Amphetamines, 41–42
Anticipatory coping, 10–11, 379, see also Coping
Appraisal
 of coping problems, 11–12, 214
 of high-risk situations, 276–280
 of severity of problem, 299–300
Appraisal-focused coping, 268–269
Arylcyclohexylamines, 44–45
Assertiveness, see Social Competence
Assessment, see Measures
Attitudes to substance use, see Expectations
Autonomic nervous system, 26, 27, 29
Availability of drugs and substance use, 172

B

Barbiturates, 42–43
Behavioral coping, see also Coping; Coping strategies; Cognitive coping
  versus cognitive coping, 283
  and contextual factors, 238
  definition and measurement of, 226
  effectiveness in relapse prevention, 229, 252–254, 260
  opiate use, 283
  of predictors, 233
  strategies of self quitters, 250
Benzodiazepines, 42–43
  and women, 150
Biphasic effects of substance use, 6, 376
Buffering interaction of coping variables, 82–87

C

Cannabinoids, 43–44, see also Marijuana
Catecholamines
  and opioids, 50
  and stress response, 29, 49
Causal modelling, 124–127, 137–139
Cessation of substance use, 19–21, 221–223, see also Relapse; Stages of substance use
  and coping behavior, 19–20, 221–222, see also Relapse
  and demographic variables, 248–249
  elements in self-change, 322–323, 337
  maintenance stage, 337–338
  and model for smoking, 223–225
  personality, 223
  relapse rates, 221, 223
  stages of, 370
  unaided quitters, 244–245
Cholesterol and stress, 30
Cigarette smoking
  and advertising, 319
  biological model of use, 236
  cessation, 223–240, 243–265, 322–323, 337–340, see also Cessation of substance use
  component analysis of, 353–358
  coping model of use, 236
  health risk, 95
  initiation, 63, 74–92, 95–112, 119–136
  maintenance, 63, 98–99
  modeling effects on, 100
  motivation for, 13–14
  pharmacological smoking, 13
  prediction, 76–82, 91
  prevalence of, 321–327
  prevention, 101–104, 109–112
  and refusal skills, 96, 101–114
  and relapse, 223
  and self-change, 295, 298–301, 312–314
  and social influence, 95–114
  social smoking, 13
  stages of change, 325, 337, see also specific stages
  and stress, 320–321
Cocaine, 42
Cognitive coping, see also Coping strategies
  versus behavioral coping, 229, 368, 283
  classification of, 226, 249
  definition, 9, 16, 226
  effectiveness in relapse prevention, 200, 229, 251–254
  in high-risk situation, 254–256, 273–274
  as predictor of substance use, 79, 83, 85, 91
  predictors of, 232, 233, 257–260
  and relapse prevention, 244, 229–230, 237
  and self-efficacy, 283–284
  as strategies of unaided quitters, 250
  subject characteristics, 257
  transsituational consistency, see Coping, transsituational consistency
  treatment effects, 231
  and unexpected situations, 232
Cognitive impairment and substance use, 271
Confidence, see Self-confidence; Self-efficacy
Contemplation stage of behavior change, see also Stages of change
  and decisional balance, 330–332
  definition, 326, 337
  processes of change, 330–332, 334–336
  and self-efficacy, 330–332
  and temptation, 330–332
Coping, see also Behavioral coping; Cognitive coping; Coping strategies; Stress coping; Temptation coping skills
  alternative coping strategies, 171–174

SUBJECT INDEX

classification of, 8–10, 16, 69–74, 106–107, 162–163, 202–203, 207, 226, 249–250, 268–269, 307, 323–324
cognitive versus behavioral, 229, 268, 283
commonalities across problem behaviors, 308, 311–315
correlation with selection of agent, 159–162
definition, 268
determinants of, 238–239, 257–260
dysfunctional, 153, 157–162, 164, 166–167
effectiveness of, 229–230, 235, 237, 252–254, 260–264, 377
failure, 286–288
field-dependence, 151
in high-risk situation, 251–252, 254–256, 257, 268, 273–274, 280–284
initiation of substance use, 63–65, 67–92
measures, 69–70, 207–208, 297
and motivation, 380–381, 259, 260, 310
versus no coping, 228–230, 254, 260
personality traits, 338
and preparedness, 232
processes of change, 328, 338–339, *see also* Processes of change
psychological distress, 346
and relapse, 224–231, 244, 287
selection of, 11–13
and self-change, 300, 305–308, 311–315
self-assessment, 248
self-efficacy, 283–284
social versus nonsocial, 143
and stages of change, 329–334
and time since cessation, 281–282
transsituational consistency, 234–235, 239, 377–378
treatment effects on, 231–232, 286
and vigilance, 238
Coping strategies, *see also* Coping
acceptance, 207, 213, *see also* Coping strategies, passive coping
achievement thoughts, 249–250
aggression, 70–74, 81
assertiveness, 9–10, 16, 81–92
avoidance, 149–250, 273–274, 288
and self-efficacy, 283–284
catharsis, 144, 207, 215–216
cognitive restructuring, 8–9, 16, 70–74, 79, 207, 268–269, 281–282
cognitive avoidance, 8, 207, 226, 268–269, 273–274, 281–282, 283–284, 288
consumption, 226
decision making, 9–10, 16, 18, 77–78, 85, 91–92, 273, 375
delay, 226
developing alternatives, 249–250, 268–269, 281–282
direct action, 9, 16, 70, 207, 213–214
distraction, 9, 16, 70, 80, 85, 144, 207, 213–214, 226
downward comparison, 8–9, 16
efficacy enhancement, 8–9, 16
entertainment, 70–74, 80
escape, 226
exercise, 70–74, 79–80, 226
help seeking, 9–10, 249–250, 268–269, 281–282
minimization, 8–9, 16
passive coping, 144, 174, 180, *see also* Coping strategies, acceptance
pleasure seeking, 9–10
prayer, 144, 174, 180, 188, 191
problem solving, 9–10, 16, 70–74, 79, 207, 268–269, 281–282
relaxation, 9, 16, 70–74, 80–81, 144, 207, 217, 226
religion, 9–10, 16, 70–74, 81, 144, 174, 180, 188, 191, 207, 214, 218
restructuring, 9, 16, 70
self-instruction, 249–250, 255–256
self-punitive cognitions, 226
social concern cognitions, 249–250
social support, 9, 16, 70–74, 79, 144, 152–155, 158–166, 174, 207, 215–216
stimulus control, 300, 312–314
substance use, 4, 13–21, 172, 176, 199–200, 213, 217–219, 268, 272–273, 279, 290, 320–321, 348, 361, 374
thoughts of consequences, 8–9, 16, 226, 249–250
willpower, 8–9, 16, 226, 230, 237, 381
withdrawal, 9–10, 16, 157
Coping with anger, 155–156
Coping with depression, 155–156
Coping with psychological distress, 346–347

Corticosteroids, *see also* Adrenal gland
and opioids, 50
role in general adaptation syndrome, 28

D

Defect model of substance use, 117, 118
Demographic factors, *see also* Epidemiology of substance use
assessment, 246
classification, 276–284
coping, 257
measures of, 121
prediction of coping style, 280–284
and prevention, 136
and substance use, 134
Dependence, 367–368, *see also* Substance use
as biological aspect of substance use, 33–38, 367–369
and psychological factors, 35–36, 367–370
Depression, *see also* Affect; Negative affect; Coping with depression
and substance use, 155–156, 272–273
Disease model of substance use, *see* Substance use, biological aspects of
Drug abuse, *see also* Substance use
definition, 33
Drug use, *see* Substance use
Drugs of abuse, 33–48, *see also* Substance use

E

Eating, *see also* Coping strategies, consumption; Obesity; Weight problems
and endogenous opioid peptides, 50–51
and stress, 50–51
and substance use, 51
Economic stress, 171, 177–178, 189–192
Educational level
measures of, 205
as predictor of substance use, 172, 175–176, 189–195
Emergency response, 27, *see also* General adaptation syndrome
Emotional distress syndrome, *see* Psychological distress
Emotion-focused coping, 151, 200, 268–269, 319

Employment status, as predictor of substance use, 172, 175–176, 189–195
Endorphines, *see* Opioids, endogenous
Epidemiology of substance use, 143–144, 147–168, 171–197, 209–212, 216, *see also* Age; Employment status; Educational level; Marital status; Sex difference
Epinephrine, 27, 29, *see also* Adrenal gland; Norepinephrine
actions of, 27, 29
and stress, 29
Estrone, and stress response, 29
Events, *see* Stressful life events
Expectations
and pay-off matrix, 375
of substance use, 14, 174, 176, 218, 374–375
Exposure orientation, 369, *see also* Adaptive orientation

G

Gender differences, *see* Sex differences
General adaptation syndrome, 27–28

H

Halo effect, 301
Helplessness, 171, 173, 187, *see also* Personal control
Heroin use, *see also* Opiate use
sex differences, 147, 157–158
High-risk situation (for relapse), *see also* Relapse crises; Relapse situations; Temptation situations
coping in, 254–256, 273–274, 287, 372–375
decision making in, 273
description of, 254–255
outcome of, 251–252, 260–264
self-assessment, 246–248, 280–284
and substance use cessation, 244
and time elapsed since cessation, 259–260
Hormones, *see* specific hormones
Hypnotics, 42
Hypochondria, 205, 209, 212

I

Illicit drugs, 284–286
Immotive stage of behavior change

SUBJECT INDEX

and decisional balance, 330–336
definition, 326, 337
self-efficacy in, 330–336
Inhalants, 45
Initiation of substance use, 17–18, 63–65, 67–92, 95–98, 372–373
Insulin, 29
Interventions
  cessation programs
    behavioral coping in, 231
    influence on coping, 231–232
    problem solving, 269–270
    processes of change, 338–339
    reappraisal therapy, 269
    relapse, 248, 339
    relapse prevention hotline, 224–225, 235
    and self-change, 358–360
    service delivery, 167–168
    and stages of change, 339
    stress management, 236
  prevention programs
    adolescents, 372–373
    coping skills in, 377
    Decision Skills Curriculum, 87–92
    methodological problems, 373
    refusal skills training, 101–102, 109–110
    social competence in, 132–137

J

Job stress
  and alcohol, 193–194
  measures, 177–178
  and substance use, 193–195

L

Life events, *see* Stressful life events
Lysergic acid diethylemide (LSD), 44

M

Maintenance of substance use, 18–19, 98–99, 143–144
Marijuana, 158–160, *see also* Cannabinoids
  sex difference in preference, 156–157
Marital status, as predictor of substance use, 172, 175–176, 188
Marital stress
  and alcohol, 192–193, 217
  and substance use, 171, 192–193

Mate-dependent coping, 158, 163–165
Measures
  Affect Balance Scale, 69
  Assertiveness Inventory, 69, 81
  attitudinal inventory for drug use, 130
  beliefs, 246
  Coping Behavior Inventory, 269
  coping skills and self-management, 297
  Daily Coping Inventory, 201–203
  Decisional Balance Scale, 327
  Duncan Index of Occupational Status, 205, 210
  Factorial Coping Measure, 69
  General Health Questionnaire, 211
  Health Locus of Control, 70, 81
  high-risk situations, 246–248
  Personality Research Form, 205, 216
  Processes of Change Questionnaire, 327, 349
  Psychological Distress Questionnaire, 349
  self-efficacy, 122, 246, 328
  self-esteem, 82
  Sick Role Tendency, 205, 209
  situational antecedents to relapse, 225–226
  Situational Competency Test, 270, 275
  Social Readjustment Rating Scale, 20, 273, *see also* Stressful life events
  social skills, 105–109
  Stanford Social Ecology Laboratory, 302–303
  Stress Reaction Scales, 69
  substance use, 74
  Syracuse Scales of Social Relations, 129–130
  Taped Situations Test, 105–109
  Weight Control Questionnaire, 349
Motivation
  and perception of problem, 299–300
  and self-change, 298, 300, 310

N

Naloxone, 48, 50
Narcotics, *see* Opioids
National Household Survey, 347
National Institute on Drug Abuse, 148–149
Negative affect
  and coping style, 4–6, 13, 15, 18, 256, 289
  and high-risk situations, 246–248, 254
  and opiate addiction, 269

Negative affect (*continued*)
  versus positive affect and relapse, 268, 270
  and relapse, 224, 228, 236–237, 272–273, 276, 279, 288, 345–346
Negative feedback model, 312
Nicotine, 40–41, *see also* Cigarette smoking
  and stress, 49
Nonspecific psychological distress syndrome, 346, *see also* Psychological distress
Norepinephrine, 27, 29, *see also* Epinephrine; Adrenal gland
  actions of, 29
  and stress, 29

O

Obesity, *see also* Weight problems
  problems of change, 352
  self-change, 296–301
  and self-management, 296, 298–301, 315
Opiate use
  as coping, 268, 273, *see also* Heroin; Opiates
  and avoidance, 274
  and behavioral coping, 271
  and cognitive impairment, 272–273
  comparison with other drugs, 271, 274
  and depression, 272–273
  and life planning, 272
  and social support, 271
  and stress, 48, 50–52
  theories of addiction, 267–268
Opioids
  and alcohol, 49
  cessation, 270–291
  dependence and tolerance, 47
  endogenous, 26, 30–31, 45–48
  ongoing use, 147–168
  pharmocologic effects, 38–39, 46–47
  structure and mode of action, 53–54
  tolerance, 39
Overdose
  and coping behavior, 159, 161–162, 168
  and substance used, 157–158, 164

P

Peer pressure, *see* Social influence
Perceived stressfulness, 172, *see also* Stress
Personal control, 172–173, 175

Personality type, and substance use, 214, 216–217
Phencyclidine, 44, 150
Physical exercise, as predictor of substance use, 79, 83
Physical health
  effect of stress on, 199–200
  measures, 179–180, 205–207
  and substance use, 188, 191–193, 212, 216–217
Positive affect, 4–6, 13, 15, 228, 279, 285
  and relapse, 228
Positive events, and predictors of substance use, 77–78, 84
Power, need for, 173, 180, 189, 196
Preparedness, and relapse crisis, 232
Problem-focused coping, 151, 200, 268–269, 319
Problem-solving therapy
  effectiveness, 237
  and relapse, 269–270
  and self-change, 299
Processes of change
  component analysis of cigarette smoking
    by process, 356–358
    by stage, 353–356
  component analysis of psychological distress
    by process, 356–358, 362
    by stage, 353–356
  component analysis of weight control
    by process, 356–358
    by stage, 353–356
  as coping, 328, 338–339
  and coping effectiveness, 324
  description, 323, 329, 349
  measure of processes across problems, 350
  and personality characteristics, 338
  and psychological therapies, 358–359, 361
  questionnaire, 327, 349
  and recent quitters, 330–336
  and relapsers, 330–336
  and self-change, 356–360
  and stages of change, 325, 338–339
Psychedelic drugs, 44
Psychoanalytic theory, 368
Psychological distress, *see also* Stress
  component analysis, 353–358
  and coping, 346–347

SUBJECT INDEX 405

prevalence, 346–347
and processes of change, 347
questionnaire, 349
and relapse, 345–346
Psychosocial stress, *see* Stress

R

Race, and adolescent substance use, 76
Rebound, physiological, 35, 39
Recent quitters
  decisional balance in, 330–333
  definition, 326, 337–338
  and processes of change, 330–336
  and self-efficacy, 330–333
  and social support, 338
Refusal skills, *see also* Social competence
  assessment, 102–106
  and cigarette smoking, 96–114
  and coping, 119
  intervention, 101–102, 109–110
  social skills, 112–113
Relapse
  affective antecedents, 224, 227–228, 236, 254–256, 279, 288
  and avoidance, 288
  and coping, 250–256, 269, 277, 287, 289
  and demographic variables, 248–249
  and high-risk situations, 268, 276
  and life events, 273
  models, 236
  and negative events, 224, 228, 236–237, 272–273, 276, 279, 288, 345–346
  and positive affect, 279–280
  and positive feedback loop, 290
  prevention versus termination, 270
  and psychological distress, 345–346
  rates, 221, 223
  relapse crises, 224
  relapse-prevention hot line, 224–225, 235
  and self-change, 295
  self-control model, 243–244
  and self-efficacy, 280, 282, 288–290
  and situational antecedents, 227, 232–234
  and social pressure, 276, 279
  theories, 280
  and triggers, 288
  and withdrawal, 227, 279–280, 289, 373

Relapse crises, *see also* High-risk situations; Relapse situations; Temptation situations
  antecedents, 227–228
  definition, 224
  situational factors
    assessment, 246
    and coping, 238, 257
    precipitants, 244–245
    time since cessation, 232
    transsituational consistency in, 234–235
    unexpected situation as, 232
    withdrawal, 227
Relapse situations, *see also* High-risk situations; Relapse crises; Temptation situations
  classification, 274
  definition, 244
  descriptions, 254–255
  measures, 246
  perceptions, 280–287
  time elapsed since cessation, 259–260
Relapsers
  cigarette smoking control program, 339–340
  decisional balance, 330–334
  definition and description, 326, 338
  and processes of change, 330–336
  and self-efficacy, 330–334
Relaxation, *see also* Coping strategies, relaxation
  and alcohol, 144
Resources, *see also* Coping
  external, 181, *see also* Coping
  internal, 174, *see also* Personal control
  personal, measures, 179–181
  as predictor of substance use, 171, 175–176, 185–188
Restorative coping, 10–11, 379, *see also* Coping
Role play assessment
  and cigarette smoking, 101, 104–109, 111–112
  validity, 105

S

Self-administration of drugs, 33
Self-change
  and alcohol, 301–315

Self-change *(continued)*
  assessment of coping strategies, 297, 305
  and cognitive coping, 299
  and decision-making process, 312
  effectiveness, 298–301, 305, 310–315
  factors influencing success, 322–323
  implications for professional treatment, 314–315
  and motivation, 298, 310
  obesity, 296–301
  and problem solving, 299
  processes of change, 356–360
  and psychotherapy, 359, 361
  and relapse, 295
  social support, 310
Self-confidence
  measures, 179
  predictor of substance use, 188–196
Self-efficacy
  age, 132
  definition, 120
  measures, 122, 181, 195–196, 246
  predictor of substance use, 82
  social skills, 120, 127
Self-esteem
  measures, 179
  predictor of substance use, 82
Self-help, *see also* Self-change
  self-help manual, 360
Self-instruction, *see also* Cognitive coping
  and high-risk situations, 255–256
  self-quitting and, 250
Self-stimulation, intracranial, 50
Sex differences
  adolescent substance use, 76
  appraisal of coping, 214–215, 218
  coping mechanisms, 144, 147–168, 283–284
  drug use behavior, 149–150, 156, 157–159
  need for power, 173, 189, 196
  personal control, 175
  as predictor of substance use, 125, 172, 175–176, 183, 188–195
  relapse, 248
Skill training, 64
Smoking, *see* Cigarette smoking
Social competence
  definition, 63
  and initiation of substance use, 64–65, 117–142
  measures, 121–124
  predictor of substance use, 121–127
  prevention of substance use, 120–128, 131–139
  and relapse-prevention model, 243
  and substance use, 243
Social influence, cigarette smoking, 96–114, *see also* Social pressure
Social learning theory
  and addiction, 371
  definition, 120
  performance-based modeling, 127
  and prevention of substance use, 118, 369
Social pressure, *see also* Social influence
  relapse, 276, 279
Social skills
  and age, 132
  and coping, 274
Social support, 9, 16, 21
  and alcohol use, 154, 165, 194
  and coping, 144, 152–155, 174, 207, 215–216
  measures of, 181
  and opiate use, 273
  predictor of substance use, 79, 191, 194
  and recent quitters, 308
  and self-change, 299, 310, 314
  social support–stress paradigm, 152–155
Stages of change, *see also* specific stages
  cessation, *see* Cessation of substance use, stages of
  coping and, 329–334
  and decisional balance, 330–334, 336–337
  description of, 352–357, 370, 372
  factors influencing progress, 334–337, 339
  and self-efficacy, 330–337
Stages of coping, 15–21, 370–372, *see also* specific stages and substances
Stages of substance use, 15–21, 370–372, *see also* specific stages
  cessation, *see* Cessation of substance use, stages of
  coping processes, 15–21
  initiation, 17–18, 370
  maintenance, 18–19, 370
  relapse, 20–21, 370

Strain, 179
Stress, *see also* Affect; Negative affect; Psychological distress; Stress response; Stressful life events; specific stressors
 categories of, 4
 cigarette smoking, 320–321
 and coping, 320, 369
 demographic factors and perception of stress, 175
 and drug abuse, 3–5
 drug metabolism, 32
 and eating, 50–51
 economic, *see* Economic stress
 job, *see* Job stress
 levels of stressors, 4
 management, 88
 marital, *see* Marital stress
 measures, 69, 70
 and opiate use, 272–273, 290
 perceived stressfulness, 172, 175
 perception, 5, 11
 physiological effects
  enzymes, 32, 48
  organ systems, 31
 reduction, 92
 self-change, 369
 and substance use, 3–5, 48–53, 67–92, 143–144, 152–155, 272–273, 290, 320–321, 369, 372
 theories of addiction, 268–279, 368–369
 urinary pH, 52
 women, 150, 152–155
Stress coping, 4, 6, 63, 143, 152–155, *see also* Coping
 definition of, 6
 generalized life stressors, 4–8
 as model of substance use, 119, 121, 126–127, 368
 and relapse, 228
 and substance use, 8, 17–21, 227, 238
Stress-reduction model, *see also* Tension reduction hypothesis
 and smoking, 235, 236
Stress responses, *see also* stress
 autonomic nervous system, 27–29
 drug metabolism, 32
 endocrine effects, 27–31
 model of substance use, 119, 121, 126–127
 organ system effects, 31–32
 and withdrawal, 52
Stressful life events
 changing–stabilizing qualities of, 202, 206–207
 controllability, 206–207, *see also* Personal control
 daily events
  measures, 201–203, 206, 212–213
  occurrence, 214, 216
  substance use, 217, 374
 desirability, 202, 206–207, 213, 217
 meaningfulness, 202, 206
Substance use, *see also* individual agents
 adolescent attitudes toward, 130
 affect management, 227–236
 and age, 132
 availability, 172
 behavioral aspects, 37–38, 367–369
 biological aspects, 33–38, 367–369, *see also* Dependence; Tolerance; Withdrawal
 causal modeling, 124–127
 cessation maintenance model, 223–225
 classification of specific agents, 33
 conditioned responses, 36
 dependence, *see* physical dependence
 drug abuse, definition, 33
 drug differences, 271, 274–276
 economic stress, 191–192
 environment, 132
 expectation of, *see* Expectations
 high-risk situations, 273–274
 initiation, 63–65, 119–136, 172–197
 job stress, 193–195
 marital stress, 192–193
 measures of, 76–92, 96–109, 177, 206–207
 pharmacology of specific drugs, 35–38
 prevalence in adolescents, 74–87, 99–101, 119
 Psychological Distress Scale, 345–346
 reasons for, 33
 and resources, 171, 185–186
 sex differences, *see* Sex differences
 and social competence, 117–139
 stages of, *see* Stages of substance use
 and stress, 3–5, 25–26, 48–53, 76–79, 199–200, *see also* Stress
 theories of addiction, 268–279

Substance use (*continued*)
  tolerance, *see* Tolerance
  and transition proneness, 136
  withdrawal, *see* Withdrawal
Symptoms, *see* Physical health

T

Temptation-coping skills, 4, 6, 12, 17–21, 63
  anticipatory strategies, 10–11
  effectiveness, 237
  and opiates, 279–280
  relapse, 223–225
  in relapse crises, 224, 228–229, 235
  restorative strategies, 10–11
Temptation situations, *see also* High-risk situations; Relapse crises; Relapse situations
  coping strategies, 250–256
  description of, 244
  survival rate, 252–254
  time elapsed since cessation, 259–260
  types of, 254–255
Tension reduction hypothesis, 199–200, 212, 216–217, 369–370
  alcohol, 14, 183, 192, 199–200, 212, 216–218, 369–370
Testosterone, and stress response, 29
Thyroid hormone, and stress response, 29
Tobacco, *see* Cigarette smoking; Nicotine
Tolerance, *see also* specific substances
  as biological aspect of substance use, 33–35, 367–369
  psychological factors, 35–36, 367–370
Tranquilizers, *see* individual agents

Transactional model of stress and coping, 200–203
Transsituational consistency in coping, 234–235, 239
Transtheoretical model of change, *see also* Stages of behavior; Processes of change
  description, 323–324, 378
  development of, 323
Treatment, *see* Intervention

V

Vasopressin, and stress, 29
Vulnerability
  measures, 179
  and substance use, 186, 189–195

W

Weight problems, *see also* Obesity
  component analysis of, 353–358
Withdrawal, *see also* specific substances
  antecedent of relapse crises, 227
  as biological aspect of substance use, 33–35, 367–369
  and coping mechanisms, 143–144, 245
  as model of relapse, 236
  psychological factors, 35–36, 367–370
  and relapse, 279–280, 289, 373
  and stress, 52
Women, *see also* Sex differences
  coping mechanisms, 144, 147–168
  drug use behavior, 149–150, 156
  smoking cessation, 225
  substance use, 147–168
Work stress, *see* Job stress